Control of
Communicable
Diseases
in Man

Control of Communicable Diseases in Man

Twelfth Edition 1975

ABRAM S BENENSON
Editor

An Official Report of the
American Public Health Association

The American Public Health Association
1015 Eighteenth Street NW
Washington, DC 20036

Interdisciplinary Books, Pamphlets & Periodicals
For the Professional & the Layman

Library of Congress Cataloging in Publication Data

American Public Health Association.
   Control of communicable diseases in man.

Published in 1918 under title: The control of communicable
  diseases.
   Includes index.
   1. Communicable diseases — Prevention. I. Benenson, Abram
S., 1914-   II. Title
[DNLM: 1. Communicable disease control. WC100 C764
RA 643.A5 1975   614.4   75-28217
ISBN 0-87553-077-X

Copyright © 1975 by American Public Health Association

Printed in the United States of America
   Text: R.J. Carroll Co., Inc., Harrisonburg, VA
   Covers: Rose Printing Co., Inc., Tallahassee, FL
   Typography: Suburban Typographers, Rockville, MD
    Set In: Century Schoolbook
Library of Congress Catalog Number: 75-28217
International Standard Book Number: 0-87553-077-X

Third Printing, May 1976

50M975; 50M1175; 35M576

Cover Design: Four basic aspects of communicable disease
                control are symbolized — grain: proper nu-
                trition; flask: research; syringe: prevention
                and treatment; hand and soap: sanitation.

R. LeROY CARPENTER, MD
Commissioner of Health
Northeast Tenth at Stonewell
Oklahoma City, OK

JAMES CHIN, MD
Chief, Infectious Disease Section
California State Department of Health
2151 Berkeley Way
Berkeley, CA

ALBERT Z. KAPIKIAN, MD
Head, Epidemiology Section
Laboratory of Infectious Diseases
National Institute of Allergy and Infectious Diseases
National Institutes of Health
Bethesda, MD

SAMUEL L. KATZ, MD
Professor and Chairman
Department of Pediatrics
Duke University School of Medicine
Durham, NC

DONALD R. PETERSON, MD
Professor of Epidemiology, University of Washington
School of Public Health and Community Medicine
Department of Epidemiology and International Health
Seattle, WA

JAY P. SANFORD, MD
Dean, School of Medicine
Uniformed Services University of the Health Sciences
6917 Arlington Road
Bethesda, MD

ROBERT E. SHOPE, MD
Professor of Epidemiology
Department of Epidemiology and Public Health
Yale University School of Medicine
60 College Street
New Haven, CT

JAMES H. STEELE, DVM
Professor of Environmental Health
University of Texas at Houston
School of Public Health
P.O. Box 20186
Houston, TX

WILLIAM D. TIGERTT, MD
    Professor of Pathology and of Experimental Medicine
    University of Maryland School of Medicine
    Baltimore, MD
FRANKLIN H. TOP, SR., MD
    Department of Preventive Medicine and Environmental Health
    College of Medicine
    Institute of Agricultural Medicine
    The University of Iowa
    Iowa City, IA
ROBERT J. WILSON, MD
    Chairman and Scientific Director
    Connaught Laboratories Limited
    1755 Steeles Avenue West
    Willowdale, Ontario, Canada

LIAISON REPRESENTATIVES

W. CHARLES COCKBURN, MD
    World Health Organization
COLONEL ROBERT T. CUTTING, MC, USA
    U.S. Department of Defense
H. BRUCE DULL, MD
    U.S. Public Health Service
N.J.B. EVANS, MB B.Chir.
    Department of Health and Social Security, London, England
SAMUEL L. KATZ, MD
    American Academy of Pediatrics
W.A. LANGSFORD, MD
    The Australian Department of Health, Canberra, A.C.T. Australia
WILLIAM F. McCULLOCH, DVM
    Conference of Public Health Veterinarians
J.A. McKIEL, MD
    Department of National Health and Welfare, Canada
DANIEL REID, MD
    Scottish Home and Health Department, Edinburgh, Scotland
BICHAT A. RODRIGUES, MD
    Pan American Health Organization
HENRY D. SMITH, MD
    Association of State and Territorial Health Officers
C.N. DEREK TAYLOR, MD
    Department of Health, New Zealand

TABLE OF CONTENTS

xi

xiii

PREFACE TO THE TWELFTH EDITION

The Twelfth Edition of *Control of Communicable Diseases in Man* continues the practice established by the American Public Health Association in 1917 to present essential facts needed for the control of the communicable diseases of man. It is intended to provide a central source of necessary information for the management of patients so that they are not the source of an outbreak and survive, and as a supplement to, not a replacement of, textbooks. Treatment indications are given, with details only for those diseases in which delay in instituting proper therapy may be hazardous to the patient.

With the passage of time, improvements in socio-economic and environmental conditions and in immunization practices have greatly reduced the incidence and distribution of the diseases of yesteryear. There has been a dramatic decline in the incidence of paralytic poliomyelitis and smallpox; on the other hand, cholera, until recently a disease restricted to a small part of the world, has spread to involve three continents and is now a continuing threat to the rest of the world.

While all the included diseases exist somewhere on the globe, the western physician has had no personal contact and usually no instruction in most of these infectious diseases. Modern jet travel has eliminated the barriers of distance and time and may bring an infected individual from some remote area of the globe into any physician's consulting room. This pocket manual attempts to present the basic facts on recognition, diagnosis, mechanisms of spread, and control to help this physician and any associated health workers recognize and manage the situation.

The changes in the contents of this manual and in the recommendations which have taken place over the past 58 years largely reflect the increase in factual knowledge of the diseases, their etiological agents and their epidemiological patterns. The committee was saddened during the preparation of this edition by the death of a man who contributed more than any other single individual to the understanding of infectious diseases. Dr. Karl F. Meyer died on April 28, 1974 at age 89. Educated as a veterinarian, he personally contributed much of the knowledge presented on brucellosis, eastern equine encephalitis, western equine encephalitis, botulism, typhoid fever, coccidioidomycosis, ornithosis and other chlamydial diseases, leptospirosis, rabies and many others. He was the undisputed expert in the United States on plague and his observations dominate that chapter in this book. An active participant in the affairs of the American Public Health Association and recipient of both its Sedgwick and Lasker Awards, K.F. had contributed directly to previous editions of this publication by reviewing pertinent chapters. We mourn the loss of this giant who continued almost to the day of his death to advance our knowledge on the control of communicable diseases of man, particularly, but not only, those transmissible from animals.

This manual considers communicable diseases known to exist in any part of the globe. While the American Public Health Association is responsible for the publication of this book, its production is a model of international cooperation with active participation of the World Health Organization and the Pan American Health Organization, as well as the major English speaking countries; New Zealand has participated in its preparation for the first time. While the point of view is American with primary concern for the problems encountered by the official and unofficial agencies in the United States involved in the control of communicable disease, our practices should be consistent with those in other countries. Global problems require internationally coordinated efforts. The results of World Health Organization activities in this direction are becoming manifest, particularly the success of the smallpox eradication program. WHO has established a group of international collaborating centers, forming a world-wide network of institutions which can provide their national counterparts with the services of consultation, collection and analysis of information, assistance in the establishment of standards, production and distribution of standard or reference material, exchange of information, training, and organization of collaborative research. Centers are maintained on enteric, gonococcal, meningococcal, staphylococcal and streptococcal infections; whooping cough; leprosy; plague; treponematosis; tuberculosis; filariasis; leishmaniasis; malaria; schistosomiasis; trypanosomiasis; arboviruses; enteroviruses; influenza; mycoplasma; respiratory virus diseases other than influenza; human rickettsioses; smallpox; trachoma; brucellosis; leptospirosis; rabies; cell cultures; and vector biology and control. WHO should be approached for further details of the services available.

Since the usual practitioner in the United States may not be abreast of the most recent therapeutic measures for exotic diseases, the therapy recommended for each disease is included in paragraph 9B7. Some of these drugs are not stocked in domestic pharmacies; the Director of the Center for Disease Control of the U.S. Public Health Service has established a service whereby rarely used therapeutic and immunoprophylactic agents may be obtained. Many of these are stocked in international air terminal quarantine stations to expedite shipment and rapid receipt. The release of vaccinia immune and zoster immune globulin is controlled by a group of physician-consultants situated in various parts of the country. The telephone number of the closest consultant can be obtained by contacting the quarantine officer at international air terminals, or physicians may call the Center for Disease Control at (404) 633-3311, [night calls (404) 633-2176)]. Drugs for the treatment of parasitic diseases are obtained by telephoning the Center for Disease Control. The items which are available from this source are specified under the appropriate disease discussions.

This edition retains the previous format and sometimes even the words originally written by previous editors, Haven Emerson and John E. Gordon. However, every chapter has been updated, based on new information reported in the published literature and in standard texts. New chapters have been added on amebic meningoencephalitis, arthropod-borne viral arthritis and rash, epidemic hemorrhagic conjunctivitis, food poisoning due to *Vibrio parahaemolyticus* and to *Bacillus cereus*, viral gastroenteritis, Lassa fever, molluscum contagiosum, non-gonococcal urethritis, verruca vulgaris, and yersiniosis; anisakiasis, babesiosis, Marburg virus disease and monkeypox are presented as chapter addenda. The separate chapter or rheumatic fever, a complication of streptococcal infections, has been deleted. The nomenclature of the disease entities follows that of the Eighth Revision of the *International Classification of Diseases* except where completely inconsistent with prevailing American usage, (e.g., infection by *Cryptococcus neoformans* is identified as cryptococcosis rather than European blastomycosis). The names of etiological organisms are those listed in the 1974 edition of *Bergey's Manual of Determinative Bacteriology* (Eighth Edition).

The final version of this edition represents the composite efforts of a group selected for their expertise in various classes of infectious diseases, supplemented by generous and valuable comments submitted by the representatives of national and international agencies responsible for disease control. The task of adjudicating between conflicting suggestions fell on the editor, who accepts the responsibility for having rejected any suggestions which subsequently were proved to have been correct.

Purposes of the manual—The aim is to provide an informative text for public health workers of official and voluntary health agencies, to include physicians, dentists, veterinarians, sanitary engineers, public health nurses, social workers, health educators and sanitarians; and for physicians, dentists and veterinarians in private practice who are concerned with the control of communicable diseases. The book is also designed for military physicians and others serving with the armed forces at home and abroad, and for health workers stationed in foreign countries. It contributes to plans for anticipating the health risks attendant on natural and man-made disasters, and serves as a guide to control of the disease situations such emergencies create. School administrators and students of medicine and public health also will find the material useful. The need for a handy reference determines the format of the manual and its pocket size.

A second general purpose is to serve public health administrators as a guide and as a source of materials in preparing regulations and legal requirements for the control of the communicable diseases, in developing programs for health education of the public, and in the administrative acts of official health agencies toward management of communicable disease. The needs of field workers have been given special attention.

The intent is to present factual knowledge in brief fashion and to advance opinion consistent with those facts as a basis for intelligent management of communicable disease, unhampered by local custom and not restricted to prevailing practices. Recommendations for standard administrative or technical procedures are avoided. The emphasis is on principle, because local conditions and interrelated problems commonly require variation in practices from state to state within the United States, and between countries. Because differences in procedure are often due to incomplete knowledge of recent advances and of practices proved successful under other and similar conditions, the attempt has been made to keep facts and opinions reasonably current by revising the manual every five years.

Scope and Contents—The presentation is standardized. Each disease is briefly identified with regard to clinical nature, laboratory diagnosis, and differentiation from allied or related conditions. Occurrence, infectious agent, reservoir, mode of transmission, incubation period, period of communicability, and susceptibility and resistance are next presented. Methods of control are described under the following four headings:

A. **Preventive measures:** Applicable generally to individuals and groups when and where the particular disease may occur in sporadic, endemic or epidemic form, and whether or not the disease is an active threat at the moment, e.g., vaccination against smallpox, chlorination of water supplies, pasteurization of milk, control of rodents and arthropods, animal control, immunization, and health education of the public.
B. **Control of patient, contacts, and the immediate environment:** Those measures designed to prevent infectious matter present

in the person and the environment of the infected individual from being conveyed in a way to spread the disease to other persons, arthropods or animals; and also the means when indicated, to keep contacts under surveillance during the assumed period of incubation of the disease, and carriers under control until they are found to be free of the infectious agent. Specific treatment is outlined to limit the period of communicability and to minimize morbidity and mortality.

C. **Epidemic measures:** Those procedures of emergency character designed to limit the spread of a communicable disease which has developed widely in a group or community or within an area, state or nation, such measures being unnecessary or not justified when the disease occurs sporadically among widely separated individuals or separated by considerable intervals.

D. **International measures:** Such controls of international travelers immigrants, goods, animals, and animal products, and their means of transport, as may arise from provisions of international health regulations, conventions, intergovernmental agreements or national laws; also, any controls that may protect populations of one country against the known risk of infection from another country where a disease may be present in endemic or epidemic form.

Reporting of Communicable Diseases —The first step in the control of communicable disease is its rapid identification, followed by notification to the local health authority that a case of communicable disease exists within the particular jurisdiction. Administrative practice as to what diseases are to be reported and how they should be reported varies greatly from one region to another because of different conditions and different frequencies of disease. This manual presents a basic scheme of reporting directed toward practical working procedure rather than ideal practice. The purpose is to provide necessary and timely information to permit the institution of appropriate control measure as well as to encourage uniformity in morbidity reporting, so that data within a country and between nations can be compared.

A system of reporting functions at four stages. The first is collection of the basic data in the local community where disease occurs. The data are next assembled at district, state or provincial level. The third stage is the collection of total information under national auspices. Finally, for certain prescribed diseases, report is made by the national health authority to the World Health Organization.

Consideration is here limited to the first stage of a reporting system—the collection of the basic data at the local level; first, because that is the fundamental part of any scheme, and second because this manual is primarily for local health workers. The basic data sought at local level are of two kinds (Definition 37, Report of a disease, p. 384).

1. Report of Cases: Each local health authority, in conformity with regulations of higher authority, will determine what diseases are to be reported, as a routine and regular procedure, who is responsible for reporting, the nature of the report required, and the manner in which reports are forwarded to the next superior jurisdiction.

    Physicians are required to report all notifiable illnesses which come to their attention; in addition, the statutes or regulations of many localities require reporting by hospital, householder, or other person having knowledge of a case of a reportable disease.

    Case Report of a communicable disease provides minimal identifying data of name, address, diagnosis, age, sex, and date of report for each patient and in some instances, suspects; dates of onset and of diagnosis are useful. The right of privacy of the individual must be respected.

    Collective Report is the assembled number of cases, by diagnosis, occuring within a prescribed time and without individual identifying data—e.g., 20 cases of malaria, week ending October 6.

2. Report of Epidemics: In addition to requirement of individual case report, any unusual or group expression of illness which may be of public concern (Definition 11, Epidemic) should be reported to the local health authority by the most expeditious means, whether subject to routine report or not specific in the list of diseases officially reportable in the particular locality; and whether a well-known or an indefinite or unknown clinical entity (see Class 4 below).

The communicable diseases listed in this manual are distributed among the following five classes, according to practical benefit presumably to be derived from reporting. These classes are referred to by number throughout the text, under Section 9B1 of each disease. The purpose is to provide a scheme on the basis of which each health jurisdiction may determine its list of regularly reportable diseases.

Class I: Case Report Universally Required by International Health Regulations

This class is limited to the *diseases subject to the International Health Regulations* (1969) (quarantinable diseases)—cholera, plague, smallpox and yellow fever, and to the *diseases under surveillance by WHO*—louse-borne typhus fever and relapsing fever, paralytic poliomyelitis, influenza and malaria.

Obligatory case report to local health authority by telephone, telegraph, or other rapid means; in an epidemic situation, collective reports of subsequent cases in a local area on a daily or weekly basis may be requested by the next superior jurisdiction—as for example, in an influenza epidemic. The local health authority forwards the initial report to next superior jurisdiction by expeditious means if it is the first recognized case in the local area or is the first case outside the limits of a local area already reported; otherwise, weekly by mail or telegraphically in unusual situations.

Class 2: Case Report Regularly Required Wherever the Disease Occurs

Two subclasses are recognized, based on the relative urgency for investigation of contacts and source of infection, or for starting control measures.

A. Case report to local health authority by telephone, telegraph, or other rapid means. These are forwarded to next superior jurisdiction weekly by mail, except that the first recognized case in an area or the first case outside the limits of a known affected local area is reported by telegraph; examples—typhoid fever, diphtheria.

B. Case report by most practicable means; forwarded to next superior jurisdiction as a collective report, weekly by mail; examples, brucellosis, leprosy.

Class 3: Selectively Reportable in Recognized Endemic Areas

In many states and countries, diseases of this class are not reportable. Reporting may be prescribed in particular regions, states or countries by reason of undue frequency or severity. Three subclasses are recognized; A and B (below) are primarily useful under conditions of established endemicity as a means leading toward prompt control measures and to judge the effectiveness of control programs. The main purpose of C (below) is to stimulate control measures or to acquire essential epidemiological data.

A. Case report by telephone, telegraph, or other rapid means in specified areas where the disease ranks in importance with Class 2A; not reportable in many countries; example—tularemia, scrub typhus.
B. Case report by most practicable means; forwarded to next superior jurisdiction as a collective report by mail weekly or monthly; not reportable in many countries; examples—bartonellosis, coccidioidomycosis.
C. Collective report weekly by mail to local health authority; forwarded to next superior jurisdiction by mail weekly, monthly, quarterly, or sometimes annually; examples—clonorchiasis, sandfly fever.

Class 4: Obligatory Report of Epidemics—No Case Report Required

Prompt report of outbreaks of particular public health importancee by telephone, telegraph, or other rapid means; forwarded to next superior jurisdiction by telephone or telegraph. Pertinent data include number of cases, within what time, approximate population involved, and apparent mode of spread; examples—food poisoning, infectious keratoconjunctivitis.

Class 5: Official Report Not Ordinarily Justifiable

Diseases of this class are of two general kinds: those typically sporadic and uncommon, often not directly transmissible from man to man (chromoblastomycosis); or of such epidemiological nature as to offer no practical measures for control (common cold).

Diseases are often made reportable but the information gathered is put to no practical use. This frequently leads to deterioration in the general level of reporting, even for diseases of much importance. Better case reporting usually results when official reporting is restricted to those diseases for which control services are provided or potential control procedures are under evaluation, or epidemiological information is needed for a definite purpose.

ACKNOWLEDGEMENTS

Grateful acknowledgement is hereby made to all the experts, both within and without the American Public Health Association, who have prepared and critically reviewed sections in their area of expertise. The conscientious efforts of the editorial committee and of the national and international liaison representatives, who not only contributed their own effort but called on the experts in their various countries, provided information to make the final product of greatest value. Special recognition must be made of the participation of Dr. Tom F. Whayne, my associate editor; without his support and efforts, I could not have accepted the responsibility for this edition. Appreciation must also be made to the staff of the Department of Community Medicine of the University of Kentucky, whose tasks were often complicated by the need to publish this edition, and to the administration of the University of Kentucky for the support provided by them for the preparation of this edition.

Abram S. Benenson, M.D.

ACTINOMYCOSIS

1. **Identification**—A chronic suppurative or granulomatous disease most frequently localized in jaw, thorax or abdomen, rarely limited to skin and subcutaneous tissues; septicemic spread with generalized disease may occur rarely. The lesions are firmly indurated granulomata; they spread slowly to contiguous tissues and break down focally to form multiple draining sinuses which penetrate to the surface. Discharges from sinus tracts may contain "sulfur granules", which are colonies of the infectious agent.

Diagnosis is confirmed by anaerobic culture.

2. **Occurrence**—An infrequent disease of man, occurring sporadically throughout the world. All races, both sexes, and all age groups may be affected; greatest frequency from 15 to 35 years of age; the ratio of males to females is approximately two to one. Also occurs in cattle, swine, horses and other animals.

3. **Infectious agent**—*Actinomyces israelii* is the usual pathogen of man and *A. bovis* that of animals with rare isolation from man. *A. naeslundii, A. eriksonii* and *Arachnia propionica (Actinomyces propionicus)* also have been reported to cause disease in man, but may be in normal oral flora. All species are gram-positive nonacid-fast anaerobic to micro-aerophilic organisms.

4. **Reservoir**—The natural reservoir of *A. israelii* is man. In the normal oral cavity *A. israelii* grows as a saprophyte in and around carious teeth, in dental plaques, and in tonsillar crypts, without apparent penetration or cellular response in adjacent tissues. Sample surveys in U.S.A., Sweden and other countries have demonstrated *A. israelii* microscopically in granules from crypts of 20% of extirpated tonsils; and isolation in anaerobic culture from as many as 30-48% of specimens of saliva or material from carious teeth. No external environmental reservoir such as straw or soil has been demonstrated.

5. **Mode of transmission**—Presumably the agent passes by contact from man to man as a part of the normal oral flora. From the oral cavity the fungus may be swallowed, inhaled or introduced into jaw tissues by injury or at the site of neglected or irritating dental defects. The source of clinical disease is endogenous. Transmission by human bite has been reported but is rare.

6. **Incubation period**—Irregular; probably many years after

1

colonization in the oral tissues, and days or months after precipitating trauma and actual penetration of tissues.

7. Period of communicability — Time and manner in which *A. israelii* becomes a part of the normal oral flora unknown. Except for the rare instances of human bite, not related to exposure to an infected person.

8. Susceptibility and resistance — Natural susceptibility is low. Immunity following attack has not been demonstrated.

9. Methods of control —

   A. *Preventive measures:* None, except that maintenance of good dental hygiene will reduce risk of infection around teeth.

   B. *Control of patient, contacts, and the immediate environment:*

   1) *Report to local health authority:* Official report not ordinarily justifiable, Class 5 (see Preface).
   2) *Isolation:* None.
   3) *Concurrent disinfection:* None.
   4) *Quarantine:* None.
   5) *Immunization of contacts:* None.
   6) *Investigation of contacts:* Not profitable.
   7) *Specific treatment:* No spontaneous recovery. Prolonged administration of penicillin in high doses is usually effective; tetracycline antibiotics are second choice and are often effective. Surgical drainage of abscesses is often necessary.

   C. *Epidemic measures:* Not applicable, a sporadic disease.

   D. *International measures:* None.

AMEBIASIS

1. Identification — Amebiasis is an infection with the protozoan parasite *Entamoeba histolytica*. The organism exists in two forms: the hardy, infective cyst and the more fragile, potentially invasive, trophozoite. The parasite may act as a commensal or invade the tissues, giving rise to intestinal or extra-intestinal disease. Most infections are asymptomatic, but *E. histolytica* must always be treated as a potential pathogen. Intestinal disease varies from acute, fulminating dysentery with fever, chills, and blood or mucoid diarrhea (amebic dysentery), to mild abdominal discomfort with diarrhea containing blood or mucus alternating with periods of constipation or remission. Amebic granulomata (ameboma), sometimes mistaken for carcinoma, may occur in the wall of the large intestine in patients with intermittent dysentery or colitis of long duration. Dissemination via the blood stream may occur, producing abscess of the liver or less commonly of the lung or brain. Ulceration of the skin, most frequently in the perianal region, may occur by direct extension from intestinal lesions.

Diagnosis is by direct microscopic demonstration of trophozoites or cysts in fresh fecal specimens, smears obtained by proctoscopy, aspirates of abscesses, or tissue sections. Organisms from these sources also may be cultured on special media. Special care should be taken for the proper collection and handling of specimens. Examination of the specimens should be done by a trained microscopist, since the organism must be differentiated from the nonpathogenic *Entamoeba hartmanni.* Use of reference laboratory facilities may be required. Serological tests are useful adjuncts in diagnosing all forms of amebiasis with the exception of the asymptomatic cyst passer, and are of particular importance in extra-intestinal disease. X-rays and/or radiographic liver scans are helpful in diagnosing amebic liver abscess.

The differential diagnosis includes shigellosis, appendicitis, balantidiasis, diverticulitis, giardiasis, and strongyloidiasis. Amebiasis can mimic ulcerative colitis and special care should be taken to distinguish the two diseases.

2. Occurrence—*Entamoeba histolytica* infection is cosmopolitan. The prevalence of infection in many areas of the world has not been established, but prevalence rates vary widely from place to place. They are higher in areas with poor sanitation and health education such as parts of the tropics and in mental institutions. The proportion of infected persons who have clinical disease may be low.

3. Infectious agent—*Entamoeba histolytica,* a protozoon not to be confused with *E. hartmanni* and *E. coli.*

4. Reservoir—Man. Usually a chronically ill or asymptomatic cyst passer.

5. Mode of transmission—In epidemics mainly by contaminated water containing cysts from feces of infected persons. Endemic spread is by hand-to-mouth transfer of fresh feces, by contaminated raw vegetables, by flies, by soiled hands of food handlers, and perhaps by water. Patients with acute amebic dysentery pose only limited danger to others because of the fragility of trophozoites.

6. **Incubation period**—Variable, from a few days to severa months or years. Commonly 2 to 4 weeks.

7. **Period of communicability**—During the period of cyst pas sing, which may continue for years.

8. **Susceptibility and resistance**—Although susceptibility to in fection is general, many persons harboring the organism do not de velop disease. Host differences such as race and age have been de scribed as affecting susceptibility of individuals to infection. Im munity to reinfection has not been clearly demonstrated.

9. **Methods of control**—

A. *Preventive measures:*
1) Improvement of living environment.
2) Sanitary disposal of human feces.
3) Protection of public water supplies against fecal con tamination; avoid cross-connections between public an private auxiliary water supplies and back-flow con nections in sewer systems. Sand filtration of water re moves nearly all cysts and diatomaceous earth filters re move them completely. Chlorination of water as gen erally practiced does not destroy cysts. Small quantitie of water as in canteens or Lyster bags are best treate with high concentrations of chlorine or iodine. Wate should be boiled where necessary.
4) Education of the general public in personal hygiene, pa ticularly sanitary disposal of feces and handwashin after defecation and before preparing or eating foo Dissemination of information regarding the risl involved in eating unpeeled or uncooked vegetables ar in drinking water of questionable purity.
5) Fly control and protection of foods against fly co tamination by screening and other appropriate means.
6) Supervision by health agencies of the health and san tary practices of persons preparing and serving food public eating places and general cleanliness of tl premises involved. Routine examination of fo handlers as a control measure is impractical.
7) Disinfectant dips for fruits and vegetables are of u proved value in preventing transmission of *histolytica*.
8) There is no satisfactory chemoprophylactic agent.

B. *Control of patient, contacts, and the immediate environmen.*
1) *Report to local health authorities:* In selected enden

areas (U.S.A.); in many states and countries not reportable, Class 3C (see Preface).

2) *Isolation:* None. Known cyst passers should be excluded from preparing, processing and serving food until treatment has been completed. Such persons should not work in areas where fecal-oral transmission might readily occur.

3) *Concurrent disinfection:* Sanitary disposal of feces.

4) *Quarantine:* None.

5) *Immunization of contacts and source of infection:* Not applicable.

6) *Investigation of contacts and source of infection:* Household members and other suspected contacts should have microscopic examination of feces and serological tests. One fecal examination may not be sufficient. Modes of transmission should be searched for, particularly via water contamination or an asymptomatic carrier.

7) *Specific treatment:* Acute amebic dysentery is best treated with metronidazole (Flagyl); which is, however, contraindicated in first trimester of pregnancy. Emetine hydrochloride or dehydroemetine followed by a combination of a tetracycline and di-iodohydroxyquin (Diodoquin) is an alternative treatment. Extra-intestinal amebiasis should be treated with metronidazole, or a combination of emetine hydrochloride and chloroquine (Aralen). Acutely ill patients may be too sick to take an oral preparation, in which case the more toxic emetine hydrochloride must be given. Abscesses may require surgical aspiration but medical treatment should be given first. Asymptomatic carriers may be treated with di-iodohydroxyquin (Diodoquin) or diloxanide furoate (Furamide).

C. *Epidemic measures:* Any group of cases from a single area or in an institution requires prompt epidemiologic investigation to determine source of infection and mode of transmission. If a common vehicle is indicated, such as water or food, appropriate measures to correct the situation should be taken. If epidemiologic evidence points to person-to-person transmission, emphasis should be on personal cleanliness, sanitary disposal of feces, and fly control.

D. *International measures:* None.

PRIMARY AMEBIC MENINGOENCEPHALITIS

1. **Identification**—A disease of humans essentially confined to the central nervous system caused by free-living amebae that ordinarily are found in water, soil, and decaying vegetation. They exist either as cysts that are resistant to environmental forces or as trophozoites which are probably the invasive stage; their growth may be enhanced by fecal contamination of water.

Two genera, *Naegleria* and *Acanthamoeba* have been implicated as causing human disease. Cases of meningoencephalitis caused by *Naegleria* organisms present a typical syndrome of fulminating meningoencephalitis with severe frontal headache, nausea, vomiting, high fever, nuchal rigidity and somnolence with death on the fifth or sixth day. The disease occurs in active young people of both sexes with no underlying illness. Pathologic findings, which are quite uniform, include moderate cerebral edema, severe hemorrhage and necrosis of the olfactory tracts, fibrino-purulent meningeal reaction with acute and chronic inflammatory cells, and inflammation and necrosis of the superficial cerebral grey matter, not involving the white matter. The greatest concentrations of amebae usually occur in the Virchow-Robin spaces. Almost all reported cases of primary amebic meningoencephalitis have been infections with *N. fowleri*. *Acanthamoeba* may produce disease characterized by insidious onset and a prolonged course or by a picture simulating aseptic meningitis. These organisms have not as yet been isolated from human brain, but characteristic cysts have been seen in stained tissue sections.

Diagnosis is made by microscopic examination of fresh spinal fluid wet mount preparations in which motile amebae may be seen or by culture on agar seeded with *Escherichia coli*. Amebae may be misidentified as macrophages or "gitter cells" if microscopic examination is made under a low power objective. The trophozoites may become flagellated after a few hours in water. *N. fowleri* is differentiable from non-pathogenic *N. gruberi* by serological tests.

2. **Occurrence**—A newly recognized disease first reported in Australia in 1965. Subsequently cases have been diagnosed in Czechoslovakia, Britain, Ireland, Belgium, New Zealand, India, and Africa. In the U.S.A., it has been reported from Florida, Texas, Virginia, Georgia, Pennsylvania, New York, and California.

3. **Infectious agents**—*Naegleria fowleri* and species of the genus *Acanthamoeba*.

4. **Reservoir**—None known for *N. fowleri* or *Acanthamoeba*.

5. **Mode of transmission**—Most cases attributed to *Naegleria*

have occurred a few days after healthy persons swam in warm fresh or brackish water. Stagnant ponds are particularly suspect but cases have occurred following swimming in warm mineral springs or swimming pools and in children who had played in mud holes. Human infection probably occurs directly via the cribriform plate as a result of contamination of the nasopharynx with water containing the amebae. Most cases have occurred during the hottest time of the year. Several cases of *Acanthamoeba* have been reported as hospital-acquired or -related infections of the brain. Patients gave no history of swimming and usually had an underlying chronic disease. Since the cysts are very hardy, it is conceivable that at times the disease may be airborne but this has never been documented.

6. **Incubation period** — From 3-7 days in documented cases.

7. **Period of communicability** — Transmission from man to man has not been documented.

8. **Susceptibility and resistance** — Unknown. Free living amebae of the genera *Hartmanella* and *Acanthamoeba* have been identified in the respiratory tract of healthy individuals. *Naegleria* has never been demonstrated in a carrier state. When disease occurs, it is usually rapidly fatal. More than 60 cases, mostly in children and young adults, have been reported in the world's literature.

9. **Methods of control** —

A. *Preventive measures* —

1) Protection of the nasopharynx from contamination by water containing *N. fowleri*. Practically, this is difficult or impossible to accomplish since the disease is uncommon and can be acquired from a wide variety of aquatic bodies and swimming pools.
2) Education of the public as to the dangers of swimming in lakes and ponds, where cases have been known to occur, and of forcing such water in the nasopharynx.
3) Swimming pools can be freed of amebae by a salt content of 0.7% while 10 ppm chlorine has been ineffective.

B. *Control of patient, contacts, and the immediate environment* —

1) *Report to local health authority:* This is a recently described disease and not reportable in most countries. Class 3B. (see Preface).
2) *Isolation:* None.
3) *Concurrent disinfection:* Incriminated pools treated with NaC1 to 0.7% concentration.
4) *Quarantine:* None.

5) *Immunization of contacts:* Not applicable.
6) *Investigation of contacts and source of infection:* History of swimming within the week prior to onset of symptoms may suggest the source of infection.
7) *Specific treatment: Naegleria* organisms are sensitive to amphotericin B; rare recovery has followed drug administered intravenously, intrathecally and by a ventricular reservoir. *Acanthamoebae* are sensitive to sulfonamides.

C. *Epidemic measures* — Multiple cases may occur following exposure to an apparently single source of infection. Any grouping of cases warrants prompt epidemiological investigation. Post implicated swimming areas to warn public of potential hazard.

D. *International measures* — None.

೧೪

ANCYLOSTOMIASIS (HOOKWORM DISEASE)
(Uncinariasis, Necatoriasis)

1. **Identification** — A chronic, debilitating disease with a variety of vague symptoms varying greatly according to the degree of anemia. The blood-letting activity of the nematode, along with malnutrition, leads to hypochromic microcytic anemia, a major cause of disability. Children with heavy, long term infection may be retarded in mental and physical development. Death is infrequent either in acute or chronic stages, and then usually in association with other infections. Light hookworm infections generally produce few or no clinical effects.

Infection is confirmed by finding hookworm eggs in feces; species recognition is through microscopic examination of adult worms or larvae cultured from the feces.

2. **Occurrence** — Widely endemic in those tropical and subtropical countries where disposal of human feces is inadequate, and soil, moisture, and temperature favor development of infective larvae. May also occur in temperate climates in similar environmental conditions (e.g., mines). *Necator americanus* is the prevailing species throughout most of tropical Africa and America;

Ancylostoma duodenale prevails in Mediterranean countries, including the Nile Valley. Both forms occur in many parts of Asia, Africa, Central and South America, the West Indies, and the South Pacific.

3. **Infectious agents**—*Necator americanus* and *Ancylostoma duodenale,* and less commonly in S.E. Asia, *A. ceylanicum.*

4. **Reservoir**—Man—an infected person discharging eggs in the feces; also dogs and cats discharging eggs of *A. ceylanicum.*

5. **Mode of transmission**—Eggs in feces are deposited on the ground and, under favorable conditions of moisture, temperature and type of soil, hatch; larvae develop to the 3rd stage, becoming infective in 7 to 10 days. Infection of man occurs when the infective larvae penetrate the bare skin, usually of the foot; in so doing they characteristically produce a dermatitis (ground itch). Infection with *Ancylostoma* may be acquired by the oral route. The larvae normally enter the skin and pass via lymphatics and blood stream to the lungs, enter the alveoli, migrate up the trachea to the pharynx, are swallowed, and reach the small intestine, where they attach to the intestinal wall, develop to maturity and produce eggs in 6 to 7 weeks, earlier (3-4 weeks) in *A. ceylanicum.*

6. **Incubation period**—Symptoms may develop after a few weeks to many months, depending on intensity of infection and nutrition of the host. Pulmonary infiltration, cough, and tracheitis may occur during the lung migration phase of infection.

7. **Period of communicability**—Infected persons are potential spreaders of infection for several years in the absence of treatment. Under favorable conditions, larvae remain infective in soil for several weeks.

8. **Susceptibility and resistance**—Universal; some immunity is thought to develop with infection.

9. **Methods of control**—

  A. *Preventive measures:*
    1) Prevention of soil contamination by installation of sanitary disposal systems for human feces, especially sanitary privies in rural areas. Night soil and sewage effluents are hazardous, especially where they are used as fertilizer.
    2) Education of the public as to dangers of soil contamination, and in preventive measures, including wearing shoes.

  B. *Control of patient, contacts, and the immediate environment:*
    1) *Report to local health authority:* Official report

ordinarily not justifiable, Class 5 (see Preface).

2) Isolation: None.

3) Concurrent disinfection: Sanitary disposal of feces to prevent contamination of soil.

4) Quarantine: None.

5) Immunization of contacts: None.

6) Investigation of contacts: Each infected contact and carrier is a potential or actual spreader of the disease.

7) Specific treatment: Tetrachlorethylene, bephenium, thiabendazole or pyrantel pamoate; toxic reactions are infrequent and therapy can be repeated if necessary; communicability is shortened. If present, ascariasis in young children should be treated before tetrachlorethylene is administered. Bephenium hydroxynaphthoate (Alcopar) is preferred to tetrachlorethylene for *A. duodenale* infections. Protein and iron supplementation of the diet is desirable.

C. Epidemic measures: Surveys for prevalence in highly endemic areas, health education in sanitation of the environment, in personal hygiene and the advisability of wearing shoes, and provision of facilities for excreta disposal for patients under treatment.

D. International measures: None.

ANGIOSTRONGYLIASIS
(Eosinophilic meningitis, Eosinophilic meningoencephalitis)

1. Identification — A disease of the central nervous system due to a nematode; meninges are predominantly involved. Invasion may be asymptomatic or mildly symptomatic; more commonly is characterized by severe headache, stiffness of neck and back, and various paresthesias. Temporary facial paralysis occurs in 5% of patients. Low-grade fever may be present. The worm has been found in the eye. Cerebrospinal fluid usually exhibits pleocytosis with 25-100% eosinophils; blood eosinophilia is not always present. Illness may last a few days to several months. Deaths have rarely been reported.

Diagnosis, especially in endemic areas, is suggested by

eosinophils in the cerebrospinal fluid. Differential diagnosis includes tuberculous meningitis, coccidioidal meningitis, cerebral cysticercosis, hydatidosis, and gnathostomiasis.

2. **Occurrence**—The disease is endemic in Hawaii, Tahiti, many other Pacific islands, and in Eastern Asia, including Vietnam, Thailand, Malaysia, Indonesia, Taiwan, and the Philippines. The nematode is found as far east as Hawaii, as far north as Japan, as far south as northern Australia, and as far west as Madagascar.

3. **Infectious agent**—*Angiostrongylus cantonensis*, a nematode (lungworm of rats). The third-stage larvae are infective.

4. **Reservoir**—The rat.

5. **Mode of transmission**—Ingestion of raw or insufficiently cooked snails, slugs or land planarians, which are intermediate or transport hosts harboring infective larvae. Prawns, fish and land crabs that have consumed snails or slugs transport the larvae, which remain infective. Lettuce and other similar vegetables contaminated by mollusks may serve as a source of infection.

6. **Incubation period**—Usually 1-3 weeks, though it may be longer or shorter.

7. **Period of communicability**—Not transmitted from man to man.

8. **Susceptibility and resistance**—Susceptibility to infection is general. Malnutrition and debilitating diseases may contribute to an increase in severity and even a fatal outcome.

9. **Methods of control**—

A. *Preventive measures:*
   1) Rat control.
   2) Thorough cooking of all foods. Boiling of snails, prawns, fish and crabs for 3-5 minutes or freezing at -15° C for 24 hours is effective in killing the larvae.
   3) Thorough cleansing of lettuce and other greens to eliminate mollusks and their products.
   4) Education of the general public in preparation of seafoods and both aquatic and terrestrial snails.

B. *Control of patient, contacts, and the immediate environment:*
   1) *Report to local health authority:* Official report not justifiable, Class 5 (see Preface).
   2) *Isolation:* None.
   3) *Concurrent disinfection:* Not necessary.
   4) *Quarantine:* None.
   5) *Immunization of contacts:* Not applicable.

    6) Investigation of contacts and source of infection: The
    source of food involved and its preparation should be
    investigated.
    7) Specific treatment: None.

C. Epidemic measures: Any grouping of several cases from a
single source or in an institution warrants prompt epidemiologic investigation.

D. International measures: None.

GNATHOSTOMIASIS is caused by the third-stage larva of
Gnathostoma spinigerum, a nematode parasite of cats and dogs.
Following ingestion of inadequately processed or cooked fish, the
third stage larvae migrate through the tissues of man and other
animals, forming transient inflammatory lesions or abscesses in
various parts of the body. Larvae may invade the brain, producing
focal cerebral lesions associated with eosinophilic pleocytosis.
Most common in Thailand.

ANTHRAX

(Malignant pustule, Malignant edema, Woolsorters' disease, Rag-
pickers' disease, Charbon)

1. Identification — An acute bacterial disease usually affecting
the skin, but may rarely involve the lungs or gastrointestinal tract.
Itching of an exposed skin surface occurs early, followed by a lesion
which becomes macular, then vesiculated, and in 2-6 days develops
into a depressed black eschar. At times the eschar is surrounded by
mild to moderate edema, sometimes with small secondary vesicles
("pearl wreath"). Pain is unusual, and if present is related to edema
or secondary infection. Untreated infections may spread to regional
lymph nodes and the bloodstream with an overwhelming
septicemia. Untreated cutaneous anthrax has a fatality rate of from
5 to 20%, but with effective antibiotic therapy, few deaths occur.
The usual lesion evolves through typical local changes even after
the initiation of antibiotic therapy.

    Initial symptoms of inhalation anthrax are mild and non-specific,
resembling common upper respiratory infection; acute symptoms
of respiratory distress, fever and shock follow in from 3 to 5 days,

with death shortly thereafter. Gastrointestinal anthrax is more difficult to recognize, except that it tends to occur in explosive outbreaks; abdominal distress is followed by fever, signs of septicemia and death in the typical case.

Laboratory confirmation is by direct demonstration of the causative organism in blood, lesions or discharges by culture or by inoculation of mice, guinea pigs or rabbits. Fluorescent antibody techniques can be used for identification of the bacillus in vesicular fluid smears, cultures, or tissue sections; gram-stained smears are often helpful.

2. **Occurrence**—Infrequent and sporadic in humans in U.S.A. and most industrial countries. Primarily an occupational hazard of industrial workers who process hides, hair (especially from goats), bone and bone products, and wool, and of veterinarians and agricultural workers who handle infected animals. Endemic in those agricultural regions of the world where anthrax in animals is common. New areas of infection in livestock may develop through introduction of animal feed containing contaiminated bone meal. Altered environmental conditions such as floods or droughts may provoke epizootics by bringing dormant anthrax spores to the surface of the soil.

3. **Infectious agent**—*Bacillus anthracis.*

4. **Reservoir**—No true reservoir. The spores of *B. anthracis,* which resist environmental factors and disinfection, remain viable in contaminated areas for many years after the source-animal infection has terminated.

5. **Mode of transmission**—Infection of skin is by contact with tissues of animals (cattle, sheep, goats, horses, pigs and others) dying of the disease; or contaminated hair, wool, hides, and soil associated with infected animals. Inhalation anthrax results from inhalation of spores. Gastrointestinal anthrax arises from ingestion of contaminated undercooked meat; there is no evidence that milk from infected animals transmits anthrax. The disease spreads among herbivorous animals through contaminated soil and feed and among omnivorous and carnivorous animals through contaminated meat, bone meal or other feeds. Biting flies and other insects are suspected of serving as mechanical vectors. Vultures have spread the organism from one area to another. Accidental infections may occur among laboratory workers.

6. **Incubation period**—Within 7 days, usually 2 to 5.

7. **Period of communicability**—No evidence of transmission from man to man. Articles and soil contaminated with spores may remain infective for years.

8. Susceptibility and resistance — Uncertain; some evidence of inapparent infection among persons in frequent contact with the infectious agent; second attacks are undocumented.

9. Methods of control —

  A. *Preventive measures:*
  1) A cell-free vaccine, available in the U.S.A. from the Center for Disease Control, Atlanta, GA (see Preface) for high-risk persons, is effective in preventing cutaneous and probably inhalation anthrax; it is recommended for veterinarians and for persons handling potentially contaminated industrial raw materials.
  2) Education in personal cleanliness, in modes of anthrax transmission and in care of skin abrasions for employees handling potentially contaminated articles.
  3) Dust control and proper ventilation in hazardous industries. Continuing medical supervision of employees, with prompt medical care of all suspicious skin lesions. Use protective clothing and adequate facilities for washing and changing clothes after work. Locate eating facilities away from places of work. Vaporized formaldehyde has been employed in textile mills contaminated with *B. anthracis.*
  4) Thorough washing, disinfection or sterilization of hair, wool or hides, and bone meal or other feed of animal origin, prior to processing.
  5) Hides of animals exposed to anthrax should not be sold, nor their carcasses used as food or feed supplements.
  6) Conduct postmortem examination of animals dying of suspected anthrax, with care not to contaminate soil or environment with blood or infected tissues. Burn carcasses or bury deeply with anhydrous calcium oxide (quick-lime), preferably at site of death. Decontaminate soil seeded with bodily discharges.
  7) Promptly treat all animals suspected of exposure to anthrax with penicillin or tetracyclines.
  8) Annual vaccination of animals in enzootic areas.
  9) Control effluents and trade wastes of rendering plants handling potentially infected animals and those from factories that manufacture products from hair, wool or hides likely to be contaminated.

  B. *Control of patient, contacts, and the immediate environment:*
  1) *Report to local health authority:* Case report obligatory in most states and countries, Class 2A (see Preface).

Report also to appropriate livestock or agriculture authority.

2) *Isolation:* Wound isolation until lesions are bacteriologically free of anthrax bacilli. It is prudent to hold inhalation anthrax cases under strict isolation.

3) *Concurrent disinfection:* Of discharges from lesions and articles soiled therewith. Spores require steam sterilization or burning for certain destruction. Terminal cleaning.

4) *Quarantine:* None.

5) *Immunization of contacts:* None.

6) *Investigation of contacts and source of infection:* Search for history of exposure to infected animals or contaminated animal products, and trace to place of origin. If in a manufacturing plant, inspect for adequacy of preventive measures as outlined in 9A above.

7) *Specific treatment:* Penicillin is the drug of choice; tetracyclines or another broad-spectrum antibiotic may be used.

C. **Epidemic measures:** The occasional epidemics in man in U.S.A. are local industrial outbreaks among employees who work with animal products, especially goat hair; outbreaks may be related to consumption of meat from infected cattle or may be an occupational hazard of animal husbandry. For appropriate control measures, see 9A above.

D. **International measures:** Sterilization of imported bone meal before use as animal feed. Disinfection of wool, hair, hides and other products when indicated and practicable; formaldehyde has been used successfully; cobalt irradiation has also been used.

ARTHROPOD-BORNE VIRAL DISEASES
(Arboviral Diseases)

Summary

A large number of arboviruses are known to produce diseases in man, and the number is growing rapidly. These diseases present principally in four clinical syndromes: (1) an acute *central nervous system disease, usually with encephalitis,* but ranging in severity from mild aseptic meningitis to coma, paralysis and death; (2) acute *benign fevers* of short duration, many resembling dengue with and without an exanthem, although on occasion some may give rise to a more serious illness with central nervous system involvement or hemorrhages; (3) *hemorrhagic fevers,* which include acute febrile diseases with extensive hemorrhagic involvement, external or internal, frequently serious, and associated with shock and significantly high fatality rates. One of them, yellow fever, also causes liver damage and jaundice; milder clinical forms of this disease may resemble the second syndrome (benign fever) and a few patients also may have an encephalitic component; (4) *polyarthritis and rash,* usually without fever, and of variable duration, benign, or with arthralgic sequelae lasting several weeks to months.

Most of these diseases are zoonoses, accidentally acquired by man through an arthropod vector, with man an unimportant host in the cycle. In the presence of viremia and a suitable vector a few may become epidemic, with man the principal source of vector infection. There is no recognized animal reservoir for some infections. Most of the viruses are mosquito-borne, several are tick-borne and others are phlebotomine-borne (sandfly). A few are transmitted by *Culicoides* species (midges, gnats). Laboratory infections occur, some by arerosols.

Though the agents differ, common epidemiologic factors in the transmission cycles, chiefly relating to the vector, characterize these diseases and therefore are important in control. Consequently, the selected diseases under each clinical syndrome are arranged in four groups: mosquito-borne, tick-borne, phlebotomine-borne and unknown. Diseases of major importance are described individually or in groups where clinical and epidemiological similarities exist. These diseases are presented in the accompanying table; some of the less important or less well-studied are not discussed in the text.

Viruses believed to be associated with human disease are listed in the Table by type of vector as reasonably established or suspected, the predominant character of recognized disease, and the geographical area where found. In some instances observed cases are too few to be certain of the usual clinical reaction. Some have been recognized only through laboratory-acquired exposure. None is included where evidence of human infection is based solely on serological survey; otherwise the number would be much greater.

Approximately 80 viruses presently classified as arboviruses produce disease in man. Most of these are further classified by hemagglutination or complement fixation into antigenic groups, of which

DISEASES IN MAN CAUSED BY ARTHROPOD-BORNE VIRUSES

Virus Group	Name of Virus	Vector	Disease in Man	Where Found
TOGAVIRUSES Group A	*Chikungunya	Mosquito	Fever, hemorrhagic fever, arthralgia	Africa, Southeast Asia, Philippines
	*Eastern equine	Mosquito	Encephalitis	Americas
	*Mayaro (Uruma)	Mosquito	Fever	South America
	*Mucambo	Mosquito	Fever	South America
	*O'nyong-nyong	Mosquito	Fever, arthralgia	Africa
	*Ross River	Mosquito	Arthritis, rash	Australia
	Sindbis	Mosquito	Fever	Africa, India, Southeast Asia, Philippines, Australia
(*Alphaviruses*)				
Group B	*Venezuelan equine	Mosquito	Fever, encephalitis	South America, Mexico, U.S.A.
	*Western equine	Mosquito	Encephalitis	Americas
	Banzi	Mosquito	Fever	Africa
	Bat salivary gland (Rio Bravo)	Unknown	Encephalitis, aseptic meningitis	U.S.A.
	*Bussuquara	Mosquito	Fever	South America
	*Dengue 1, 2, 3, and 4	Mosquito	Fever, rash, hemorrhagic fever	Africa, Asia, Pacific Islands, South America, Caribbean area, Australia, New Guinea
(*Flaviviruses*)	*Central European encephalitis	Tick	Encephalitis	Europe

Diseases in Man Caused by Arthropod-Borne Viruses (Continued)

Virus Group	Name of Virus	Vector	Disease in Man	Where Found
	Ilheus	Mosquito	Fever, encephalitis	South America, Central America
	*Japanese (B)	Mosquito	Encephalitis	Asia, Pacific Islands
	Kunjin	Mosquito	Fever	Australia, Sarawak
	*Kyasanur Forest	Tick	Hemorrhagic fever	India
	*Louping ill	Tick	Encephalitis	Great Britain
	*Murray Valley	Mosquito	Encephalitis	Australia, New Guinea
	Negishi	Unknown	Encephalitis	Japan
	*Omsk hemorrhagic	Tick	Hemorrhagic fever	U.S.S.R.
	*Powassan	Tick	Encephalitis	Canada, U.S.A.
Togaviruses— Group B continued	*Russian spring-summer (tick-borne encephalitis)	Tick	Encephalitis	Europe, Asia
	Spondweni	Mosquito	Fever	Africa
	*St. Louis	Mosquito	Encephalitis	Americas, Jamaica,
	Usutu	Mosquito	Fever	Africa
	Wesselsbron	Mosquito	Fever	Africa, Asia
	*West Nile	Mosquito	Fever, encephalitis, rash	Africa, India, Middle East, Europe
	*Yellow fever	Mosquito	Hemorrhagic fever	Africa, South and Central America

* Asterisked Groups and Viruses are discussed in the text. See Index for page numbers.

Diseases in Man Caused by Arthropod-Borne Viruses

Virus Group	Name of Virus	Vector	Disease in Man	Where Found
BUNYAVIRUSES				
Group C*	Zika	Mosquito	Fever	Africa, Southeast Asia
	Apeu	Mosquito	Fever	South America
	Caraparu	Mosquito	Fever	South America
	Itaqui	Mosquito	Fever	South America
	Madrid	Mosquito	Fever	South America
	Marituba	Mosquito	Fever	South America
	Murutucu	Mosquito	Fever	South America
	Oriboca	Mosquito	Fever	South America
	Ossa	Mosquito	Fever	South America
	Restan	Mosquito	Fever	South America
Bunyamwera group	*Bunyamwera	Mosquito	Fever	Africa
	Germiston	Mosquito	Fever	Africa
	Guaroa	Mosquito	Fever	South America, Panama
	Ilesha	Mosquito	Fever	Africa
	Wyeomyia	Unknown	Fever	South America, Panama
Bwamba group	*Bwamba	Mosquito	Fever	Africa
California group	*California	Mosquito	Encephalitis	U.S.A., Canada
	*LaCrosse	Mosquito	Encephalitis	U.S.A., Canada
	Tahyna	Mosquito	Fever	Europe
Guama group	Catu	Mosquito	Fever	South America
	Guama	Mosquito	Fever	South America
	Candiru	Unknown	Fever	South America
Sandfly fever group* (Phlebotomus fever)	Chagres	Phlebotomine	Fever	Central America
	Naples type	Phlebotomine	Fever	Europe, Africa, Asia
	Punta Toro	Phlebotomine	Fever	Panama

*Asterisked Groups and viruses are discussed in the text. See Index for page numbers.

Diseases in Man Caused by Arthropod-Borne Viruses (Continued)

Virus Group	Name of Virus	Vector	Disease in Man	Where Found
	Sicilian type	Phlebotomine	Fever	Europe, Africa, Asia
Simbu group	Shuni	Mosquito	Fever	Africa
	*Oropouche	Mosquito	Fever	South America
Ungrouped	Crimean hemorrhagic-Congo	Tick	Hemorrhagic fever	Europe, Africa
	Dugbe	Tick	Fever	Africa
	Ganjam	Tick	Fever	India
	Nairobi sheep disease	Tick	Fever	Africa
	Rift Valley	Mosquito	Fever	Africa
	Thogoto	Tick	Meningitis	Africa, Europe
ORBIVIRUSES				
Changuinola group	*Changuinola	Phlebotomine	Fever	Central America
Kemerovo group*	Kemerovo	Tick	Fever	Europe
	Tribec-Lipovnik	Tick	Fever	Europe
Ungrouped	*Colorado tick fever	Tick	Fever	U.S.A.
RHABDOVIRUSES				
Vesicular stomatitis group	*Vesicular stomatitis, Indiana & New Jersey	Phlebotomine	Fever	North and Central America
	Chandipura	Mosquito	Fever	India
	Piry	Mosquito	Fever	South America
NOT CLASSIFIED	Nyando	Mosquito	Fever	Africa
	Quaranfil	Tick	Fever	Africa

*Asterisked groups and viruses are discussed in the text. See Index for page numbers.

A and B are the largest and best known. Both groups A and B contain agents causing predominantly encephalitis and agents causing predominantly other febrile illnesses. Group A contains only mosquito-borne viruses, group B both mosquito-borne and tick-borne agents and some agents without recognized vectors. Viruses of group C and several other groups produce principally febrile diseases. Several human pathogens for which no common antigens have been demonstrated necessarily remain in a miscellaneous category.

∞

ARTHROPOD BORNE VIRAL ARTHRITIS AND RASH
I. Mosquito-borne

A. EPIDEMIC POLYARTHRITIS AND RASH

1. Identification — An acute, self-limited disease characterized by arthritis, primarily in the small joints of the extremities, which lasts from 2 days to 8 months. In many patients arthritis is followed in one to ten days by a maculo-papular rash, which though rarely vesicular, may cover much of the skin surface. Petechiae and enanthem are rare. Fever is usually absent. Lymphadenopathy, paresthesias and tenderness of palms and soles are present in a small percentage of cases. Serologic tests show a rise in titer to group A arboviruses, but the virus has not been isolated.

2. Occurrence — Major outbreaks have occurred in Murray Valley, Northern Territory, and Queensland in Australia and sporadic cases in the coastal regions of Australia and New Guinea.

3. Infectious agent — Group A arbovirus, probably the Ross River virus.

4. Reservoir — Unknown.

5. Mode of transmission — Probably transmitted by Culicine mosquitoes.

6. Incubation period — 10 to 11 days.

7. Period of communicability — No evidence of transmission from man to man.

8. Susceptibility and resistance — Recovery is universal and followed by lasting immunity; second attacks are unknown. Inapparent infections are common, especially in children.

9. **Methods of control—**

A. *Preventive measures:*
 1) The general measures applicable to mosquito-borne viral encephalitides (9A-1 through 5 and 9A-7, pp. 24 and 25).

B. *Control of patient, contacts, and the immediate environment:*
 1) *Report to local health authority:* Not a reportable disease, Class 3B (see Preface).
 2) *Isolation:* None.
 3) *Concurrent disinfection:* None.
 4) *Quarantine:* None.
 5) *Immunization of contacts:* None.
 6) *Investigation of contacts:* Place of residence of patient during fortnight previous to onset. Search for unreported or undiagnosed cases; bleed febrile or asymptomatic family members and carry out a viremia test using suckling mice.
 7) *Specific treatment:* None.

C. *Epidemic measures:* Same as for arthropod-borne viral fevers (see 9C 1-3, p. 30).

D. *International measures:* None. WHO Collaborating Centres (see Preface).

ARTHROPOD-BORNE VIRAL ENCEPHALITIDES

I. Mosquito-borne
EASTERN EQUINE, WESTERN EQUINE, CALIFORNIA, JAPANESE, MURRAY VALLEY, AND ST. LOUIS ENCEPHALITIS

1. Identification—A group of acute inflammatory diseases of short duration, involving parts of the brain, spinal cord and meninges. Signs and symptoms are similar, but vary in severity and rate of progress. Mild cases often occur as aseptic meningitis. Severe infections are usually marked by acute onset, headache, high fever, meningeal signs, stupor, disorientation, coma, spasticity, tremors, occasionally convulsions (especially in infants) and spastic, but rarely flaccid, paralysis. Fatality rates range from 5 to 60%, that of Japanese and eastern equine types being highest. With most viruses, conspicuous sequelae are rare except in infants; more evident with eastern equine and Japanese; no parkinsonism. Mild leucocytosis is usual; leucocytes in spinal fluid range from 50 to 200 per cu. mm., occasionally 1,000 or more in infants.

Specific identification is by demonstrated antibody titer rises between early and late specimens of serum by neutralization, complement fixation and hemagglutination inhibition. Group reactions may occur. Virus may be isolated by inoculation of suckling mice or tissue culture with the brain tissue of fatal cases, rarely with blood or cerebrospinal fluid; histopathological changes are not specific for individual viruses.

The diseases require differentiation from the tick-borne encephalitides, encephalitic and non-paralytic poliomyelitis, rabies, mumps meningo-encephalitis, lymphocytic choriomeningitis, aseptic meningitis due to enteroviruses, herpes encephalitis, post-vaccinal or postinfection encephalitides, bacterial, protozoal, leptospiral and mycotic meningitides or encephalitides; also from the von Economo type of encephalitis (encephalitis lethargica), of unknown etiology, frequently seen just before and after 1920, but now rarely reported. Venezuelan equine and West Nile viruses, primarily producing arthropod-borne viral fever (pp. 30-33), are sometimes responsible for encephalitis.

2. **Occurrence** — Eastern equine encephalitis is recognized in eastern and north central U.S.A. and adjacent Canada, in scattered areas of Central and South America and in the Caribbean Islands; western equine in western or central U.S.A. and Canada and in scattered areas further east; Japanese in western Pacific Islands from Japan to the Philippines and in many areas of eastern Asia from Korea to Indonesia and India; Murray Valley in parts of Australia and New Guinea; St. Louis in most of U.S.A. and also in Trinidad, Jamaica, Panama, and Brazil; California encephalitis is a forest acquired disease in the U.S.A. and Canada. Cases occur in temperate latitudes in summer and early fall, and are commonly limited to areas and years of high temperature and many mosquitoes; these diseases tend to persist endemically in hot, irrigated valley regions, are irregularly noted in dry farming areas, and may also be seasonal in tropical countries, depending on rainfall and vector population.

3. **Infectious agents** — Each disease is caused by a specific virus in one of three groups: eastern equine and western equine in group A togaviruses; Japanese, Murray Valley and St. Louis in group B togaviruses; LaCrosse and possibly others in the California group.

4. **Reservoir** — The true reservoir or means of winter carry-over is unknown; possibly in birds, rodents, bats, reptiles, amphibians or surviving mosquito eggs or adults, possibly differing for each virus.

5. **Mode of transmission** — By the bite of infective mosquitoes.

Most important vectors are: for eastern equine in U.S.A., probably *Culiseta melanura* from bird to bird and one or more *Aedes* species from birds or animals to man; for western equine in western U.S.A., *Culex tarsalis*; for Japanese, *C. tritaeniorhynchus*, and also *C. gelidus* in tropics; for Murray Valley, probably *C. annulirostris*; for St. Louis in U.S.A., *C. tarsalis*, the *C. pipiens-quinquefasciatus* complex, and *C. nigripalpus*; for California, *Aedes canadiens*, and *A. triseriatus*. Mosquitoes usually acquire the infection from wild birds or rodents, but pigs are of some importance for Japanese; for others, occasionally a mammal such as the horse. LaCrosse virus is transovarially transmitted in *A. triseriatus*.

6. **Incubation period** — Usually 5 to 15 days.

7. **Period of communicability** — Not directly transmitted from man to man. Virus is not usually demonstrable in the blood of man after onset of disease. Mosquitoes remain infective for life. Viremia in birds usually lasts 2 to 5 days but may be prolonged in bats, reptiles and amphibia, particularly if interrupted by hibernation. Horses develop active disease with the two equine viruses and with Japanese, but viremia is rarely present for long periods or in high titer; therefore, man and horses are uncommon sources of mosquito infection.

8. **Susceptibility and resistance** — Susceptibility to clinical disease is usually highest in infancy and old age; inapparent or undiagnosed infection is more common at other ages. Susceptibility varies with virus; e.g., St. Louis tends to spare young children. Infection results in homologous immunity. In highly endemic areas adults are largely immune to local strains by reason of mild and inapparent infection; susceptibles are mainly children.

9. **Methods of Control** —

   A. *Preventive measures:*
      1) Destruction of larvae and elimination of breeding places of known or suspected vector mosquitoes.
      2) Killing mosquitoes by space and residual spraying of human habitations. (See Malaria 9A1, p. 191).
      3) Screening of sleeping and living quarters; use of mosquito bed nets.
      4) Avoiding exposure to mosquitoes during hours of biting, or by using repellents. (See Malaria 9A4, p. 192).
      5) Education of the public as to mode of spread and control.
      6) Mouse brain-inactivated vaccine for children is used against Japanese encephalitis in Japan and experimentally in a few other countries, including Taiwan.

Tissue culture vaccines are under development; no licensed vaccines for others. For those under continued intensive exposure Eastern Equine Encephalitis Vaccine, Inactivated, Dried, is available on an investigational basis from the Center for Disease Control, Atlanta, Georgia (see Preface).
7) Passive protection of accidentally exposed laboratory workers by human or animal immune serum.

B. *Control of patient, contacts, and the immediate environment:*
   1) *Report to local health authority:* Case report obligatory in most states of U.S.A. and in some other countries, Class 2A (see Preface). Report under the appropriate disease; or as encephalitis, other forms; or as aseptic meningitis, with etiology or clinical type specified when known.
   2) *Isolation:* None; virus not usually found in blood, secretions or discharges during clinical manifestations.
   3) *Concurrent disinfection:* None.
   4) *Quarantine:* None.
   5) *Immunization of contacts:* None.
   6) *Investigation of contacts and source of infection:* Search for missed cases and the presence of vector mosquitoes; test for viremia in both febrile and asymptomatic family members; primarily a community problem (see 9C)
   7) *Specific treatment:* None.

C. *Epidemic measures:*
   1) Identification of disease among horses or birds and recognition of human cases in the community have epidemiological value by indicating frequency of infection and areas involved. Immunization of horses probably does not limit spread of the virus in the community.
   2) Fogging or spraying from aircraft with suitable insecticides has shown promise for aborting urban epidemics of St. Louis encephalitis.

D. *International measures:* Insecticide spraying of airplanes arriving from recognized areas of prevalence. WHO Collaborating Centers (see Preface).

II. Tick-borne
   RUSSIAN SPRING-SUMMER ENCEPHALITIS, CENTRAL
   EUROPEAN ENCEPHALITIS, LOUPING ILL, POWAS-
   SAN ENCEPHALITIS

1. **Identification**—A group of diseases clinically resembling mosquito-borne encephalitides, except that the Russian spring-summer type often is associated with flaccid paralysis, particularly of the shoulder girdle, and with residua. Central European encephalitis (diphasic milk fever or diphasic meningo-encephalitis) has a longer course, averaging 3 weeks; initial febrile stage is unassociated with symptoms referable to central nervous system; a second phase of fever and meningo-encephalitis follows 4 to 10 days after apparent recovery; fatality and severe residua are less frequent than for the Russian spring-summer disease. Louping ill in man also has a diphasic pattern and is relatively mild.

Specific identification is by serological tests or by isolation of virus from blood during acute illness by inoculation of suckling mice or tissue culture. Common serological tests cannot be expected to differentiate members of this group, but do distinguish the group from most other similar diseases.

2. **Occurrence**—Disease of the central nervous system from this virus complex is distributed spottily over much of the USSR, other parts of eastern and central Europe, Scandinavia and Great Britain. In general, the spring-summer type has a more eastern or Asian distribution; diphasic meningo-encephalitis predominates in Europe, while louping ill is present in Scotland, Northern England, and Ireland. Powassan virus is present in Canada and the U.S.A. Seasonal incidence depends on activity of the tick vectors. *Ixodes persulcatus* is usually active in spring and early summer, while *I. ricinus* continues activity into late summer or early autumn. Areas of highest incidence are those where man has intimate association with large numbers of infected ticks, generally in rural or forested areas, but also in some urban populations. Local epidemics of Central European encephalitis have occurred among persons consuming raw milk from goats or sheep, thus the name diphasic milk fever. Laboratory infections are common, some with serious sequelae, others fatal.

3. **Infectious agents**—Minor antigenic differences exist, more with Powassan than others, but viruses in these diseases are closely related and form a complex within group B togaviruses.

4. **Reservoir**—The tick or a combination of tick and mammal appears to be the true reservoir; transovarian tick passage of some

USSR viruses has been demonstrated. Sheep and deer are the hosts most involved in louping ill. Rodents and sometimes other mammals and birds, rarely man, give rise to tick infections in Europe and Asia.

5. **Mode of transmission**—By the bite of infective ticks, or by consumption of milk from certain infected animals. *Ixodes persulcatus* is the principal vector in eastern USSR and *I. ricinus* in western USSR and other parts of Europe; the latter is also the vector of louping ill of sheep in Scotland. *I. cookei* is the principal vector in eastern Canada and U.S.A. Larval ticks usually ingest virus by feeding on rodents, sometimes other mammals and birds. Adult ticks may acquire infection from man. Raw milk may be a vehicle for diphasic meningo-encephalitis.

6. **Incubation period**—Usually 7 to 14 days.

7. **Period of communicability**—Not directly transmitted from man to man. A tick infected at any stage remains infective for life. Viremia in a variety of vertebrates may last for several days; in man up to a week or 10 days.

8. **Susceptibility and resistance**—Both sexes and all ages are susceptible. The age pattern varies widely in different regions and is influenced by opportunity for exposure to ticks, consumption of milk from infected animals, or by previously acquired immunity. Infection, whether inapparent or overt, leads to immunity.

9. **Methods of Control**—

A. *Preventive measures:*
1) See Tick-borne Rickettsial Fevers 9A1 and 2, for measures against ticks (p. 268).
2) Formalinized virus vaccines have been used extensively in the USSR with reported safety and effectiveness.
3) Boil or pasteurize milk from susceptible animals in areas where diphasic meningo-encephalitis occurs.

B. *Control of patient, contacts, and the immediate environment:*
1) *Report to local health authority:* In selected endemic areas; in most countries not a reportable disease, Class 3B (see Preface).
2) *Isolation:* None, if patient is tick-free.
3) *Concurrent disinfection:* None.
4) *Quarantine:* None.
5) *Immunization of contacts:* None.
6) *Investigation of contacts and source of infection:* Search for missed cases, presence of tick vectors and animals excreting virus in milk.

7) *Specific treatment:* None.

C. *Epidemic measures:* See Tick-borne Rickettsial Fevers (p. 267).

D. *International measures:* WHO Collaborating Centers (see Preface).

ARTHROPOD-BORNE VIRAL FEVERS

I. Mosquito-borne

A. DENGUE FEVER

(Breakbone fever)

1. Identification—An acute febrile disease characterized by sudden onset, fever for about 5 days and rarely more than 7, intense headache, retro-orbital pains, joint and muscle pains, and rash. Early general erythema occurs in some cases. The rash usually appears 3 to 4 days after onset of fever and is either maculopapular or scarlatiniform. Petechiae may appear on the feet or legs, in the axillae, or on the palate on the last day of fever or shortly thereafter. Dark-skinned races frequently have no visible rash. Recovery may be associated with prolonged fatigue and depression. Leucopenia and lymphadenopathy are usual. Epidemics are explosive but the fatality rate is exceedingly low.

Differential diagnosis includes all diseases listed under Arthropod-Borne Hemorrhagic Fevers (see pp. 37-46) Colorado tick fever, the sandfly fevers, influenza, rubella, and others.

Hemagglutination-inhibition, complement-fixation or neutralization tests are diagnostic aids. Virus is isolated from blood by inoculation of suckling mice or by tissue culture techniques.

2. Occurrence—Dengue viruses are now endemic in most countries of tropical Asia (Sri Lanka, India, Bangladesh, Burma, Thailand, Laos, Cambodia, North and South Vietnam, Malaysia, Singapore, Indonesia, New Guinea and the Philippines). Since 1971, epidemics of dengue fever have involved much of Polynesia and more recently, Micronesia; it appears to be endemic in Tahiti. Dengue viruses are endemic in many of the islands of the Caribbean . and in several Central and South American countries. Recently, they have been recovered from West Africa. Epidemics can occur wherever vectors are present and virus is introduced, whether in urban or rural areas.

3. Infectious agent—The viruses of dengue fever include immunological types 1, 2, 3, and 4—group B togaviruses. The same viruses are responsible for hemorrhagic fever (see Arthropod-borne Viral Hemorrhagic Fevers, pp. 37-46).

4. Reservoir—Man, together with the mosquito, is one reservoir; the monkey-mosquito complex may be a reservoir in Western Malaysia.

5. Mode of transmission—By the bite of infective mosquitoes, *Aedes aegypti, A. albopictus,* or one of the *A. scutellaris* complex, infected by biting an infectious human or possibly a monkey.

6. Incubation period—3 to 15 days, commonly 5 to 6 days.

7. Period of communicability—Not directly transmitted from man to man. Patients are usually infective for mosquitoes from the day before onset to the 5th day of disease. The mosquito becomes infective 8 to 11 days after the blood meal and remains so for life.

8. Susceptibility and resistance—Susceptibility is apparently universal, but children usually have a milder disease than adults. Homologous immunity is of long duration; heterologous immunity, though present, is brief and may permit mild, undiagnosed febrile illness.

9. Methods of Control—

   A. Preventive measures:
     1) Community survey to determine density of vector mosquitoes, to identify breeding places, and to promote and implement plans for their elimination.
     2) Education of the public on personal measures for protection against mosquitoes, including use of repellents and bed nets (see Malaria 9A3 and 4, p. 192).

   B. Control of patient, contacts, and the immediate environment:
     1) Report to local health authority: Obligatory report of epidemics; no case report, Class 4 (see Preface).
     2) Isolation: Patients should be kept in screened rooms for at least 5 days after onset, or in quarters treated with an effective insecticide.
     3) Concurrent disinfection: None.
     4) Quarantine: None.
     5) Immunization of contacts: None.
     6) Investigation of contacts: Determine place of residence of patient during fortnight previous to onset and search for unreported or undiagnosed cases.
     7) Specific treatment: None.

C. Epidemic measures:
1) Search for and destroy *Aedes* species of mosquitoes in places of human habitation.
2) Use of mosquito repellents by persons exposed through occupation or other necessity to bites of vector mosquitoes.
3) Fogging or airplane spraying with a suitable insecticide has shown promise for aborting urban epidemics.

D. International measures: Enforcement of international agreements designed to prevent spread of the disease by man, monkey, and mosquito and transfer via ships, airplanes and land transport from areas where an epidemic exists. WHO Collaborating Centres (see Preface).

∞

B. BUNYAMWERA, BWAMBA, CHIKUNGUNYA, MAY-ARO O'NYONG-NYONG, RIFT VALLEY, VENEZUELAN EQUINE, WEST NILE, GROUP C VIRAL FEVERS, OROPOUCHE, AND OTHERS

1. Identification — A group of febrile illnesses usually lasting a week or less, many of which are dengue-like (see table for mosquito-borne viruses). Usual onset is with headache, malaise, arthralgia or myalgia and occasionally nausea and vomiting; generally some conjunctivitis and photophobia. Fever may or may not be diphasic (saddleback). Rashes are common in West Nile, chikungunya and o'nyong-nyong. Hemorrhages sometimes occur in chikungunya fever in Southeast Asia and India; leucopenia is common; convalescence frequently prolonged. Meningo-encephalitis occasionally complicates West Nile and Venezuelan equine virus infections. Several group C viruses are reported to produce weakness in the lower limbs. Rarely fatal, except for encephalitis from Venezuelan equine. Epidemics of chikungunya, o'nyong-nyong, Venezuelan equine, and Oropouche may involve thousands of patients.

Serological tests differentiate other fevers of viral or unknown origin, but chikungunya, o'nyong-nyong, and others in group A are difficult to distinguish from one another. Specific diagnosis is possible by virus isolation from blood during the febrile period by inoculation of suckling mice or tissue culture; Venezuelan equine also may be isolated from nasopharyngeal washings. Laboratory infections occur with many of these viruses.

2. Occurrence—West Nile virus is present in Egypt, Israel, India, France and probably is widespread in parts of Africa and the northern Mediterranean area. Chikungunya virus is found in Africa, India, Southeast Asia and the Philippine Islands; Rift Valley, o'nyong-nyong, Bwamba and Bunyamwera fevers thus far have been identified only in Africa. Mayaro and group C fevers occur in tropical South America, Panama and Trinidad, while Venezuelan equine and other closely related viruses (Mucambo) are observed in Venezuela, Florida, Middle America and Mexico; Oropouche fever is found in Trinidad and Brazil; Kunjin virus in Australia. Seasonal incidence depends on vector prevalence. Recognized occurrence is primarily rural or forest, though occasionally chikungunya occurs in explosive urban outbreaks.

3. Infectious agents—Each disease is due to an independent virus of the same name as the disease. West Nile, Banzi, Kunjin, Spondweni, and Zika viruses are in group B togaviruses; the closely related chikungunya and o'nyong-nyong along with Mayaro, Mucambo, and Venezuelan equine viruses, are in group A togaviruses. Group C viruses are Apeu, Caraparu, Itaqui, Madrid, Marituba, Murutucu, Oriboca, Ossa and Restan. Oropouche is in the Simbu group. Others in smaller groups are listed in the preceding table.

4. Reservoir—Unknown for some viruses in the group. All appear to be tropics-dependent and to require a continuous vertebrate-mosquito cycle. Horses are a source of mosquito infection for Venezuelan equine encephalitis; birds for West Nile; sheep, other domestic ruminants, game, monkeys and rodents for Rift Valley, and rodents for group C.

5. Mode of transmission—In most instances by bite of an infective mosquito; for chikungunya, Aedes aegypti and possibly others; West Nile, Culex univittatus in Egypt and C. pipiens molestus in Israel; o'nyong-nyong, Anopheles species; Mayaro, Mansonia and Haemagogus species; Bunyamwera, Aedes species; group C viruses, species of Aedes, and Culex (Melanoconion). Viruses of the Venezuelan equine complex have been isolated from a number of genera and species, many of which may be infected in the laboratory, including Mansonia, Psorophora, Aedes, Culex, Haemagogus, Sabethini and Anopheles. For Rift Valley in sheep and other animals (see par. 4 above), Aedes caballus, A. circumluteolus and A. theileri; species of Eretmapodites probably are important in forest cycles; most human infections are asso-

ciated predominantly with handling of infective material of animal origin during necropsy and butchering.

6. **Incubation period** — Usually 3 to 12 days.

7. **Period of communicability** — Not directly transmitted from man to man, except possibly for Venezuelan equine virus which is present in pharyngeal secretions. Infected mosquitoes probably transmit virus throughout life. Viremia, essential to vector infection, is present for many of these viruses during early clinical illness in man.

8. **Susceptibility and resistance** — Susceptibility appears general, in both sexes and throughout life. Inapparent infections and mild but undiagnosed disease are common. Infection leads to immunity; susceptibles in highly endemic areas are mainly young children.

9. **Methods of control** —

   A. Preventive measures:

      1) The general measures applicable to mosquito-borne viral encephalitides (9A1 through 5 and 9A7, p. 24-25). For Rift Valley, precautions in care and handling of infected animals and their products.

      2) An experimental attenuated virus vaccine (TC-83) for Venezuelan equine has been used effectively to protect laboratory workers and other adults at high risk. (Available in U.S.A. as an investigational drug from the Center for Disease Control, Atlanta, Georgia, see preface.) This vaccine is also effective in protecting horses. An experimental inactivated tissue culture vaccine also is used for Rift Valley.

   B. Control of patient, contacts, and the immediate environment:

      1) Report to local health authority: In selected endemic areas; in most countries not a reportable disease, Class 3B (see Preface).

      2) Isolation: Keep patient in screened room or in quarters treated with an insecticide for at least 5 days after onset or until afebrile.

      3) Concurrent disinfection: None.

      4) Quarantine: None.

      5) Immunization of contacts: None.

      6) Investigation of contacts: Determine place of residence of patient during fortnight previous to onset. Search for unreported or undiagnosed cases.

      7) Specific treatment: None.

   C. Epidemic measures:

      1) Community survey to determine density of vector mos-

quitoes, to identify their breeding places, and to promote their elimination.
2) Use of mosquito repellents by persons exposed because
of occupation or otherwise to bites of vectors.
3) Identification of the disease among horses (Venezuelan),
or sheep and other animals (Rift Valley), and serological
survey of birds (West Nile), or rodents (group C
viruses), have epidemiological value by indicating frequency of infection and areas involved.
4) Immunization of horses against Venezuelan equine viral
infection.

D. *International measures:* For Rift Valley fever and
Venezuelan equine, vaccinate animals and restrict movement of animals from enzootic areas to those free from disease; for others, none except enforcement of international
agreements designed to prevent transfer of mosquitoes by
ships, airplanes and land transport. WHO Collaborating
Centres (see Preface).

∞

II. Tick-borne

COLORADO TICK FEVER AND OTHER TICK-BORNE FEVERS

1. **Identification**—Colorado tick fever is an acute febrile,
biphasic, dengue-like disease, with infrequent rash. A brief remission is usual, followed by a second bout of fever lasting 2 or 3
days; neutropenia almost always occurs on the 4th or 5th day of
fever. Characteristically a mild infection, but may be severe in
children with occasional encephalitis or tendency to bleed. Deaths
are uncommon.

Laboratory confirmation is by isolation of virus by inoculation of
suckling mice or cell cultures with erythrocytes; complement-fixing
and neutralizing antibodies do not appear for 2 weeks or longer.
Clinical manifestations of other types and diagnostic methods vary
only slightly.

2. **Occurrence**—Known areas of occurrence of Colorado type are
in Western Canada and in Washington, Oregon, Idaho, Montana,
California, Nevada, Utah, Wyoming, Colorado and South Dakota in

the U.S.A. Virus has been isolated from *Dermacentor andersoni* ticks in British Columbia and New Mexico. The disease is most frequent in adult males, but also affects children and women; seasonal incidence parallels the period of greatest tick activity; endemic in occurrence and the disease is common in much of the affected area. Geographic distribution of other types are shown in the preceding table.

3. Infectious agents—The viruses of Colorado tick fever and Nairobi sheep disease and the Kemerovo, Tribec-Lipovnik, Quaranfil, Ganjam and Dugbe viruses.

4. Reservoir—For Colorado type, small mammals, ground squirrels, porcupine, chipmunk and *Peromyscus* species. Also nymphal and larval ticks, principally *D. andersoni.*

5. Mode of transmission—To man by bite of the infective adult vector tick. In Colorado type, immature ticks *(Dermacentor andersoni)* acquire infection by feeding on infected viremic animals; they remain infected through the various moults and transmit virus to man by feeding as adult ticks.

6. Incubation period—Usually 4 to 5 days.

7. Period of communicability—Not directly transmitted from man to man; the wildlife cycle is maintained by ticks, which remain infective throughout life. Virus is present in man during the course of the fever, and in Colorado tick fever, from 2 to 16 weeks or more after onset.

8. Susceptibility and resistance—Susceptibility apparently is universal. Second attacks are unknown. Experimental reinfection is unsuccessful.

9. Methods of control—

    A. *Preventive measures:*
        1) Control of ticks. (See Rocky Mountain Spotted Fever, 9A1 and 9A2, p. 268).
        2) No available vaccine.

    B. *Control of patient, contacts, and the immediate environment:*
        1) Report to local health authority: In endemic areas (U.S.A.); in most states and countries not a reportable disease, Class 3B (see Preface).
        2) Isolation: None.
        3) Concurrent disinfection: None; remove ticks from patients.
        4) Quarantine: None.

5) *Immunization of contacts:* None.
6) *Investigation of contacts and source of infection:* Identification of tick-infested areas.
7) *Specific treatment:* None.

C. *Epidemic measures:* Not applicable.

D. *International measures:* WHO Collaborating Centres (see Preface).

∞

III. Phlebotomine-borne

SANDFLY FEVER

(Pappataci fever, Phlebotomus fever, Three-day fever)

1. **Identification**—A 3 or 4 day fever clinically resembling influenza, but without inflammation of the respiratory tract. Headache, with fever of 38.3° to 39.5°C (101° to 103°F), sometimes higher, retrobulbar pain on motion of the eyes, injected sclerae, malaise, nausea, and pain in the limbs and back are characteristic. Leucopenia is usual on 4th or 5th day after onset of fever. Symptoms may be alarming, but death is unknown. Diagnosis is based on the clinical picture and the occurrence of multiple similar cases. Complete recovery may be preceded by prolonged mental depression.

Diagnosis may be confirmed by neutralization tests, using mouse-adapted viruses, or by isolation of virus from blood in newborn mice.

2. **Occurrence**—In those parts of Europe, Africa and Asia where the vector exists; also in Central and South America, where closely related viral agents are present. A disease of sub-tropical and tropical areas with long periods of hot, dry weather; in general, in a belt extending around the Mediterranean and eastward into Burma and China. Seasonal, between April and October, and prone to appear as a disease of troops and travelers from nonendemic areas.

3. **Infectious agents**—The viruses of sandfly fever; at least five related immunological types (Naples, Sicilian, Candiru, Chagres and Punta Toro) have been isolated from man and differentiated. In

addition, Changuinola virus and vesicular stomatitis virus of the Indiana type have been isolated from *Lutzomyia* species, both of which produce febrile disease in man.

4. **Reservoir**—Principal reservoir is the man-sandfly complex; an animal reservoir is suspected, but not yet demonstrated except that rodents may harbor New World sandfly fever viruses. Transovarian transmission of some viruses has been demonstrated in phlebotomines. Cattle, horses and swine are principal hosts of vesicular stomatitis virus.

5. **Mode of transmission**—By bite of an infective sandfly. The vector of the classical viruses is a small hairy, blood-sucking midge *Phlebotomus papatasii*, the common sandfly, which bites at night and has a limited flight range. Sandflies of the genus *Sergentomyia* also have been found to be infected and may be vectors. Members of the genus *Lutzomyia* or *Brumptomyia* are involved in Central and South America.

6. **Incubation period**—Up to 6 days, usually 3 to 4 days, rarely less.

7. **Period of communicability**—Virus is present in the blood of an infected person at least 24 hours before and 24 hours after onset of fever. Phlebotomines become infective about 7 days after biting an infected person and remain so for life.

8. **Susceptibility and resistance**—Susceptibility is essentially universal; homologous acquired immunity is possibly lasting. Relative resistance of native populations in sandfly areas is probably attributable to infection early in life.

9. **Methods of control**—

   A. *Preventive measures:* Control of sandflies is the important consideration. (See Cutaneous Leishmaniasis 9A1, p. 171).

   B. *Control of patient, contacts, and the immediate environment:*
      1) *Report to local health authority:* In selected endemic areas; in most countries not a reportable disease, Class 3C (see Preface).
      2) *Isolation:* None; prevent access of sandflies to infected individual for the first few days of illness by very fine screening or mosquito bed nets (10-12 mesh per cm. or 25-30 mesh to the inch, aperture size not more than 0.08 cm or 0.035 inches) and/or by spraying quarters with an insecticide.
      3) *Concurrent disinfection:* None; destruction of sandflies in the dwelling.

    4) Quarantine: None.
    5) Immunization of contacts: Not currently available.
    6) Investigation of contacts and source of infection: Search
       for breeding areas of sandflies around dwellings, espe-
       cially in rubble heaps, masonry cracks, and under
       stones.
    7) Specific treatment: None.

C. Epidemic measures:
    1) Community use of insecticides to destroy sandflies in
       and about human habitations.
    2) Education of public on conditions leading to infection,
       and importance of preventing bites of sandflies by use of
       repellents while in infected areas, particularly after
       sundown.

D. International measures: WHO Collaborating Centres (see
Preface).

ARTHROPOD-BORNE VIRAL HEMORRHAGIC FEVERS

I. Mosquito-borne

  A. YELLOW FEVER

1. Identification—An acute infectious disease of short duration
and varying severity. The mildest cases are clinically indeterminate; typical attacks are characterized by a dengue-like illness, i.e.,
sudden onset, fever, headache, backache, prostration, nausea and
vomiting. As the disease progresses, the pulse slows and weakens,
though the temperature may be elevated; albuminuria becomes pronounced and anuria may occur. Leucopenia appears early and is
most pronounced about the 5th day. Common hemorrhagic symptoms include epistaxis, buccal bleeding, hematemesis, and melena.
Jaundice is moderate early in the disease, and is intensified later.
The fatality rate among indigenous populations of endemic regions
is less than 5%, but may reach 50% among non-indigenous groups or
in epidemics.

Laboratory diagnosis is by isolation of virus from blood by
inoculation of suckling mice or tissue cultures and by demonstration of a rising titer of antibodies in paired acute-phase and

convalescent sera. It is suggested but not proved by demonstration of typical lesions of the liver.

2. Occurrence—Except for a few cases in Trinidad, W.I., in 1954, no outbreak of urban yellow fever has been transmitted by *Aedes aegypti* in the Americas since 1942. Urban yellow fever outbreaks are still reported from Africa in areas contiguous to rain forest regions where jungle yellow fever is endemic. Urban yellow fever, when first introduced into a community in the Americas, tended to attack both sexes and all ages and races, whereas jungle yellow fever of tropical America now occurs predominantly among adult males 20 to 40 years of age who are exposed in the jungle.

Jungle yellow fever is enzootic in the Amazon basin, including the Colombian elanos and eastern regions of Peru and Bolivia. It has occurred from time to time in all mainland American countries from Mexico to Argentina, with the exception of El Salvador, Uruguay and Chile. In Africa it extends from the West Coast south of the Shara Desert through Angola, Zaire, and into Zambia, Botswana, Malawi, Uganda, Tanzania, Kenya, Ethiopia, the Somali Republic and the Sudan. There is no evidence that yellow fever ever has been present in Asia and probably not on the easternmost coast of Africa.

3. **Infectious agent**—The virus of yellow fever, a group B togavirus.

4. **Reservoir**—In urban areas the reservoir of infection is man and *Aedes aegypti* mosquitoes; in forest areas, vertebrates other than man, mainly monkeys and forest mosquitoes. Man has no essential role in transmission of jungle yellow fever, or in maintaining the virus.

5. **Mode of transmission**—In urban and certain rural areas, by the bite of infective *Aedes aegypti* mosquitoes. In forests of South America, by the bite of several species of forest mosquitoes of the genus *Haemagogus* and by *Aedes leucocelaenus*. In Uganda and probably other parts of Africa, *A. africanus* is the vector in the monkey population, while *A. simpsoni*, a semi-domestic mosquito, and probably other *Aedes* species transmit the virus from monkey to man. In large epidemics in Ethiopia, good epidemiological evidence incriminated *A. simpsoni* as a man-to-man vector.

6. **Incubation period**—3 to 6 days.

7. **Period of communicability**—Blood of patients is infective for mosquitoes shortly before onset of fever and for the first 3 to 5 days of illness. Highly communicable where many susceptible persons and abundant vector mosquitoes coexist. Not communicable by contact or common vehicles. The extrinsic period of incubation

before *A. aegypti* becomes infective is commonly 9 to 12 days at the usual summer temperatures. *A. aegypti* mosquitoes, once infected, remain so for life, but transovarian passage does not occur.

8. **Susceptibility and resistance** — Recovery from yellow fever is followed by lasting immunity; second attacks are unknown. Mild inapparent infections are common in endemic areas. Transient passive immunity in infants born to immune mothers may persist up to 6 months. In natural infection, antibodies appear in the blood within the first week.

9. **Methods of control** —

A. *Preventive measures:*

1) Urban yellow fever, by eradication or control of *A. aegypti* mosquitoes; vaccination when indicated (see 9A3 and 9C1 below).

2) Sylvan or jungle yellow fever, transmitted by *Haemagogus* and forest species of *Aedes*, is best controlled by vaccination, which is recommended for all persons in rural communities whose occupation brings them into forests in yellow fever areas, and for persons who intend to visit those areas. Protective clothing, bed nets and repellents are advised for persons not immunized.

3) Active immunization of all persons necessarily exposed to infection because of residence, occupation or travel. A single subcutaneous injection of a vaccine containing viable 17D strain virus, cultivated in chick embryo, is effective. Antibodies appear from 7 to 10 days after vaccination and persist for at least 17 years, probably much longer, though revaccination is still required by the end of 10 years. This is the only vaccine used in the Americas. A second method employs a living neurotropic yellow fever virus (Dakar strain prepared in mouse brain) administered by cutaneous scarification to persons 10 years of age and over. Reactions are more frequent and fatal encephalitis is an occasional complication.

B. *Control of patient, contacts, and the immediate environment:*

1) *Report to local health authority:* Case report universally required by International Health Regulations, (1969)* WHO, Class 1 (see Preface).

2) *Isolation:* None. Prevent access of mosquitoes to patient

---

*Second Annotated Edition, 1974

during first 3 days by screening sickroom or by spraying quarters with residual insecticide, or by bed net.

3) *Concurrent disinfection:* None. Home of patient and all houses in vicinity should be sprayed promptly with an effective insecticide.

4) *Quarantine:* None.

5) *Immunization of contacts:* Family and other contacts and neighbors not previously immunized should be vaccinated promptly.

6) *Investigation of contacts and source of infection:* Inquiry about all places, including forested areas, visited by patient 3 to 6 days before onset, to locate focus of yellow fever; observe all persons visiting that focus. Search of premises and place of work for mosquitoes capable of transmitting infection. Attention to mild febrile illnesses and unexplained deaths suggesting yellow fever.

7) *Specific treatment:* None.

C. *Epidemic measures:*

1) Urban or aegypti-transmitted yellow fever:

a) Vaccinate the populations beginning with persons most exposed and those living in *A. aegypti* infested parts of the area.

b) Spray all houses in community with insecticides has shown promise for controlling urban epidemics.

c) Apply larvicide to or eliminate all actual and potential breeding places of *A. aegypti.*

2) Jungle or sylvan yellow fever:

a) Immediate vaccination of all persons living in or near forested areas or entering such areas.

b) Avoidance by unvaccinated individuals of those tracts of forest where infection has been localized, and similarly by vaccinated persons for the first week after vaccination.

3) In regions where yellow fever may occur, a diagnostic viscerotomy service should be organized to collect small specimens of liver from fatal febrile illnesses of 10 days duration or less; many cases and outbreaks otherwise missed are thereby discovered.

4) In South and Central America, confirmed deaths of howler and spider monkeys in the forest are presumptive evidence of the presence of yellow fever. Confirmation by the histopathological examination of livers of

moribund or recently dead monkeys or by virus isolation is highly desirable.

5) Immunity surveys by mouse neutralization tests of wild primates captured in forested areas are useful in defining enzootic areas. Serological surveys of human populations are practically useless where yellow fever vaccine has been widely used.

D. *International measures:*

1) Telegraphic notification by governments to WHO and to adjacent countries of the first imported, first transferred, or first non-imported case of yellow fever, in an area previously free of the disease; and of newly discovered or reactivated foci of yellow fever infection among vertebrates other than man.

2) Measures applicable to ships, aircraft and land transport arriving from yellow fever areas are specified in the International Health Regulations, (1969)* WHO, Geneva.

3) Animal quarantine: Quarantine of monkeys and other wild primates arriving from yellow fever areas may be required until 7 days have elapsed after leaving such areas.

4) International travelers: A valid international certificate of vaccination against yellow fever is required by many countries for entry of travelers coming from or through recognized yellow fever zones of Africa and South America; otherwise, quarantine measures are applicable. The International Certificate of Vaccination is valid from 10 days after date of vaccination for 10 years; if revaccinated within that period from date of revaccination for 10 years.

---

*Second Annotated Edition, 1974

B. HEMORRHAGIC FEVERS OF THE PHILIPPINES AND SOUTHEAST ASIA

(Dengue Hemorrhagic Fever—DHF)

1. Identification—A severe dengue illness endemic in most of tropical Asia, characterized by abnormal vascular permeability, hypovolemia and abnormal blood clotting mechanism(s). Recognized principally in children, although adults are affected in some outbreaks. Characterized by sudden onset of high fever accompanied by facial flush and non-specific constitutional symptoms such as anorexia, vomiting, headache and abdominal pain. Hemorrhagic phenomena are seen frequently, but not always and include a positive tourniquet test, easy bruisability, bleeding at venepuncture sites, a fine petechial rash, epistaxis, or gum bleeding. Gastrointestinal hemorrhage is infrequent and more usually follows a period of uncontrolled shock. The liver is usually enlarged during the febrile stage which lasts 2-7 days. In some patients, after a few days of fever, their condition suddenly deteriorates as manifested by signs of circulatory failure such as cool, blotchy skin, circumoral cyanosis, rapid pulse and, in severe cases, hypotension or abnormally narrow pulse pressure, i.e., the dengue shock syndrome (DSS). In all cases, platelet counts are abnormally low; in severe cases there is an elevated hematocrit, low serum albumin, elevated transaminases, a prolonged prothrombin time, and low levels of C3 complement protein. The fatality rate of shock cases is 10-50%.

Serologic tests show a rise in titer against dengue viruses, usually of the anamnestic type (IgG). Primary-type antibody responses have been reported in a few cases. Virus can be isolated from blood during the acute febrile stage by inoculation of suckling mice or tissue culture. Isolation from organs at autopsy is rare.

2. Occurrence—Outbreaks have occurred in the Philippines, Burma, Thailand, Indonesia, Malaysia, Singapore, North and South Vietnam, Ceylon and India. An outbreak on Niue Island was recently recorded. DHF is observed almost exclusively among Oriental members of the population. Occurrence is limited to rainy seasons and areas of high *Aedes aegypti* prevalence; not yet observed where only *A. albopictus* is present.

3. Infectious agents—Viruses presently classed as dengue virus, types 1, 2, 3 and 4—group B togaviruses. Most shock cases are seen during the second of sequential dengue infections. Chikungunya virus may be responsible for some mild cases with hemorrhagic manifestations (not hypovolemia) in Bangkok, and for more severe hemorrhagic cases in Calcutta.

4. **Reservoir** — Unknown; probably man and *A. aegypti.*

5. **Mode of transmission** — By bite of an infective *Aedes aegypti* mosquito. Viruses have been isolated from this mosquito during epidemics. Isolations from *A. albopictus* are less common.

6. **Incubation period** — Unknown.

7. **Period of communicability** — No evidence of direct transmission from man to man.

8. **Susceptibility and resistance** — Pathogenesis may be explained by sensitization of hosts to previous dengue infections, by enhanced virulence of a particular strain or by unusual genetic susceptibility of hosts. Modal age of attack in epidemics thus far recognized is about 3 to 5 years, with a range from 4 months to the young adult years. Prevalence of dengue antibodies in the general population is high in older children and in adults. Many mild cases are recognized by serologic tests. Classical dengue has been observed in Caucasians during epidemics of hemorrhagic disease in Orientals. A host factor involved in susceptibility is strongly suspected.

9. **Methods of control** — See Arthropod-borne viral fevers, Dengue fever, 9A to 9D, pp. 29-30.

B. Control of patient, contacts, and the immediate environment:

    7) Specific treatment: The major pathophysiological abnormality in DHF/DSS is an acute increase in vascular permeability. Hypovolemic shock resulting from plasma loss leads to tissue anoxia, metabolic acidosis and death. Plasma loss may continue from 24-48 hours. Most cases respond to oxygen therapy and rapid replacement with fluid and electrolyte solution (lactated Ringer's solution at 10-20 ml/kg/hr) and plasma. The rate of fluid and plasma administration must be judged by estimates of loss. However, during early convalescence, fluid resorption may reduce the hematocrit, but this should not be mistaken as a sign of internal hemorrhage. Blood transfusions are indicated only when severe bleeding results in a true falling hematocrit. Heparin may help combat severe hemorrhage and should be used when there is specific laboratory evidence of disseminated intravascular coagulation.

    Non-hepatoxic sedatives such as chloral hydrate may be needed to treat agitated children. When DHF/DSS exists or is suspected, aspirin is contraindicated.

II. Tick-borne

A. CRIMEAN HEMORRHAGIC FEVER—CONGO AND CEN-
TRAL ASIAN HEMORRHAGIC FEVER

1. **Identification**—Sudden onset with fever, malaise, weakness, irritability, headache, severe pain in limbs and loins, and marked anorexia. Vomiting, abdominal pain, and diarrhea occur occasionally. Flush on face and chest, and injection of conjunctivae develop early. Hemorrhagic enanthem of soft palate, uvula and pharnyx, and fine petechial rash spreading from chest and abdomen to the body generally are associated with the disease; occasionally large purpuric areas are observed. There may be some bleeding from gums, nose, lungs, uterus and intestine, but in large amount only in serious or fatal cases. Hematuria and albuminuria are slight or absent. Fever is constantly elevated for 5 to 12 days and falls by lysis. Convalescence is prolonged. Other findings are leucopenia and eosinophilia. Thrombocytopenia is present but bleeding time is normal. The reported fatality rate ranges from 2% to 50%.

Diagnosis is by isolation of virus from blood by inoculation of suckling mice. Serological diagnosis is by gel diffusion precipitation and indirect hemagglutination; some sera show nonspecific neutralization with certain strains.

2. **Occurrence**—Crimean type is observed in the steppe regions of the Western Crimea, on the Kersch peninsula, and in the Rostov-Don and Astrakhan regions; the Central Asian type in Kazakstan and Uzbekistan. Most patients are agricultural workers in fallow lands or dairy workers. Seasonal occurrence is from June to September, the period of vector activity. Sporadic cases of a similar disease have been observed in several areas of Central Africa.

3. **Infectious agent**—The Crimean and central Asian viruses have been identified as the Congo virus, a Bunyavirus, originally isolated in Africa (Congo, Uganda, Nigeria and Senegal).

4. **Reservoir**—In nature, believed to be hares, birds and *Hyalomma* species of ticks in USSR.

5. **Mode of transmission**—By bite of infective adult *Hyalomma marginatum* or *H. anatolicum*. Immature ticks are believed to acquire infection from the animal hosts.

6. **Incubation period**—7 to 12 days.

7. **Period of communicability**—Not directly transmitted from man to man. An infected tick probably remains so for life.

8. **Susceptibility and resistance**—Immunity for at least 1 year.

9. **Methods of control**—

A. *Preventive measures:* See Rocky Mountain Spotted Fever (p. 268) for preventive measures against ticks. No available vaccine.

B. *Control of patient, contacts, and the immediate environment:*

   1) Report to local health authority: In selected endemic areas; in most countries not a reportable disease, Class 3B (see Preface).

   2) Isolation: None if patient is tick-free.

   3) Concurrent disinfection: Bloody discharges may be infective; decontaminate by heat or chlorine disinfectants.

   4) Quarantine: None.

   5) Immunization: None.

   6) Investigation of contacts and source of infection: Search for missed cases and the presence of infective hares and other possible vectors.

   7) Specific treatment: Convalescent serum is reported to be useful.

C. *Epidemic measures:* See Rocky Mountain Spotted Fever, p. 267.

D. *International measures:* WHO Collaborating Centers (see Preface).

B. OMSK HEMORRHAGIC FEVER AND KYASANUR FOREST DISEASE

1. Identification—These two diseases have marked similarities. Onset is sudden, with headache, fever, pain in lower back and limbs, and severe prostration; often is associated with conjunctivitis, diarrhea and vomiting by the 3rd to 4th day. A papulovesicular eruption on the soft palate is an important diagnostic sign. Usually there is no involvement of the central nervous system. Severe cases are associated with hemorrhages but with no cutaneous rash. Bleeding occurs from gums, nose, gastrointestinal tract, uterus and lungs (but rarely from the kidneys), sometimes for many days and, when serious, results in shock and death; shock also may occur without manifest hemorrhage. Estimated fatality is from 1-10%. Leucopenia and thrombocytopenia are marked. Febrile period ranges from 5 days to 2 weeks, at times with a secondary rise in the 3rd week. Convalescence tends to be slow and prolonged.

Diagnosis is by isolation of virus from blood in suckling mice or tissue cultures as long as 10 days following onset, or by serological tests.

2. **Occurrence** — In the Kyasanur Forest of the Shimoga District, Mysore State, India, principally in young adult males exposed in the forest during the dry season from January to June. The Omsk type formerly occurred in rural workers and children exposed to infected ticks in the steppe regions of the Omsk Oblast in Siberia, but recently only in the Novosibirsk region. Seasonal occurrence in each area coincides with vector activity. Laboratory infections are common with both viruses.

3. **Infectious agents** — Viruses of these two diseases are closely related. The agents belong to the Russian spring-summer-louping ill complex of group B togaviruses, and are similar antigenically to other member viruses.

4. **Reservoir** — In Kyasanur Forest disease, probably rodents and monkeys; in the Omsk disease, rodents, muskrats, and possibly ticks, since transovarian passage has been reported for other viruses of this complex.

5. **Mode of transmission** — By bite of infective ticks (especially nymphal stages), probably *Haemaphysalis spinigera* in Kyansanur Forest disease. In the Omsk type, infective ticks possibly are *Dermacentor pictus* and *D. marginatus,* although recent data implicate direct transmission from muskrat to man and suggest that ticks may not be the principal vectors.

6. **Incubation period** — Usually 3 to 8 days.

7. **Period of communicability** — Not directly transmitted from man to man. Infected ticks remain so for life.

8. **Susceptibility and resistance** — All ages and sexes are probably susceptible; previous infection leads to immunity.

9. **Methods of control** — See Tick-borne Encephalitis and Rocky Mountain Spotted Fever (pp. 27 and 268). A formalinized mouse brain virus vaccine has been reported effective for Omsk, but as yet has been inadequately tested for Kyasanur Forest disease.

ASCARIASIS

1. **Identification** — A helminthic infection of the small intestine. Symptoms are variable, often vague or absent and ordinarily mild; live worms passed in stools or vomited are frequently the first recognized sign of infection. Pulmonary signs include Loeffler's syndrome with irregular respiration, spasms of coughing, fever and pronounced blood eosinophilia. Ascaris pneumonitis is important in children. Heavy parasite burdens may cause digestive and nutritional disturbances, abdominal pain, vomiting, restlessness, and disturbed sleep. Serious complications among children, especially in insanitary areas of tropical countries, include bowel obstruction and, occasionally, death due to migration of adult worms into liver, gallbladder, peritoneal cavity or appendix, and rarely, from perforation of the intestine. Deaths from other causes may be mis-attributed to this more obvious infection. Diagnosis is by identifying eggs in feces or adult worms passed rectally or by mouth.

2. **Occurrence** — Common and worldwide, with greatest frequency in moist tropical countries, where prevalence may exceed 50% of a population. Children of preschool and early school age are more frequently and more heavily infected than older children and adults. In U.S.A. the disease is most prevalent in the South.

3. **Infectious agent** — *Ascaris lumbricoides,* the large intestinal round worm of man.

4. **Reservoir** — Man.

5. **Mode of transmission** — By ingestion of infective eggs from soil contaminated with human feces containing eggs, but not directly from man to man. Eggs must undergo initial development (embryonation) for two to several weeks at ambient temperatures. Salads and other foods eaten raw are the common vehicles. Contaminated soil may be carried long distances on feet or footwear into houses and conveyances; transmission of infection by dust is also possible. Embryonated eggs are ingested, hatch in the intestinal lumen and the larvae penetrate the gut wall and reach the liver and lungs by way of the lymphatic and circulatory systems. The larvae, upon reaching the lungs, pass into air passages, ascend the bronchi, are swallowed, and eventually reach the small intestine, where they grow to maturity and mate. Eggs are passed from gravid females and are discharged in feces.

6. **Incubation period** — Worms reach maturity about 2 months after embryonated eggs are ingested by man.

7. **Period of communicability** — As long as mature fertilized

female worms live in the intestine. Most adult worms live less than 10 months; maximum life span is under 1-1/2 years. The female can produce up to 200,000 eggs a day. Embryonated eggs, under favorable conditions, remain viable in soil for months or possibly years.

8. **Susceptibility and resistance** — Susceptibility is general.

9. **Methods of control** —

A. *Preventive measures:*
   1) Provision of adequate facilities for proper disposal of feces and prevention of soil contamination in areas immediately adjacent to houses, particularly in play areas of children.
   2) In rural areas, construction of privies in such manner as to prevent dissemination of ascarid eggs through overflow, drainage, or otherwise. Treatment of night soil, such as composting, is practiced to advantage where such facilities are lacking and in areas where human feces are used as fertilizer.
   3) Education of all persons, particularly children and food handlers, in the use of toilet facilities and washing of hands after defecating. Encouragement of satisfactory hygienic habits on the part of children; in particular, they should be trained to wash their hands before handling food, and not to eat food which has been dropped on the floor.

B. *Control of patient, contacts, and the immediate environment:*
   1) *Report to local health authority:* Official report not ordinarily justifiable, Class 5 (see Preface).
   2) *Isolation:* None.
   3) *Concurrent disinfection:* Sanitary disposal of feces.
   4) *Quarantine:* None.
   5) *Immunization of contacts:* None.
   6) *Investigation of contacts and source of infection:* Individual and environmental sources of infection should be sought, particularly in persons and on premises of families affected.
   7) *Specific treatment:* Piperazine hexahydrate or piperazine salts (citrate, adipate, or phosphate), levamisole, pyrantel pamoate or thiabendazole.

C. *Epidemic measures:* Surveys for prevalence in highly endemic areas, education in sanitation of environment and in personal hygiene, and provision of treatment facilities.

D. *International measures:* None.

ASPERGILLOSIS

1. **Identification**—A variety of clinical syndromes can be produced by several *Aspergillus* species: (1) Inhalation of the fungus may cause asthmatic attacks in hypersensitive persons. (2) Saprophytic endobronchial colonization in patients with bronchitis or bronchiectasis may cause bronchial plugs and atelectasis, or a large mass of hyphae may fill a previously existing cavity (fungus ball or aspergilloma). *Aspergillus* may appear in a bacterial lung abscess or empyema. (3) *Aspergillus* pneumonia may occur, particularly in patients receiving cytotoxic or immunosuppressive therapy; it may disseminate to brain, kidneys and other organs and is usually fatal. Invasion of blood vessels with thrombosis and infarction is characteristic of pneumonic and disseminated infection. (4) Otomycosis is usually caused by *Aspergillus* species. (5) It may infect the implantation site of a cardiac prosthetic valve. (6) Rarely, the fungus may cause granulomas of the paranasal sinuses. (7) Growing on certain foods, many isolates of *A. flavus* and occasionally other species of *Aspergillus*, will produce aflatoxins. These toxins are a cause of disease in animals and fish and are carcinogenic for experimental animals, but no adverse effects on man have been proved.

Among findings that suggest a diagnosis of allergic aspergillosis are (1) isolation of *Aspergillus* from sputum and (2) demonstration, by the use of an *Aspergillus* species antigen, of any or all of the following: bronchial constriction on inhalation, serum precipitins, pulmonary eosinophilia, and immediate cutaneous reactions after a scratch test. Diagnosis of saprophytic endobronchial colonization is based on culture or microscopic demonstration of *Aspergillus* in sputum or in plugs of expectorated hyphae. Serum precipitins to *Aspergillus* antigens usually are present. Radiologic evidence of a fungus ball is often obtainable. Diagnosis of invasive aspergillosis depends upon microscopic demonstration of the fungus in infected tissue. Cultural confirmation is desirable.

2. **Occurrence**—An uncommon sporadic disease. No distinctive differences in incidence by race or sex.

3. **Infectious agent**—*Aspergillus fumigatus* and *A. flavus* are the most common causes of aspergillosis, though other species also have been implicated. *A. niger* or *A. fumigatus* cause the fungus ball; *A. niger* is the usual cause of otomycosis.

4. **Reservoir and source of infection**—Compost piles undergoing fermentation and decay are prominent reservoirs and sources of infection. Fungi also are found in hay stored when damp, in decaying

vegetation, in cereal grains, and in a variety of other foodstuffs stored under conditions which permit them to heat.

5. Mode of transmission — Inhalation of airborne spores.

6. Incubation period — Probably a few days to weeks.

7. Period of communicability — Not directly transmitted from man to man.

8. Susceptibility and resistance — The frequency of the fungus in the external environment and the usual occurrence of the disease as a secondary infection suggest a high degree of resistance by healthy persons.

9. Methods of Control —

A. *Preventive measures:* None.

B. *Control of patient, contacts, and the immediate environment:*
 1) *Report to local health authority:* Official report ordinarily not justifiable; Class 5 (see Preface).
 2) *Isolation:* None.
 3) *Concurrent disinfection:* Ordinary cleanliness. Terminal cleaning.
 4) *Quarantine:* None.
 5) *Immunization of contacts:* None.
 6) *Investigation of contacts:* Ordinarily not profitable.
 7) *Specific treatment:* Amphotericin B (Fungizone) should be tried in tissue invasive forms. Any immunosuppressive therapy in use should be reduced or discontinued. Solely endobronchial colonization should be treated by measures to improve bronchopulmonary drainage.

C. *Epidemic measures:* Not applicable — sporadic disease.

D. *International measures:* None.

BALANTIDIASIS

(Balantidiosis, Balantidial dysentery)

1. Identification — A disease of the colon characteristically producing diarrhea or dysentery, accompanied by abdominal colic, tenesmus, nausea, and vomiting. Infection often asymptomatic. Occasionally the dysentery is of amebic type and stools may contain much blood and mucus, but relatively little pus. Peritoneal and urogenital invasion are rare.

Diagnosis is by identifying the trophozoites or cysts of *Balantidium coli* in fresh feces, or trophozoites in material obtained by sigmoidoscopy.

2. Occurrence — Worldwide in distribution; the incidence of disease in man is low. Water-borne epidemics occasionally occur in areas of poor environmental sanitation. Association with hogs may result in a higher incidence.

3. Infectious agent — *Balantidium coli*, a ciliated protozoon.

4. Reservoir — Swine, man and possibly other animals.

5. Mode of transmission — Infection is by ingestion of cysts from feces of infected hosts; in epidemics, mainly by fecally contaminated water. Sporadic transmission is by water, by hand-to-mouth transfer of feces, by contaminated raw meat and vegetables, by flies, and by soiled hands of food handlers.

6. Incubation period — Unknown; may be only a few days.

7. Period of communicability — During periods of diarrhea or dysentery while infection persists. Cysts are rarely excreted.

8. Susceptibility and resistance — Man appears to have a high natural resistance. In individuals debilitated from other diseases the infection may be serious and even fatal.

9. Methods of control —

A. *Preventive measures:*
1) Sanitary disposal of feces.
2) Avoidance of contact with hog feces.
3) Protection of public water supplies against fecal contamination. Diatomaceous earth filters remove all cysts, but usual chlorination of water does not destroy cysts; the efficacy of iodine is unproved. Small quantities of water are best purified by boiling.
4) Education of the general public in personal hygiene.
5) Fly control and protection of foods against fly contamination.
6) Supervision by health agencies of food handlers.

B. *Control of patient, contacts, and the immediate environment:*
1) *Report to local health authority:* Official report not justifiable, Class 5 (see Preface).
2) *Isolation:* None.
3) *Concurrent disinfection:* Sanitary disposal of feces.
4) *Quarantine:* None.

5) *Immunization of contacts:* Not applicable.
6) *Investigation of contacts and source of infection.* Microscopic examination of feces of household members and suspected contacts. Also investigate contact with hogs.
7) *Specific treatment:* Tetracyclines eliminate infection metronidazole (Flagyl) and paromomycin (Humatin) are also effective.

C. *Epidemic measures:* Any grouping of several cases in a single area or institution requires prompt epidemiological investigation.

D. *International measures:* None.

BARTONELLOSIS
(Oroya fever, verruga peruana, Carrion's disease)

1. Identification — An illness typically occurring in 2 stages, with an interval of weeks to months usually separating an initial acute febrile period (Oroya fever) and an eruptive period (verruga peruana). The febrile Oroya fever stage is characterized by irregular fever, severe anemia, pain in bones and joints, and lympha denopathy. The eruptive stage may merge with the febrile stage verruga peruana may develop without an antecedent first stage. In any case the eruption is in crops of papules or nodules resembling hemangiomas, sometimes with many small lesions, sometimes with a few tumor-like sub-epithelial nodules. The fatality rate of un treated Oroya fever ranges from 10 to 40%, usually associated with salmonella septicemia; verruga peruana has a prolonged course but few deaths.

Diagnosis is by demonstration of the infectious agent within red blood cells during the acute stage, in sections of skin lesions during the eruptive stage, or by blood culture on special media during either stage.

2. Occurrence — Limited to mountain valleys of Peru, Ecuador and southwest Colombia, within altitudes of 2500 to 8000 ft. (750 to 2500 m.) above sea level where the vector is present; no special predilection for age, race or sex.

3. Infectious agent — *Bartonella bacilliformis.*

4. Reservoir—An infected person with the agent present in the blood. In endemic areas the asymptomatic carrier rate may reach 5%. No known animal reservoir.

5. Mode of transmission—By bite of sandflies of the genus *Phlebotomus;* species not identified for all areas; *Phlebotomus (Lutzomyia) verrucarum* is important in Peru. These insects all feed only at night.

6. Incubation period—Usually 16 to 22 days, but occasionally 3 to 4 months.

7. Period of communicability—Not directly transmitted from man to man. Infectivity of man for the sandfly is long; the infectious agent may be present in blood weeks before and up to several years after actual illness. Duration of infectivity of the sandfly is unknown.

8. Susceptibility and resistance—Susceptibility is general but the disease is milder in children than adults. Inapparent infections and carriers are known. Recovery from untreated Oroya fever almost invariably gives permanent immunity to this form; the verruga stage may recur.

9. Methods of control—

    A. Preventive measures:
        1) Control of sandflies. (See Cutaneous Leishmaniasis, p. 171).
        2) Avoid known endemic areas after sundown; otherwise apply insect repellent to exposed parts of the body.

    B. Control of patient, contacts, and the immediate environment:
        1) *Report to local health authority:* In selected endemic areas; in most countries not a reportable disease, Class 3B (see Preface).
        2) *Isolation:* None. The infected individual should be protected from bites of phlebotomines (see 9A).
        3) *Concurrent disinfection:* None.
        4) *Quarantine:* None.
        5) *Immunization of contacts:* None.
        6) *Investigation of contacts and source of infection:* Identification of sandflies, particularly in localities where the infected person was exposed after sundown during the preceding 3 to 8 weeks.
        7) *Specific treatment:* Penicillin, streptomycin, chloramphenicol, and tetracyclines are all effective in reducing fever and bacteremia. Chloramphenicol or ampicillin are the drugs of choice; they work directly against

Bartonella, but more importantly also against the frequent secondary salmonellosis.

C. *Epidemic measures:* Intensification of case finding and systematic spraying of houses with a residual insecticide.

D. *International measures:* None.

❧

BLASTOMYCOSIS, NORTH AMERICAN
(Gilchrist's disease)

1. **Identification** — Systemic blastomycosis is a chronic granulomatous mycosis, primarily of the lungs. It begins with a fever and symptoms of respiratory infection resembling influenza and progresses gradually with fever, loss of weight, cachexia with cough, and purulent sputum. Dissemination results in abscesses in skin, bone, prostate, scrotal contents and occasionally visceral organs. It is frequently fatal if untreated.

Cutaneous blastomycosis is characterized by a papule which ulcerates and spreads slowly and peripherally for months or years. The ulcer becomes irregular, crusted, and forms a granulomatous base and an elevated papilliform to verrucous border which contains minute abscesses. The center of the ulcer heals with a thin scar. The lesions are usually on exposed parts of the body such as the face, hands, wrists, or feet and ankles. Cutaneous blastomycosis ordinarily is a local manifestation of existing systemic disease.

Direct microscopic examination of unstained smears of sputum and materials from lesions shows characteristic budding forms of the fungus which can be cultured. Serological test results can be misleading because of cross reactions with histoplasmosis; complement fixation tests are often negative in cases with active disease. Blastomycin skin test is often negative and misleading.

2. **Occurrence** — Uncommon. Occurs sporadically in central and southeastern U.S.A., Canada, Africa, and rarely in Latin America. Rare in children; more frequent in males than in females. Infection of dogs is frequent; disease has also been reported in horses, cats and sea lions.

3. **Infectious agent** — *Blastomyces dermatitidis (Ajellomyces dermatitidis),* a dimorphic fungus that grows as a yeast in the tis-

sues and in enriched culture media at 37ºC., and as a mold at room temperature (25ºC).

4. **Reservoir**—Probably soil.

5. **Mode of transmission**—Conidia, typical of the mold or saprophytic growth form, probably are inhaled in spore-laden dust.

6. **Incubation period**—Probably a few weeks or less, to months.

7. **Period of communicability**—Not transmitted directly from man or animals to man.

8. **Susceptibility and resistance**—Unknown. Inapparent pulmonary infections are probable, but of undetermined frequency. No information on immunity; the rarity of the disease and of laboratory infections suggests man is relatively resistant.

9. **Methods of control**—

   A. Preventive measures: Unknown.

   B. Control of patient, contacts, and the immediate environment:
     1) Report to local health authority: Official report not ordinarily justifiable, Class 5 (see Preface).
     2) Isolation: None.
     3) Concurrent disinfection: Sputum, discharges and all contaminated articles. Terminal cleaning.
     4) Quarantine: None.
     5) Immunization of contacts: None.
     6) Investigation of contacts: Not profitable.
     7) Specific treatment: Amphotericin B (Fungizone) is the present drug of choice. Hydroxystilbamidine isethionate is an effective alternative in less severe cases.

   C. Epidemic measures: Not applicable, a sporadic disease.

   D. International measures: None.

BLASTOMYCOSIS, SOUTH AMERICAN
(Paracoccidioidal granuloma, Paracoccidioidomycosis)

1. **Identification**—A serious and at times fatal chronic mycosis, characterized by lung involvement and/or ulcerative lesions of the mucosa (oral, nasal, rectal) and of the skin. Lymphadenopathy is

frequent. In disseminated cases all viscera may be affected; the adrenal gland is especially susceptible.

Diagnosis is confirmed histologically or by cultivation of the infectious agent. Serological techniques may assist in diagnosis.

Keloidal blastomycosis (Lobo's Disease), a disease with only skin involvement, formerly confused with the South American blastomycosis, is caused by *Loboa loboi*, a fungus known only in its tissue form and not yet grown in culture.

2. **Occurrence**—Endemic in the tropical and subtropical forests of South America and, to a lesser extent, of Central America and Mexico. Workers in contact with soil such as farmers, laborers and construction workers are especially at risk. Highest incidence is in adults aged 30 to 50 years; 13 times as common in males as in females.

3. **Infectious agent**—*Paracoccidioides brasiliensis*, a dimorphic fungus.

4. **Reservoir**—Probably soil or spore-laden dust.

5. **Mode of transmission**—Presumably, but not proved to be, acquired through inhalation of contaminated soil or dust.

6. **Incubation period**—Highly variable, from 1 month to many years.

7. **Period of communicability**—Not known to be transmitted directly from man to man.

8. **Susceptibility and resistance**—Unknown.

9. **Methods of control**—

   A. *Preventive measures:* None.

   B. *Control of patient, contacts, and the immediate environment:*

      1) *Report to local health authority:* Official report not ordinarily justifiable, Class 5 (see Preface).
      2) *Isolation:* None.
      3) *Concurrent disinfection:* Of discharges and contaminated articles. Terminal cleaning.
      4) *Quarantine:* None.
      5) *Immunization of contacts:* None.
      6) *Investigation of contacts:* Not profitable.
      7) *Specific treatment:* Amphotericin B (Fungizone), given intravenously, promptly arrests spread of lesions and is drug of choice. Sulfonamides control the disease, but treatment must be continued indefinitely to prevent re-

lapse. Amphotericin B probably should be followed by treatment with sulfonamide.

C. *Epidemic measure:* Not applicable, a sporadic disease.

D. *International measures:* None.

BRUCELLOSIS

(Undulant fever, Malta fever, Mediterranean fever, Bang's disease).

1. **Identification** — A systemic disease with acute or insidious onset, characterized by continued, intermittent or irregular fever of variable duration, headache, weakness, profuse sweating, chills or chilliness, arthralgia, depression, and generalized aching. Nonpurulent meningitis and pneumonitis may occur. The disease may last for several days, many months, or occasionally several years. Orchitis and vertebral osteomyelitis are uncommon but characteristic features. Recovery is usual but disability is often pronounced. The fatality rate is 2% or less; higher for *Brucella melitensis* infections than for other species. Clinical diagnosis is often difficult and uncertain. Death is rare in persons without complications.

Laboratory diagnosis is by isolation of the infectious agent from blood, bone marrow or other tissues, or from discharges of the patient. The agglutination test is valuable, especially with paired sera to show rise in antibody titer. Tests specific for gamma-G antibody are useful, particularly in chronic cases.

2. **Occurrence** — Worldwide, especially in Mediterranean countries of Europe and North Africa, Central Asia, Mexico, and South America. Predominantly an occupational disease of those working with infected animals or their carcasses, especially farm workers, veterinarians and abattoir workers, hence more frequent among males. Sporadic cases and outbreaks occur among consumers of unpasteurized milk or milk products (especially cheese) from cows, sheep and goats. Reported incidence in the U.S.A. is less than 200 cases annually and is declining.

3. **Infectious agents** — *Brucella abortus*, biotypes 1-9; *B. canis; B. melitensis*, biotypes 1-3, and *B. suis*, biotypes 1-4.

4. **Reservoir** — Reservoirs of human infection are cattle, swine,

sheep, goats, horses and reindeer; in U.S.A., mainly swine, cattle and Alaskan caribou. *B. canis,* a problem in laboratory dog colonies and kennels, can infect animal handlers.

5. Mode of transmission — By contact with tissues, blood, urine, vaginal discharges, aborted fetuses and especially placentas, and by ingestion of milk or dairy products (cheese) from infected animals. Airborne infection may occur from animals in pens and stables; also in laboratories and abattoirs.

6. Incubation period — Highly variable and difficult to ascertain; usually 5 to 21 days, occasionally several months.

7. Period of communicability — No evidence of communicability from man to man.

8. Susceptibility and resistance — Severity and duration of clinical illness are subject to wide differences. Children are less likely to have manifest disease than are adults. Mild and inapparent infections are frequent. Duration of acquired immunity is uncertain.

9. Methods of control — Ultimate control of brucellosis in man rests in the elimination of the disease among domestic animals.

    A. Preventive measures:
1) Education of farmers and workers in slaughter houses, packing plants and butcher shops as to the nature of the disease and the danger of handling carcasses or products of infected animals.
2) Search for infection among livestock by the agglutination reaction; eliminate infected animals by segregation or slaughter. Infection among swine usually requires slaughter of the herd. Immunization of calves is recommended only in areas of high prevalence.
3) Pasteurization of milk and dairy products from cows, sheep or goats. Boiling of milk is practical and effective when pasteurization is impossible.
4) Care in handling and disposal of discharges and fetus from an aborted animal. Disinfection of contaminated areas.
5) Meat inspection and condemning of carcasses of diseased swine; not a useful procedure for cattle or goats.

    B. Control of patient, contacts, and the immediate environment:
1) *Report to local health authority:* Case report obligatory in most states and countries, Class 2B (see Preface).

   2) *Isolation:* None.

   3) *Concurrent disinfection:* Of purulent discharges.

   4) *Quarantine:* None.

   5) *Immunization of contacts:* None.

   6) *Investigation of contacts and source of infection:* Trace infection to the common or individual source, usually infected domestic goats, swine or cattle, or unpasteurized milk or dairy products from cows and goats. Test suspected animals, remove reactors.

   7) *Specific treatment:* Tetracycline (or oxytetracycline or chlortetracycline) alone is adequate for most patients. In more seriously ill patients or those with abscesses, the addition of streptomycin may enhance the efficacy of treatment. In severely ill patients, steroids may be administered to decrease systemic toxicity. Relapses occur in about 5 percent of treated patients and are not due to resistant organisms. They should be treated again with the original regimen.

C.   *Epidemic measures:* Search for common vehicle of infection, usually unpasteurized milk or milk products from an infected herd. Stop distribution or provide pasteurization.

D.   *International measures:* Control of domestic animals and animal products in international trade and transport. WHO Collaborating Centres (see Preface).

CANDIDIASIS

(Moniliasis, Thrush, Candidosis)

1. Identification—A mycosis, usually confined to the superficial layers of skin or mucous membranes and presenting clinically as oral thrush, intertrigo, vulvovaginitis, paronychia or onychomycosis. Ulcers or pseudomembranes may be formed in the esophagus, gastrointestinal tract or bladder. Hematogenous dissemination may produce lesions in other organs such as kidney, spleen, lung, liver, endocardium, eye, meninges, brain, or around a cardiac valve prosthesis.

Diagnosis requires consideration of both laboratory and clinical evidence of candidiasis. The single most valuable laboratory test is microscopic demonstration of pseudohyphae and yeast cells in infected tissue or fluid. Cultural confirmation is important, but does not prove that organism is causally related to the disease state present. Serological tests are under evaluation.

2. **Occurrence**—Worldwide but sporadic. The fungus is often part of the normal flora in man, the incidence depending on site and also upon many local and systemic factors. Oral thrush is a common, usually benign condition of the first few weeks of life. Clinical disease occurs when host defense is low. Examples of local factors contributing to superficial candidiasis would be interdigital intertrigo and paronychia on hands with excessive exposure to water, e.g., housewives, bartenders, or intertrigo in moist skin folds of obese individuals. Prominent among systemic factors predisposing to candidiasis are diabetes mellitus, therapy with broad spectrum antibiotics and supraphysiologic doses of adrenal corticosteroids, hyperalimentation, and certain immune deficiencies.

3. **Infectious agents**—*Candida albicans,* a yeast-like fungus, and occasionally other species of *Candida.*

4. **Reservoir**—Man is the important reservoir.

5. **Mode of transmission**—By contact with excretions of mouth, skin, vagina, and especially feces from patients or carriers, from mother to infant during childbirth, and by endogenous spread. Disseminated candidiasis may originate from mucosal lesions, unsterile narcotic injections, percutaneous intravenous catheters and retention catheters in the bladder.

6. **Incubation period**—Variable, 2 to 5 days in thrush of infants.

7. **Period of communicability**—Presumably for duration of lesions.

8. **Susceptibility and resistance**—The frequency of isolating a *Candida* species from sputum, throat, feces or urine in the absence of clinical evidence of infection suggests a low level of pathogenicity or a widespread immunity. Many adults have a delayed dermal hypersensitivity to the fungus and possess humoral antibodies. Repeated clinical skin eruptions are common.

9. **Methods of control**—

   A. *Preventive measures:* Detection and treatment of vaginal thrush during third trimester of pregnancy to prevent neonatal thrush. To prevent systemic spread, early detection and local treatment of thrush in mouth, esophagus or urinary bladder of debilitated patients, especially those receiving antibiotics, immunosuppresive drugs, or adrenal corticosteroids. For persistent recurrence of vaginal thrush, preventive measures include treatment of sexual partner with topical nystatin, treatment of presumed bowel reservoir with oral nystatin.

B. Control of patient, contacts, and the immediate environment:
1) *Report to local health authority:* Official report ordinarily not justifiable, Class 5 (see Preface).
2) *Isolation:* In nurseries, segregation of patients with oral thrush.
3) *Concurrent disinfection:* Of secretions and contaminated articles.
4) *Quarantine:* None.
5) *Immunization of contacts:* None.
6) *Investigation of contacts:* Not profitable in sporadic cases.
7) *Specific treatment:* Ameliorating underlying causes of candidiasis often facilitates cure, e.g., removal of indwelling venous catheters. Topical nystatin is useful in many forms of superficial candidiasis. Intravenous amphotericin B is the drug of choice for visceral candidiasis; oral 5-fluorocytosine is a possible alternative in milder cases, provided the isolated organism is susceptible.

C. Epidemic measures: Epidemics are largely limited to thrush in nurseries for the newborn. Cultures should be taken from the mouths of infants during the first 2 days of life. If *C. albicans* is demonstrated, clinical thrush can be confidently predicted. Such infants and those with oral thrush should be segregated, and increased emphasis given to general cleanliness. Concurrent disinfection and terminal cleaning should be practiced; compare to epidemic diarrhea in hospital nurseries (p. 99).

D. International measures: None.

∞

CAPILLARIASIS

Two forms of capillariasis have been recognized, both of which are relatively new diseases, i.e., intestinal capillariasis and hepatic capillariasis.

A. INTESTINAL CAPILLARIASIS

1. **Identification**—A clinical syndrome due to a nematode parasite, *Capillaria philippinensis*, first described in Manila in 1963. Clinically, the disease is an enteropathy with massive protein loss and a malabsorption syndrome which lead to progressive weight loss and extreme emaciation. Fatal cases are characterized by the presence of large numbers of parasites in the small intestine with ascites and pleural transudate.

Diagnosis is made on clinical findings plus the identification of eggs and/or larval or adult parasites in the stool. The eggs resemble those of *Trichuris trichiura* from which they must be differentiated. Jejunal biopsy may reveal the worms in the lumen and in the mucosa of the intestine.

2. **Occurrence**—Intestinal capillariasis is endemic in the Philippine Islands and has been found in Thailand. It has reached epidemic proportions on Luzon where more than one thousand cases had been diagnosed by 1967. In some villages a third of the population was found to be infected.

3. **Infectious agent**—*Capillaria philippinensis*, a nematode parasite inhabiting the small intestine.

4. **Reservoir**—Unknown. Various animals, including the goat, water buffalo, dog, and pig have been suspected. Fish in lagoons on Luzon have been shown to serve as intermediate hosts.

5. **Mode of transmission**—The life cycle and mode of transmission remain unknown. Studies have shown that infective larvae developed in fish fed on the nematode eggs, and monkeys fed these fish became infected; autoinfection also occurred. A history of ingestion of raw or inadequately cooked fish is frequently obtained. Males between the ages of twenty and forty-five years appear to be particularly at risk.

6. **Incubation period**—Unknown; based on monkey studies, a month or more.

7. **Period of communicability**—Unknown.

8. **Susceptibility and resistance**—Susceptibility appears to be

general in those geographic areas in the Philippines in which the parasite is prevalent. Attack rates are often high. Fatality rates of 10% have been reported, but sub-clinical cases also occur.

9. **Methods of control** —

   A. *Preventive measures:*
      1) Though the mode of transmission has not been definitely demonstrated, raw fish should not be eaten and all foods of animal origin, especially fish, should be thoroughly cooked.
      2) Provision of adequate facilities for the disposal of feces.

   B. *Control of patients, contacts, and the immediate environment:*
      1) *Report to local health authority:* Case report by most practicable means. Class 3 (see Preface).
      2) *Isolation:* None.
      3) *Concurrent disinfection:* None. Sanitary disposal of feces.
      4) *Quarantine:* None.
      5) *Immunization of contacts:* None.
      6) *Investigation of contacts:* All members of family group, including feces examination.
      7) *Specific treatment:* Thiabendazole (Mintezol) may be effective, but prolonged therapy is necessary.

   C. *Epidemic measures:* Prompt investigation of cases and contacts with treatment of cases as indicated. Education in cooking of fish to remove a source of infection.

   D. *International measures:* None.

B. HEPATIC CAPILLARIASIS

1. **Identification** — A disease of mammals due to a nematode parasite, *Capillaria hepatica*. Commonly a parasite of rats in which infection rates as high as 86% have been reported; also occurs less frequently in dogs, shrews, voles, pigs, monkeys, beavers, and other wild carnivores and omnivores. Infection has been reported in thirty-three species of mammals in North America. The first human infection was recorded in 1924. Though widely distributed geographically, it remains a rare disease in man.

Adult worms in the liver produce eggs which remain in the parenchyma until the death of the animal host. When the host dies and the infected organ decomposes, the eggs embryonate and become infective. When eaten by a susceptible host, including man, they hatch in the small intestine, and liberate larvae which migrate through the wall of the gut and eventually reach the portal system and establish a genuine infection. In the liver they are filtered out, reach maturity and again produce eggs. Spurious infection of humans occurs when contaminated livers containing the eggs are eaten, either raw or cooked, prior to embryonation (requires 2 to 4 weeks outside the host); eggs appear in the stool, but since they do not hatch, the infection is not established.

Symptoms are often quite severe and most cases reported in the literature have terminated fatally. The liver may be grotesquely enlarged, with marked ascites, weight loss and emaciation in terminal cases. Eosinophilia is a common finding. Diagnosis is made by demonstrating eggs of the parasite in a liver biopsy or at autopsy.

2. Occurrence—Hepatic capillariasis has been reported from North America, India, Turkey, South Africa, Hawaii, Mexico, and Brazil.

3. Infectious agent—*Capillaria hepatica*, a nematode worm.

4. Reservoir—Many species of rodents and other mammals harbor the parasite in nature.

5. Mode of transmission—Human infection occurs when embryonated eggs are eaten in contaminated food, water, or dirt.

6. Incubation period—3 to 4 weeks.

7. Period of communicability—Not directly transmitted from man to man.

8. Susceptibility and resistance—Susceptibility is universal.

9. Methods of control—

   A. Preventive measures:
     1) Prevent eating of dirt.
     2) Protection of water supplies and food from contamination with soil.

   B. Control of patients, contacts, and the immediate environment:
     1) Report to local authority: Optional report, Class 3 C (see Preface).
     2) Isolation: None.
     3) Concurrent disinfection: None.

4) Quarantine: None.
5) Immunization of contacts: None.
6) Investigation of contacts: Not applicable.
7) Specific treatment: None is known.

C. Epidemic measures: Not applicable.

D. International measures: None.

CARDITIS, VIRAL

1. Identification — An acute or subacute myocarditis or pericarditis, which occurs as a primary disease and may occasionally complicate various viral infections. The most frequently identified causative agents are enteroviruses of the Coxsackie groups.

The myocardium is particularly affected in young children, in whom fever and lethargy may be followed rapidly by heart failure, with pallor, cyanosis, dyspnea, tachycardia and enlargement of heart and liver. Heart failure may be progressive and fatal, or recovery may take place over a few weeks; some cases run a relapsing course over months and may show residual heart damage. In adults, pericarditis is the commonest manifestation, with acute chest pain, disturbance of heart rate and rhythm, and often dyspnea. The disease may complicate pleurodynia (see pp. 231-233).

Specific diagnosis is made by isolation of the infectious agent (e.g., coxsackievirus) from feces, pericardial fluid or postmortem heart tissue. Serologic studies can be supportive, but are not conclusive without isolation of an agent.

2. Occurrence — An uncommon disease, mainly sporadic but commoner during epidemics of Coxsackie group B virus infection. Institutional outbreaks with high fatality in the newborn have been described in maternity units.

3. Infectious agents — Various group B coxsackieviruses (types 1, 2, 3, 4, 5); occasionally group A coxsackieviruses (types 1, 4, 9, 16, 23); also poliovirus in severe infections. Influenza, mumps, measles, rubella, varicella-zoster, vaccinia, smallpox, Colorado tick fever and other arboviruses, lymphocytic choriomeningitis virus, and echovirus 6 (see Index for page location) have been isolated from patients with carditis.

4. Reservoir, 5. Mode of transmission, 6. Incubation period, 7. Period of communicability, 8. Susceptibility and resistance, and 9. Methods of control — Depend on the specific infectious agent.

∞

CAT-SCRATCH DISEASE

(Cat-scratch fever, Benign inoculation lymphoreticulosis)

1. Identification — A subacute, self-limited infectious disease characterized by malaise, granulomatous lymphadenitis, and variable degrees and patterns of fever. Usually preceded by a cat scratch in which a primary lesion often develops, followed by regional lymph node involvement. Suppuration occurs in about 1/4 of patients; pus obtained from lymph nodes is bacteriologically sterile. Recurrent and chronic forms are rare; rashes, erythema nodosum, thrombocytopenia, Parinaud's oculoglandular syndrome (conjunctivitis with enlargement of homolateral preauricular node), and encephalitis are reported rarely.

Diagnosis is based on a consistent clinical picture and histopathological characteristics of involved lymph nodes; investigational skin test antigens are not recommended for regular use because of the risk of transmitting hepatitis virus or other unidentified agents. Pasteurellosis, a bacterial infection with *Pasteurella multocida*, acquired by animal bite, may cause a similar clinical picture.

2. Occurrence — Worldwide but uncommon; occurs in all seasons. Striking increase in cases in some winters has been reported in northern U.S. and Canada. Sexes equally affected; more frequent in children and young people. Familial clustering occurs.

3. Infectious agent — Unknown.

4. Reservoir — Probably one of several animals, usually with inapparent infection, most frequently the cat.

5. Mode of transmission — Infected animals suspected of transmitting infection to man by scratching, biting, licking, or other means. Minor trauma after insect bites, or contact with splinters or thorns is suspected as the mode of transmission in the absence of known direct contact with animals.

6. Incubation period — Usually 7 to 14 days from inoculation to primary lesion; possibly as short as 2 days.

7. Period of communicability — Unknown for reservoir hosts. Not directly transmitted from man to man.

8. Susceptibility and resistance — Unknown.

9. Methods of control —

    A. *Preventive measures:* Unknown.

    B. *Control of patient, contacts, and the immediate environment:*
        1) Report to local health authority: Official report not ordinarily justifiable, Class 5 (see Preface).
        2) Isolation: None.
        3) Concurrent disinfection: Of discharges from purulent lesions.
        4) Quarantine: None.
        5) Immunization of contacts: None.
        6) Investigation of contacts: Examination of family contacts for similar illness.
        7) Specific treatment: None.

    C. *Epidemic measures:* Not applicable.

    D. *International measures:* None.

CHANCROID
(Ulcus Molle, Soft chancre)

1. Identification — An acute, localized, self-limited autoinoculable genital infection characterized clinically by painful necrotizing ulcerations at site of inoculation, often accompanied by painful inflammatory swelling and suppuration of regional lymph nodes, frequently unilateral. Extragenital lesions have been reported.

Diagnostic aids: Microscopic examination of stained exudate from edges of lesions, culture of pus from buboes, and biopsy.

2. Occurrence — No particular differences in incidence according to age, race or sex except as determined by sexual habits. Most common in tropical and subtropical regions, especially in seaports where incidence may be higher than that of syphilis; in temperate zones uncommon or even rare.

3. **Infectious agent** — *Haemophilus ducreyi*, the Ducrey bacillus.

4. **Reservoir** — Man.

5. **Mode of transmission** — Direct sexual contact with discharges from open lesions and pus from buboes; suggestive evidence of asymptomatic infections in women. Rare instances of professionally acquired lesions on hands of physicians and nurses; accidental inoculation of children is known. Indirect transmission rare. Prostitution, sexual promiscuity and uncleanliness favor transmission.

6. **Incubation period** — From 3 to 5 days, up to 14 days; if fissures or abrasions of mucous membranes are present, as short as 24 hours.

7. **Period of communicability** — As long as infectious agent persists in original lesion or in discharging regional lymph nodes usually until healed; in most instances a matter of weeks.

8. **Susceptibility and resistance** — Susceptibility is general; no evidence of natural resistance.

9. **Methods of control** —

A. *Preventive measures:* Thorough washing of genitalia with soap and water promptly after intercourse, otherwise preventive measures are those of syphilis (pp. 316-317).

B. *Control of patient, contacts, and the immediate environment.*
   1) *Report to local health authority:* Case report obligatory in many states and countries, Class 2B (see Preface).
   2) *Isolation:* None; avoid sexual contact until all lesions are healed.
   3) *Concurrent disinfection:* None; stress personal cleanliness.
   4) *Quarantine:* None.
   5) *Immunization of contacts:* Not applicable; prompt treatment on recognition or clinical suspicion of disease.
   6) *Investigation of contacts:* Search for sexual contacts of 2 weeks before and after onset. Women without visible signs may be carriers.
   7) *Specific treatment:* Sulfonamides. Streptomycin or tetracyclines only if infectious agent is sulfonamide resistant, since either may mask syphilis.

C. *Epidemic measures:* Persisting levels of occurrence or an increased incidence are indications for more rigid application of measures outlined in 9A. or 9B.

D. *International measures:* (see Syphilis, 9D, p. 318).

CHICKENPOX—HERPES ZOSTER
(Varicella—Shingles)

1. **Identification**—Chickenpox is an acute generalized viral disease of sudden onset with slight fever, mild constitutional symptoms and an eruption of the skin which is maculopapular for a few hours, vesicular for 3 to 4 days, and leaves a granular scab. Lesions tend to be more abundant on covered than on exposed parts of the body; may appear on scalp, high in the axilla, on mucous membranes of the mouth and upper respiratory tract, and on the conjunctiva; commonly occur in successive crops, with several stages of maturity present at the same time; may be so few as to escape observation. Mild, atypical and inapparent infections occur. Rarely fatal, a primary viral pneumonia is the commonest cause of death in adults and septic complications and encephalitis in children.

Herpes zoster is a local manifestation of recurrent, recrudescent or reactivation infection with the same virus. Vesicles with an erythematous base are restricted to skin areas supplied by sensory nerves of a single or associated group of dorsal root ganglia. Lesions may appear in crops in irregular fashion along nerve pathways, are usually unilateral, and are deeper seated and more closely aggregated than chickenpox; histologically they are identical. Severe pain and paresthesia are common. Occurs mainly in older adults although there is some evidence that almost 10% of children being treated for a malignant neoplasm are prone to develop herpes zoster. Occasionally a varicelliform eruption follows some days after zoster, and rarely a secondary eruption of zoster type after chickenpox.

Laboratory tests, such as visualization of the virus by electron microscopy, isolation of virus in tissue culture, or the demonstration of a rise in complement-fixing serum antibody, are useful but not readily available. Multinucleate giant epithelial cells may be detected in Giemsa stained scrapings of the base of a lesion; these are not found in vaccinia or variola lesions.

2. **Occurrence**—Worldwide. Infection with varicella-zoster virus is nearly universal. In metropolitan communities, about 3/4 of the population have had chickenpox by age 15. Zoster occurs more commonly in older people. In temperate zones chickenpox occurs most frequently in winter and early spring.

3. **Infectious agent**—The varicella—zoster virus (V-Z virus).

4. **Reservoir**—An infected person.

5. **Mode of transmission**—From person to person by direct contact, droplet, or airborne spread of secretions of respiratory

tract of infected persons. Indirectly through articles freshly soiled by discharges from vesicles and mucous membranes of infected persons. In contrast to vaccinia and variola, scabs from varicella lesions are not infective. One of the most readily communicable of diseases, especially in the early stages of the eruption. Susceptibles may contract chickenpox from patients with herpes zoster.

6. **Incubation period** — From 2 to 3 weeks; commonly 13 to 17 days.

7. **Period of communicability** — As long as 5 days before the eruption of chickenpox, and not more than 6 days after the last crop of vesicles. Patients with altered immunity may continue to develop new lesions and contagiousness is thus prolonged.

8. **Susceptibility and resistance** — Susceptibility to chickenpox is universal among those not previously infected; ordinarily a more severe disease of adults than of children. One infection confers long immunity; second attacks are rare. Infection apparently remains latent and may recur years later as herpes zoster in a proportion of older adults, sometimes in children.

Patients with leukemia may suffer severe, prolonged or fatal chickenpox. Adults with cancer, especially of lymphoid tissue with or without steroid therapy, may have an increased frequency of zoster, both localized and disseminated.

9. Methods of control —

A. *Preventive measures:*
1) Protect patients with immuno-deficient conditions such as leukemia against exposure. Gamma globulin from zoster convalescent patients, while generally scarce, is effective in preventing disease. (see 9B below.)
2) Cases reported as chickenpox in persons over 15 years, or at any age during an epidemic of smallpox, should be investigated to eliminate the possibility of smallpox.

B. *Control of patient, contacts, and the immediate environment:*
1) *Report to local health authority:* Official report is not ordinarily justifiable. Case report of chickenpox in adults (Class 3B, see Preface) may be required where smallpox is endemic.
2) *Isolation:* None; exclusion from school for 1 week after eruption first appears and avoidance of contact with susceptibles.
3) *Concurrent disinfection:* Articles soiled by discharges from the nose and throat and from lesions.
4) *Quarantine:* None.

5) *Protection of contacts:* Specific immune serum globulin from zoster-convalescent patients (Zoster Immune Globulin—ZIG) may prevent or modify disease in close contacts of cases. Limited amounts of ZIG are available from the Center for Disease Control, Atlanta, Georgia, for certain high-risk patients exposed to chickenpox.

6) *Investigation of contacts:* Of no practical importance except where there is suspicion of smallpox.

7) *Specific treatment:* none.

C. **Epidemic measures:** None.

D. **International measures:** None.

CHOLERA

1. **Identification**—A serious acute intestinal disease characterized by sudden onset, profuse watery stools, vomiting, rapid dehydration, acidosis and circulatory collapse. Death may occur within a few hours of onset. Fatality rates in untreated cases may exceed 50%; with proper treatment they are below 1%. Mild cases with only diarrhea are common, especially in children. Inapparent and wholly asymptomatic infections are many times more frequent than clinically recognized cases, especially in El Tor cholera.

The diagnosis is confirmed by culturing cholera vibrios from feces or vomitus, or by demonstrating a significant rise in titer of specific antibodies in paired sera taken in the acute and convalescent stage, provided vaccine has not been given.

2. **Occurrence**—During the 19th century pandemic cholera repeatedly spread from its traditional home in Bengal and other parts of India to most parts of the world. During the first half of the 20th century the disease was largely confined to Asia although a severe epidemic occurred in Egypt in 1947.

Since 1961, cholera has spread extensively from a focus in Sulawesi in Indonesia through most of Asia and the Middle East into Eastern Europe and Africa and from North Africa into the Iberian Peninsula and, in 1973, into Italy. The disease has had a tendency to persist in most of the affected countries.

Except for 2 laboratory-acquired cases in 1966, there were no reports of indigenous cholera in the Western Hemisphere between

1911 and 1972. In 1973, however, a case occurred in Texas with no known source. Cases among air travelers have occurred in other parts of the world, e.g., Bahrain to Australia and New Zealand 1972, resulting in more than 40 cases and one death. Individual cases have occurred among travelers in many other areas, including Western Europe and Canada.

3. **Infectious agent** — *Vibrio cholerae*, the comma vibrio; classical and El Tor biotypes may be either Inaba and Ogawa serotypes. The diseases caused by these variants are clinically indistinguishable. In any single epidemic one particular variant tends to be dominant.

4. **Reservoir** — Man.

5. **Mode of transmission** — Transmission occurs through ingestion of water contaminated with feces or vomitus of patients, and to a lesser extent, feces of carriers, food contaminated by water, soiled hands, or flies. Spread from person-to-person by direct contact is of relatively minor importance, if it occurs at all.

6. **Incubation period** — From a few hours to 5 days, usually 2 to 3 days.

7. **Period of communicability** — Unknown, but presumably for the duration of the stool-positive carrier state, which usually lasts for a few days after recovery. However, the carrier state may persist for several months. A rare chronic biliary infection lasting for years has been observed, associated with intermittent shedding of vibrios in the stool. Effective antibiotics, e.g., tetracycline, shorten the period of communicability.

8. **Susceptibility and resistance** — Susceptibility is variable and poorly understood; gastric achlorhydria increases risk of disease. Clinical cholera is usually confined to the lowest socioeconomic groups. Even in severe epidemics attack rates rarely exceed 1 or 2%, although inapparent infection rates are much higher. Infection results in significant serological response in agglutinating, vibriocidal and antitoxic antibodies; their presence is associated with resistance to clinical disease. In endemic areas, most persons acquire antibodies by early adulthood. Partial active immunity (about 50% protection) to overt disease is induced by cholera vaccines, but the duration is short-lived (a few months) and does not prevent asymptomatic infection. Specific immunity to the Inaba serotype protects against Ogawa infections but not the reverse; there are no known immunological differences between the classical and El Tor biotypes.

9. **Methods of Control—**

   A. *Preventive measures:*
      1) Sanitary disposal of human feces, together with ready availability and use of handwashing facilities.
      2) Protection and purification of water supplies (see Typhoid Fever 9A1, p. 351).
      3) Boiling of milk or pasteurization of milk and dairy products (see Typhoid Fever 9A4, p. 351).
      4) Sanitary supervision of processing, preparation, and serving of foods, especially those eaten moist and/or raw; special attention to provision and use of handwashing facilities by food-handlers.
      5) Destruction of flies, control of fly breeding and screening to protect foods from fly contamination (see Typhoid Fever 9A3, p. 351).
      6) Education of the public in personal hygiene, especially thorough handwashing before eating and after defecation.
      7) Active immunization is of relatively little value as a practical control measure and ordinarily is not recommended because it is expensive, stimulates only transient immunity, and confers a false sense of security to both recipients and health administrators.

   B. *Control of patient, contacts, and the immediate environment:*
      1) *Report to local health authority:* Case report universally required by International Health Regulations (1969)*, WHO, Geneva, Class 1 (see Preface).
      2) *Isolation:* Hospitalization is desirable for patients experiencing acute symptoms, but strict isolation is not necessary. Crowded cholera wards can be operated without hazard to staff and visitors if attendants will practice scrupulous cleanliness. Hospital staff and visitors are usually not at risk, assuming effective handwashing and basic procedures of cleanliness are practiced. Fly control may be helpful. Measures that unnecessarily prohibit or otherwise compromise the movement of people, foods, or other goods are usually not justified.
      3) *Concurrent disinfection:* Of feces and vomitus, and of articles used by patients with carbolic acid or other disinfectant; disinfection of hands each time after handling articles contaminated by feces. Terminal cleaning.

---

* Second Annotated Edition, 1974.

4) *Quarantine:* None.

5) *Management of contacts:* Surveillance of contacts for 5 days from last exposure and longer if their feces are known to contain cholera vibrios. Chemoprophylaxis of family contacts with tetracycline or furazolidone is recommended. Immunization of contacts is not indicated.

6) *Investigation of contacts and source of infection:* Search for the vehicle(s) of transmission. Investigate possibilities of infection from polluted drinking water or from contaminated food. Because there is no practical way to find all infected cases in a community, a search for unreported cases is only recommended among contacts or those exposed to a possible common source.

7) *Specific treatment:* Prompt fluid therapy using adequate volumes of electrolyte solutions to correct dehydration, acidosis and hypokalemia is required. For patients in shock, isotonic intravenous fluids containing 25-48 mEq/l of HCO_3^- and 10-15 mEq/l of K^+ (such as Ringer's lactate) or Dacca solution (NaCl 5 gm, $NaHCO_3$ 4 gm, KCl 1 gm per liter) are given as rapidly as possible. After effective circulation has been restored by intravenous fluids, (5 to 10% of body weight depending on degree of dehydration) liquids containing glucose (20 grams per liter), sodium chloride (3.5 grams per liter), $NaHCO_3$ (2.5 grams per liter) and KCl (1.5 grams per liter) are well absorbed from the intestinal tract and should be given by mouth to complete rehydration and to maintain fluid and electrolyte balance. Tetracycline and other antimicrobial agents reduce the volume of intravenous fluids required by limiting the duration and volume of the diarrhea; antibiotics also shorten the period of excretion of vibrios.

C. *Epidemic measures:*

1) Ensure the availability and proper use of adequate treatment facilities.

2) Adopt emergency measures to assure a safe water supply; boil water used for drinking, cooking, or washing dishes or food containers unless water supply is treated adequately, e.g., by chlorination, and is protected from contamination thereafter.

3) Initiate a thorough investigation designed to find the vehicle and circumstances (time, place, person) of transmission and plan control measures accordingly.

4) Assure careful supervision of food and drink. After cooking or boiling, protect against contamination as by flies and unclean human handling.

5) Control flies by limiting fly breeding, by use of appropriate insecticides and by screening kitchens and eating places. (see Typhoid Fever 9A3, p. 351).

6) Vaccine is inappropriate in this epidemic situation and should not be used. Immunization of high risk or exposed groups with reliable vaccine may be indicated.

D. *International measures:*

1) Telegraphic notification by governments to WHO and to adjacent countries of the first imported, first transferred or first non-imported case of cholera in an area previously free of the disease.

2) Measures applicable to ships, aircraft and land transport arriving from cholera areas are specified in International Health Regulations (1969),* WHO, Geneva.

3) International travelers: Evidence of immunization is no longer recommended by WHO as a requirement in travel from country to country in any part of the world and is not required by the U.S.A., though some individual countries may continue to require vaccinations. Travelers may be required to submit to a stool examination when they have come from an infected area within the incubation period of cholera (5 days).

4) WHO Collaborating Centres (see Preface).

CHROMOBLASTOMYCOSIS
(Chromomycosis, Dermatitis verrucosa)

1. Identification—A chronic spreading mycosis of the skin and subcutaneous tissues, usually of a lower extremity. Hematogenous spread to the brain has been reported. Progression to contiguous tissues is slow, over a period of years, with eventual large verrucous or even cauliflower-like masses, and lymph stasis. Rarely a cause of death.

Microscopic examination of scrapings or biopsies from lesions re-

---

* Second Annotated Edition, 1974.

veals characteristic brown hyphae or thick-walled, rounded brown cells. Confirmation of the diagnosis should be attempted by culture of the fungus.

2. **Occurrence**—Worldwide distribution as sporadic cases in widely scattered areas, but mainly Central America, Caribbean Islands, South America, South Pacific Islands, Australia, Madagascar and South Africa. Primarily a disease of rural tropical regions, probably because of more frequent penetrating wounds of feet not protected by shoes. The disease is most common in men aged 30 to 50 years; females are rarely infected.

3. **Infectious agents**—*Phialophora verrucosa, Fonsecaea (Phialophora) pedrosoi, F. compacta* and *Cladosporium carrionii. (C. trichoides* causes brain abscesses but not the typical lesions of chromoblastomycosis. Its tissue form is mycelial without the formation of the sclerotic cells typical of chromoblastomycosis).

4. **Reservoir**—Presumably wood, soil, or vegetation.

5. **Mode of transmission**—Traumatic contact with contaminated wood or other materials.

6. **Incubation period**—Unknown; probably months.

7. **Period of communicability**—Not directly transmitted from man to man.

8. **Susceptibility and resistance**—Unknown, but rarity of disease and absence of laboratory infections suggest man is relatively resistant.

9. **Methods of control**—

A. *Preventive measures:* Protection against small puncture wounds, as by wearing shoes or protective clothing.

B. *Control of patient, contacts, and the immediate environment:*
   1) *Report to local health authority:* Official report not ordinarily justifiable, Class 5 (see Preface).
   2) *Isolation:* None.
   3) *Concurrent disinfection:* Of discharges from lesions and articles soiled therewith.
   4) *Quarantine:* None.
   5) *Immunization of contacts:* Not applicable.
   6) *Investigation of contacts:* Not profitable.
   7) *Specific treatment:* Early experience with 5-fluorocytosine has been favorable. Calciferol or local injections of amphotericin B also may be tried.

C. *Epidemic measures:* Not applicable, a sporadic disease.

D. *International measures:* None.

CLONORCHIASIS
(Chinese liver fluke disease)

1. Identification — A trematode disease of the bile ducts. Clinical reaction may be slight or absent in light infections. Symptoms result from local irritation of bile ducts by the flukes, from toxemia and possibly from secondary bacterial invaders. Loss of appetite, diarrhea, and a sensation of abdominal pressure are common early symptoms. Bile duct obstruction, rarely producing jaundice, may be followed by cirrhosis, enlargement and tenderness of liver, and progressive ascites and edema. Eosinophilia (5 to 40%) is frequent. A chronic disease, sometimes of 30 years or longer duration, but not often a direct or contributing cause of death.

Direct diagnosis is by finding the characteristic fluke eggs in feces or by duodenal drainage; to be differentiated from heterophyid and opisthorchid flukes.

2. Occurrence — Highly endemic in Southeast China, where it is present throughout the country except in the northwest; widespread in Japan, endemic in Taiwan and South Korea and in Vietnam, principally the Red River Delta. In other parts of the world imported cases may occur in immigrants from Asia.

3. Infectious agent — *Clonorchis sinensis,* the Asiatic liver fluke.

4. Reservoir — Man, cat, dog, hog, and other animals are reservoir hosts of adult flukes.

5. Mode of transmission — Man is infected by eating freshwater fish, containing encysted larvae. During digestion, larvae are freed from cysts, and migrate via the common bile duct to biliary radicles. Eggs deposited in the bile passages are evacuated in feces. Eggs in feces contain a fully developed miracidium; when ingested by a susceptible snail of the family *Amnicolidae,* they hatch in its intestine and penetrate vascular spaces. Cercariae develop and emerge into water; on contact with a second intermediate host (40 species of freshwater fishes—*Cyprinidae),* cercariae penetrate the host and encyst, usually in muscle, occasionally on underside of scales. The complete life cycle, from man to man, requires at least three months.

6. Incubation period — Undetermined; flukes reach maturity within 16 to 25 days after encysted larvae are ingested.

7. Period of communicability — Infected individuals may pass viable eggs for as long as 30 years. Not directly transmitted from man to man.

8. Susceptibility and resistance — Susceptibility is universal. No resistance with age; in endemic areas highest prevalence is at age 55 to 60 years.

9. Methods of control—

A. *Preventive measures:*

1) Thorough cooking of all freshwater fish.
2) In endemic areas, education of the public as to dangers of eating raw or improperly cooked fish and the necessity for sanitary disposal of feces.

B. *Control of patient, contacts, and the immediate environment:*

1) *Report to local health authority:* Official report not ordinarily justifiable, Class 5 (see Preface).
2) *Isolation:* None.
3) *Concurrent disinfection:* Sanitary disposal of feces.
4) *Quarantine:* None.
5) *Immunization of contacts:* Not applicable.
6) *Investigation of contacts and source of infection:* Of the individual case, unprofitable. A community problem (see 9C below).
7) *Specific treatment:* Chloroquine phosphate 0.5 gm twice daily for 3 days, then 0.5 gm daily for 30 days is reported to be effective.

C. *Epidemic measures:* Locate source of infected fish. Shipments of dried or pickled fish are the likely source in nonendemic areas.

D. *International measures:* Control of fish or fish products imported from endemic areas.

COCCIDIOIDOMYCOSIS
(Valley fever; Desert fever; Desert rheumatism; Coccidioidal granuloma)

1. Identification—An internal mycosis which begins as a respiratory infection.

A. *Primary Infection:* May be entirely asymptomatic or resemble an acute influenzal illness with fever, chills, cough and pleural pain. About one-fifth of clinically recognized cases (an estimated 5% of all primary infections) develop erythema nodosum, a complication most frequent in white females and rarest in Negro males. Primary infection may (1) heal completely without detectable residuals, (2) leave fibrosis or calcification of pulmonary lesions, (3) leave a persistent thin-walled cavity, or (4) and most rarely, progress to the disseminated form of the disease comparable to progressive primary tuberculosis.

B. *Progressive Primary Coccidioidomycosis (Coccidioidal granuloma):* A progressive, highly fatal and uncommon granulomatous disease characterized by lung lesions and single or aggregated abscesses throughout the body, especially in subcutaneous tissues, skin, bone, peritoneum, testes, thyroid and central nervous system. Coccidioidal meningitis resembles tuberculous meningitis. A granulomatous disease, "paracoccidioidal granuloma" (see pp. 55-57), has no relationship to coccidioidomycosis.

The fungus may be demonstrated by microscopic examination of sputum or by culture. Reactivity to skin test with coccidioidin appears usually within 2 to 3 days after onset of symptoms but may not develop for up to 3 weeks; precipitin and complement-fixation tests are usually positive within the first 3 months of clinical disease. Serial skin and serological tests may be necessary to confirm a recent infection.

2. Occurrence—Primary infections are extremely common in scattered highly endemic arid and semiarid areas of the Western Hemisphere: in U.S.A. from California to west Texas; in northern Argentina, Venezuela, Mexico, and Central America. Dusty fomites from endemic areas can transmit infections elsewhere; infections occur in persons who have merely traveled through endemic areas. Affects all ages, both sexes and all races. Infection most frequent in summer, especially after wind and dust storms. An important disease among migrant workers and military recruits in endemic areas. Coccidioidal granuloma has the geographic distribution of coccidioidomycosis.

3. Infectious agent—*Coccidioides immitis,* a dimorphic fungus; grows in soil and in culture media as a mold that reproduces by arthrospores; in tissues and under special conditions of culture it grows spherical cells which reproduce by endospore formation.

4. Reservoir—Soil; a fungus that propagates in soil, especially in and around rodent burrows, in regions where temperature, moisture and soil requirements are satisfactory; infects man, cattle, cats, dogs, horses, burros, sheep, swine, wild desert rodents, coyotes, chinchillas, llamas, and other species.

5. Mode of transmission — Inhalation of spores from soil and in laboratories from culture media. Accidental inoculation of infected pus into the skin can result in local granuloma formation.

6. Incubation period — One to 4 weeks in primary infection. Coccidioidal granuloma develops insidiously, most often preceded by unrecognized symptoms of primary pulmonary infection.

7. Period of communicability — Not directly transmitted from man or animal to man. After 7 to 10 days *C. immitis* on casts or dressings may rarely change from the parasitic to the infective saprophytic form.

8. Susceptibility and resistance — A general susceptibility to primary infection is indicated by high prevalence of positive coccidioidin reactors in endemic areas; recovery apparently is followed by solid immunity. More than half of patients with symptomatic infection are between 15 and 25 years of age; males are affected much more frequently than females, probably because of occupational exposure. Dissemination occurs in infected Negroes and Filipinos 10 times more often than in whites.

9. Methods of control —

A. *Preventive measures:* In endemic areas, planting of grass, oiling of air fields and other dust control measures. Individuals from nonendemic areas should preferably not be recruited to dusty occupations, such as road building.

B. *Control of patient, contacts, and the immediate environment:*
 1) *Report to local health authority:* Case report of recognized coccidioidal disease in selected endemic areas (U.S.A.); in many countries not a reportable disease, Class 3B (see Preface).
 2) *Isolation:* None.
 3) *Concurrent disinfection:* Of discharges and soiled articles. Terminal cleaning.
 4) *Quarantine:* None.
 5) *Immunization of contacts:* None.
 6) *Investigation of contacts:* Not profitable except in cases appearing in nonendemic areas, where residence and travel history should be obtained.
 7) *Specific treatment:* Amphotericin B (Fungizone) is beneficial in disseminated infections.

C. *Epidemic measures:* Epidemics occur only when groups of susceptibles are infected by airborne spores. Dust control measures should be instituted where practicable (see 9 above).

D. *International measures:* None.

CONJUNCTIVITIS, ACUTE BACTERIAL

1. **Identification**—A clinical syndrome beginning with lacrimation, irritation, and injection of the palpebral and bulbar conjunctivae of one or both eyes, followed by edema of lids, photophobia, and mucopurulent exudate. In severe cases, ecchymoses of bulbar conjunctiva and marginal infiltration in the cornea may occur. A non-fatal disease, the clinical course is usually 2 to 3 weeks; many patients have no more than injection of the conjunctivae and slight exudate for a few days.

Confirmation of clinical diagnosis by bacteriologic culture or microscopic examination of smear of exudate is required to differentiate from adenovirus, inclusion conjuctivitis, trachoma, echovirus, gonococcal and ideopathic conjunctivitis or Reiter's syndrome.

2. **Occurrence**—Widespread and common throughout the world, particularly in warmer climates; frequently epidemic. In U.S.A., infection with *Haemophilus aegyptius* is largely confined to southern rural areas, Georgia to California, primarily during summer and early autumn. It has been an important cause of school absenteeism. Infection with other organisms occurs throughout U.S.A., often in association with acute viral respiratory disease during cold seasons.

3. **Infectious agents**—*H. aegyptius* (Koch-Weeks bacillus) and pneumococci appear to be the most important; *H. influenzae, Moraxella lacunata,* staphylococci, streptococci, and *Corynebacterium diphtheriae* produce the disease. A gram-negative diplococcus resembling the gonococcus is responsible for epidemics with much loss of sight among young children in North Africa and the Middle East.

4. **Reservoir**—Man. Carriers of *H. aegyptius* are common in many areas during inter-epidemic periods.

5. **Mode of transmission**—Contact with discharges from the conjunctivae or upper respiratory tract of infected persons, through contaminated fingers, clothing, or other articles. In some areas may be mechanically transmitted by eye gnats or flies, but their importance as vectors is undetermined and probably differs from area to area.

6. **Incubation period**—Usually 24 to 72 hours.

7. **Period of communicability**—During the course of active infection.

8. **Susceptibility and resistance**—Children under 5 years are

most often affected; incidence decreases with age. The debilitated and aged are particularly susceptible to staphylococcal infections. Immunity after attack is low-grade and variable, according to the infectious agent.

9. **Methods of control—**

   A. *Preventive measures:* Personal hygiene, hygienic care and treatment of affected eyes.

   B. *Control of patient, contacts, and the immediate environment:*

      1) *Report to local health authority:* Obligatory report of epidemics; no case report, Class 4 (see Preface).

      2) *Isolation:* None. Children should not attend school during the acute stage.

      3) *Concurrent disinfection:* Of discharges and soiled articles. Terminal cleaning.

      4) *Quarantine:* None.

      5) *Immunization of contacts:* None.

      6) *Investigation of contacts:* Usually not profitable.

      7) *Specific treatment:* Local application of an ointment or drops containing a neomycin-polymyxin mixture, tetracycline, erythromycin, gentamicin or a sulfonamide such as sodium sulfacetamide.

   C. *Epidemic measures:*

      1) Adequate and intensive treatment of patients and their associates.

      2) In areas where insects are suspected of mechanically transmitting infection, measures to prevent access of eye gnats or flies to eyes of sick and well persons.

      3) Insect control, according to the suspected vector.

   D. *International measures:* None.

CONJUNCTIVITIS, EPIDEMIC HEMORRHAGIC

1. **Identification**— A virus infection with sudden onset of pain or the sensation of a foreign body in the eye. The disease rapidly progresses (1-2 days) to the full clinical picture of swollen eyelids, injection of the conjunctivae, often with a circumcorneal distribu-

tion, seromucous discharge and subconjunctival hemorrhages. Epithelial, but not subepithelial, keratitis and anterior uveitis may be present. Commonly both eyes are involved and the hemorrhages, which commence in the region of the upper fornix, may vary in size from petechiae to large ecchymoses. Preauricular adenopathy is frequently present. Some patients experience systemic symptoms, most commonly those of an upper respiratory infection. The disease is self limiting, uninfluenced by antibiotics, with the ocular signs and symptoms resolving in 1-2 weeks.

Lumbosacral radiculomyelitis, commencing a few days to a month after the conjunctivitis and commonly leaving some residual weakness of the lower limbs, has been observed in a small number of patients in India. Neurological complications have not been reported elsewhere.

Laboratory confirmation of the diagnosis is by the detection of virus in conjunctival scrapings by electron microscopy or culture or by demonstrating, during the course of the illness, a rise in neutralizing antibodies to one of the two causal viruses.

2. **Occurrence** — Since first recognized in Ghana in 1969, and Indonesia in 1970, outbreaks have been observed in many African and Asian and some European countries in a pandemic spread. No cases have, as yet, been reported from Australia, New Zealand or North or South America.

3. **Infectious Agents** — A picornavirus. Two serologically distinct types have been found in association with epidemics; the most prevalent type has been designated as enterovirus 70.

4. **Reservoir** — Man.

5. **Mode of transmission** — Transmission occurs by direct or indirect contact with discharge from infected eyes and possibly by droplet infection from those with virus in the throat. Mechanical transmission by flies or other agents has not been excluded. Person to person transmission is most noticeable in families. Large epidemics have been associated with overcrowding and low standards of hygiene.

6. **Incubation period** — Probably 1 to 2 days.

7. **Period of communicability** — Unknown, but assumed to be for the period of active disease.

8. **Susceptibility and resistance** — Infection can occur at all ages. Reinfections and/or relapses have been reported. The role and duration of the immune response is not yet clear.

9. **Methods of Control** —

   A. *Preventive measures:* Personal hygiene; avoid overcrowding. Strict asepsis in ophthalmic clinics.

B. Control of patient, contacts, and the immediate environment:

1) *Report to local health authority:* Obligatory report of epidemics; no case report, Class 4 (see Preface).
2) *Isolation:* Desirable to restrict contact with cases while disease is active e.g., children should not attend school.
3) *Concurrent disinfection:* Of conjunctival discharges and articles soiled by them. Terminal cleaning.
4) *Quarantine:* None.
5) *Immunization of contacts:* None.
6) *Investigation of contacts:* Locate other cases.
7) *Specific treatment:* None.

C. Epidemic measures:

1) Organize adequate facilities for the diagnosis and symptomatic treatment of cases.
2) Improve standard of hygiene and limit overcrowding wherever possible.

D. International measures: WHO Collaborating Centres (see Preface).

CONJUNCTIVITIS, INCLUSION

(Neonatal inclusion blennorrhea, Swimming pool conjunctivitis, Para trachoma, "Sticky eye")

1. Identification—In the newborn, an acute papillary conjunctivitis with abundant mucopurulent exudate. In children and adults an acute follicular conjunctivitis with pre-auricular lymphadenopathy, often with superficial corneal involvement. In the newborn the acute stage usually subsides spontaneously in a few weeks but the disease may persist for as long as a year. In adults there may also be a chronic phase with minimal exudate and symptoms which sometimes persist for a year or longer. The agent infects the urethral epithelium in men and the cervix in women and is sometimes associated with a mild urethritis or cervicitis. Specific treatment results in rapid recovery.

Laboratory confirmation is made by the demonstration of typical intra-cytoplasmic inclusion bodies in the epithelial cells of Giemsa stained conjunctival or genital scrapings, by specific immuno-fluorescent staining or by isolation of the agent in chick embryo yolk sac or cell culture.

Neonatal inclusion conjunctivitis is distinguished clinically from more serious gonococcal ophthalmia neonatorum (see p. 135) by the latter's shorter incubation period (3 days).

2. **Occurrence** — Sporadic eye cases are reported throughout the world in sexually active adults and their newborn offspring. Small epidemics are reported in North America, Europe and Japan.

3. **Infectious agent** — *Chlamydia (Bedsonia) trachomatis* which includes several antigenic types (TRIC agents).

4. **Reservoir** — Man.

5. **Mode of transmission** — The agent is transmitted during sexual intercourse; the genital discharges of infected persons are infectious. Eye infection in the newborn is by direct contact with infected birth passages. Adults become infected by the trans-mission of genital secretions to the eye, usually by the fingers. Out-breaks have been reported in non-chlorinated swimming pools pre-sumably contaminated with genito-urinary exudates. Eye-to-eye transmission may occur rarely.

6. **Incubation period** — 5 to 12 days.

7. **Period of communicability** — While genital infection persists; this can be longer than 10 months in the female.

8. **Susceptibility and resistance** — There is no evidence of resistance to re-infection with the inclusion conjunctivitis agent although the severity of the disease may be decreased. No racial immunity has been shown.

9. **Methods of control** —

A. *Preventive measures:* Difficult to apply in view of the inapparent nature of genital infections. General preventive measures are those for the venereal diseases (Syphilis 9A, p. 316). Instillation of silver nitrate or penicillin into the eye soon after birth does not prevent neonatal infection.

B. *Control of patient, contacts, and the immediate environment:*
1) *Report to local health authority:* Case report of neonatal cases obligatory in most states and many countries, Class 2B, (see Preface).
2) *Isolation:* For the first 48 hours after commencing treat-ment.
3) *Concurrent disinfection:* Aseptic techniques and hand washing by personnel appear to be adequate to prevent nursery transmission.

    4) Quarantine: None.

    5) Immunization of contacts: Not applicable.

    6) Investigation of contacts: All sexual consorts of adult cases and of mothers of neonatally infected infants should be examined and treated. Since infection is common in sexually promiscuous adults, all contacts should be investigated for gonorrhea and syphilis at the same time.

    7) Specific treatment: For both ocular and genital infections the tetracyclines or erythromycin are effective, given by mouth in full doses for 3 to 5 weeks. Oral sulfonamides are also effective but carry a high risk of untoward reactions. Local application of chemotherapeutic agents to the eye is relatively ineffective in adults. Treatment of choice for neonatal infection is topical tetracycline ointment; alternately sulfacetamide drops.

C. Epidemic measures: Sanitary control of swimming pools; ordinary chlorination suffices. Individuals contaminating swimming pools are difficult to trace.

D. International measures: WHO Collaborating Centres (see Preface).

CRYPTOCOCCOSIS
(Torulosis, European blastomycosis, Busse-Buschke's disease)

1. Identification — A mycosis usually presenting as a subacute or chronic meningoencephalitis. Infection of lung, kidney, prostate, bone or liver occurs, often with few local symptoms. Skin may show acneiform lesions, ulcers or subcutaneous tumor-like masses. Occasionally, *Cryptococcus neoformans* seems to be an endobronchial saprophyte in patients with lung disease of other origin.

Diagnosis of cryptococcal meningitis is aided by microscopic examination of spinal fluid mixed with India ink. Urine or pus also may contain encapsulated budding forms. Serologic tests for antigen in serum and cerebrospinal fluid are sometimes helpful. Diagnosis is confirmed by culture or histopathology. Media containing cycloheximide inhibit *C. neoformans* and should not be used.

2. **Occurrence**—Sporadic cases occur in all parts of the world. All races are susceptible; males are infected twice as frequently as females, mainly adults. Infection also occurs in cats, dogs, horses, cows, monkeys and other animals.

3. **Infectious agent**—*Cryptococcus neoformans.*

4. **Reservoir**—Saprophytic growth in the external environment. The infectious agent can be isolated consistently from old pigeon nests and pigeon droppings and from soil in many parts of the world.

5. **Mode of transmission**—Presumably by inhalation.

6. **Incubation period**—Unknown. Pulmonary disease may precede brain infection by months or years.

7. **Period of communicability**—Not directly transmitted from man to man.

8. **Susceptibility and resistance**—The frequency of *C. neoformans* in the external environment and the infrequency of disease suggest that man has an appreciable resistance. Susceptibility is increased during adrenal corticosteroid therapy and in disorders of the reticuloendothelial system, particularly Hodgkin's disease.

9. **Methods of control**—

   A. *Preventive measures:* Educate public as to danger of exposure to accumulations of pigeon droppings.

   B. *Control of patient, contacts, and the immediate environment:*
      1) *Report to local health authority:* Official report ordinarily not justifiable, Class 5 (see Preface).
      2) *Isolation:* None.
      3) *Concurrent disinfection:* Of discharges and contaminated dressings. Terminal cleaning.
      4) *Quarantine:* None.
      5) *Immunization of contacts:* None.
      6) *Investigation of contacts and source of infection:* Investigate exposure to accumulations of pigeon droppings, especially on window ledges, in aviaries, roosts and nests.
      7) *Specific treatment:* Amphotericin B (Fungizone) given intravenously is effective in many cases; 5-fluorocytosine is less effective alone, but may be efficacious in combination with amphotericin B.

   C. *Epidemic measures:* None.

   D. *International measures:* None.

CYTOMEGALICINCLUSION DISEASE

1. **Identification** — Symptomatic disease is a rare consequence of this common infection. Its most severe form occurs in the perinatal period following congenital infection. The neonate may exhibit signs and symptoms of severe generalized infection, especially involving the central nervous system and liver; lethargy, convulsions, jaundice, petechiae and purpura, hepatosplenomegaly, chorioretinitis, intracerebral calcification, and pulmonary infiltrates occur in varying degrees. Survivors may exhibit mental retardation, microcephaly, motor disabilities, hearing loss, and evidence of chronic liver disease. Death may occur *in utero;* neonatal case fatality is high for severely affected infants, but most congenital infections (approximately 1.0% of births) are inapparent.

Infection acquired later in life is generally inapparent, but may cause a mononucleosis-like syndrome distinguishable from infectious mononucleosis only by the absence of heterophile antibodies and a lower frequency of lymphadenopathy and tonsillo-pharyngitis. This may occur spontaneously, most commonly in young adults and cause up to 10% of all cases of "mononucleosis" seen among university students. A similar syndrome may follow blood transfusion, although many post-transfusion infections are clinically inapparent. Disseminated infection with pneumonitis and hepatitis may follow a primary infection or reactivation of a latent infection in immunodeficient patients.

The presence of infection is established by isolation of the virus from urine, saliva, cervical secretions, semen, breast milk, or tissue in human fibroblast cell cultures, by demonstration of typical "cytomegalic" cells in sediments of body fluids or in organs, and by demonstration of a significant rise in titer of serum antibody.

2. **Occurrence** — Infection occurs throughout the world. The prevalence of serum antibody differs between countries, varying from 40% in highly developed areas to 100% in developing countries, is similar in arctic areas and tropical regions, is inversely related to socioeconomic status within the United States, and is higher in women than in men (possibly related to pregnancy).

3. **Infectious agent** — Cytomegalovirus, a member of the herpesvirus family; includes several antigenically related strains.

4. **Reservoir** — Man is the only known reservoir. Cytomegaloviruses not infectious for man are found in many animal species.

5. **Mode of transmission** — Not completely known. Virus is excreted in urine, saliva, and may be found in cervical secretions

(more frequently as pregnancy progresses), breast milk, and semen. The fetus may acquire infection *in utero;* fetal infection occurs most commonly during a mother's primary infection, but may occasionally develop even when maternal antibody existed prior to conception. Postnatal infection occurs more commonly in infants born of mothers shedding cytomegalovirus in cervical secretions at delivery; thus transmission of the virus from the infected cervix at delivery is a major route of infection in early life. Viremia may be present in asymptomatic persons and the virus may be transmitted by blood transfusion, probably associated with leukocytes.

6. **Incubation period**—Information is incomplete. Illness following transfusion with infected blood begins 4-8 weeks following the transfusion; infections acquired during birth are first demonstrable 3-12 weeks after delivery.

7. **Period of communicability**—Virus is excreted in urine or saliva for many months and may persist for several years following primary infection. Adults appear to excrete virus for shorter periods, despite the persistence of latent infection. Excretion recurs with immunodeficiency and cervical excretion recurs during pregnancy.

8. **Susceptibility and resistance**—Infection is nearly universal. Fetuses, patients with debilitating diseases, or those on immunosuppressive drugs are more susceptible to overt disease.

9. **Methods of control** —

   A. *Preventive measures:* Unknown

   B. *Control of patient, contacts, and the immediate environment:*
      1) *Report to local health authority:* Official report not ordinarily justifiable, Class 5 (see Preface).
      2) *Isolation:* None. Patients known to be excreting virus should be isolated while in the hospital; persons with no antibodies and pregnant women should not care for them.
      3) *Concurrent disinfection:* Discharges from hospitalized patients and articles soiled therewith.
      4) *Quarantine:* None.
      5) *Immunization of contacts:* None available.
      6) *Investigation of contacts and source of infection:* None.
      7) *Specific treatment:* None.

   C. *Epidemic measures:* None.

   D. *International measures:* None.

DERMATOPHYTOSIS

(Ringworm; Dermatomycosis, Tinea, Epidermophytosis, Trichophytosis, Microsporosis)

Ringworm is a general term applied to mycotic disease of keratinized areas of the body (hair, skin and nails). Various genera and species of fungi known collectively as the dermatophytes are causative agents. The dermatomycoses are subdivided according to sites of infection.

A. RINGWORM OF THE SCALP

(Tinea capitis)

1. **Identification**—Begins as a small papule and spreads peripherally, leaving scaly patches of temporary baldness. Infected hairs become brittle and break off easily. Occasionally boggy, raised and suppurative lesions develop, called kerions. Examination of the scalp under ultraviolet light (Wood's filter) for yellow-green fluorescence is helpful in diagnosing tinea capitis caused by *Microsporum canis* and *M. audouinii. Trichophyton* species do not fluoresce.

Favus of the scalp is a variety of tinea capitis caused by *Trichophyton schoenleinii;* it is characterized by a mousy odor and by formation of small, yellowish cup-like crusts (scutulae) giving the appearance of being stuck on the scalp. Affected hairs do not break off but become gray and lusterless and eventually fall out and leave baldness which may be permanent.

Microscopic examination of scales and hair in 10% potassium hydroxide reveals characteristic arthrospores. The fungus should be cultured for confirmation of the diagnosis.

Tinea capitis is easily distinguished from piedra, a fungus infection of the hair occurring in South America and some countries of Southeast Asia. Piedra is characterized by black, hard "gritty" or white, soft pasty nodules on the hair shafts, caused by *Piedraia hortai* and *T. brigelii* respectively.

2. **Occurrence**—Tinea capitis caused by *M. audouinii* is widespread in the U.S.A., particularly in urban areas. *M. canis* infection occurs in both rural and urban areas wherever infected cats and dogs are present and is the primary causative agent in Australia. *T. mentagrophytes* and *T. verrucosum* infections occur in rural areas where the disease exists in cattle, horses, rodents and wild animals. *T. tonsurans* infections are epidemic in urban areas in southern and eastern U.S.A., Puerto Rico and Mexico.

3. **Infectious agents**—Various species of *Microsporum* and

Trichophyton. Identification of genus and species is important epidemiologically and to determine prognosis.

4. **Reservoir** — Principal reservoir of *M. audouinii, T. schoeleinii* and *T. tonsurans* is man; animals, especially dogs, cats and cattle, harbor the other organisms noted above.

5. **Mode of transmission** — Direct or indirect contact, especially with the backs of theater seats, barber clippers, toilet articles or clothing contaminated with hair from man or infected animals.

6. **Incubation period** — 10 to 14 days.

7. **Period of communicability** — As long as lesions are present and viable spores persist on contaminated materials.

8. **Susceptibility and resistance** — Children before the age of puberty are highly susceptible to *M. audouinii* and *M. canis;* all ages are subject to *Trichophyton* infections. Reinfections are seldom if ever reported.

9. **Methods of Control** —

A. *Preventive measures:*

1) In the presence of epidemics or in hyperendemic areas, heads of young children should be surveyed by ultra-violet light (Wood's filter) before entering school. Also search for spotty alopecia and well-circumscribed lesions, especially in children with unkempt hair.

2) Education of the public, especially parents, as to the danger of acquiring infection from infected children as well as from dogs, cats, and other animals.

B. *Control of patient, contacts, and the immediate environment:*

1) *Report to local health authority:* Obligatory report of epidemics; no individual case report, Class 4 (see Preface). Outbreaks in schools should be reported to school authorities.

2) *Isolation:* Impractical.

3) *Concurrent disinfection:* In mild cases, daily washing of the scalp removes loose hair. In severe cases wash scalp daily and cover hair with a cap. Contaminated caps should be boiled after use.

4) *Quarantine:* Not practical.

5) *Immunization of contacts:* None.

6) *Investigation of contacts and source of infection:* Study household contacts, and pets and farm animals for evidence of infection; treat if infected. Some animals, especially cats, may be inapparent carriers.

7) *Specific treatment:* Griseofulvin by mouth is treatment

of choice for many. Topical antifungal medications such as Whitfield's ointment may be used concurrently. Systemic antibacterial agents are useful in the treatment of secondarily infected lesions (kerions), together with use of a keratolytic cream and a cotton cover for the scalp. Examine weekly and take cultures; when negative complete recovery may be assumed.

C. *Epidemic measures:* In epidemics in schools or other institutions educate children and parents as to mode of spread, prevention and personal hygiene; enlist services of physicians and nurses for diagnosis; carry out follow-up surveys.

D. *International measures:* None.

B. RINGWORM OF THE BODY
(Tinea corporis)

1. **Identification**—An infectious disease of the skin other than of the scalp, bearded areas, and feet, characteristically appearing as flat, spreading ring-shaped lesions. The periphery is usually reddish, vesicular or pustular, and may be dry and scaly or moist and crusted. As the lesion progresses peripherally, the central area often clears, leaving apparently normal skin. Differentiation from inguinal candidiasis is necessary, since treatment differs.

Presumptive diagnosis is made by taking scrapings from the advancing lesion margins, clearing in 10% potassium hydroxide and examining microscopically for segmented, branched filaments of fungus. Final identification is by culture.

2. **Occurrence**—Worldwide and relatively frequent. Males are infected more often than females. All ages are susceptible; racial differences are minimal.

3. **Infectious agents**—Various species of *Microsporum* and *Trichophyton;* also *Epidermophyton floccosum.*

4. **Reservoir**—Man and animals.

5. **Mode of transmission**—Direct or indirect contact with skin and scalp lesions of infected persons, lesions of animals, contaminated floors, shower stalls, benches and similar articles.

6. **Incubation period**—4 to 10 days.

7. **Period of communicability**—As long as lesions are present and viable spores persist on contaminated materials.

8. **Susceptibility and resistance**—Susceptibility is widespread. Clinical manifestations are commonly exaggerated under conditions

of friction and excessive perspiration, as in axillary and inguinal regions, and when environmental temperatures and humidity are high.

9. **Methods of Control** —

    A. Preventive measures: Proper laundering (with sterilization) of towels and clothing; general cleanliness in showers and dressing rooms of gymnasiums, especially repeated washing of benches. A fungicidal agent such as cresol should be used for disinfecting benches and floors. Frequent hosing down and rapid draining of shower rooms.

    B. Control of patient, contacts, and the immediate environment:

        1) Report to local health authority: Obligatory report of epidemics; no individual case report, Class 4 (see Preface). Report infections of school children to school authority.

        2) Isolation: Infected children should be excluded from gymnasiums, swimming pools and activities likely to lead to exposure of others.

        3) Concurrent disinfection: Effective and frequent laundering of clothing.

        4) Quarantine: None.

        5) Immunization of contacts: None.

        6) Investigation of contacts and source of infection: Examination of school and household contacts and of household pets and farm animals; treat infections as indicated.

        7) Specific treatment: Griseofulvin by mouth; thorough bathing with soap and water, removal of scabs and crusts, and application of an effective topical fungicide.

    C. Epidemic measures: Education of children and of parents concerning the nature of the infection, its mode of spread and the necessity of maintaining good personal hygiene.

    D. International measures: None.

C. RINGWORM OF THE FOOT
(Tinea pedis, Athlete's foot)

1. **Identification** — Scaling or cracking of the skin, especially between the toes, or blisters containing a thin watery fluid are characteristic; most laymen recognize it as "athlete's foot." In severe cases, vesicular lesions appear on various parts of the body, especially the hands; these dermatophytids do not contain the fungus but are an allergic reaction to fungus products.

Diagnosis is verified by microscopic examination of potassium hydroxide-treated scrapings from lesions between the toes which reveal segmented branching filaments. Clinical appearances of lesions are not diagnostic.

2. Occurrence—Worldwide; a common disease. Adults more often affected than children; males more than females. No differences in racial susceptibility. Infections are more frequent in hot weather.

3. Infectious agents—*Trichophyton rubrum, T. mentagrophytes, Microsporum* species and rarely, *Epidermaphyton floccosum.*

4. Reservoir—Man.

5. Mode of transmission—Direct or indirect contact with skin lesions of infected persons or contaminated floors, shower stalls and other articles used by infected persons.

6. Incubation period—Unknown.

7. Period of communicability—As long as lesions are present and viable spores persist on contaminated materials.

8. Susceptibility and resistance—Susceptibility is variable and infection may be inapparent. Secondary attacks are frequent.

9. Methods of control—

    A. Preventive measures: Those for tinea corporis above. Education of the public on maintenance of strict personal hygiene; special care in drying areas between toes after bathing. Regular use of a dusting powder containing an effective fungicide on the feet and particularly between the toes.

    B. Control of patient, contacts, and the immediate environment:
        1) Report to local health authority: Official report not ordinarily justifiable, Class 5 (see Preface). Report high incidence in schools to school authorities.
        2) Isolation: None.
        3) Concurrent disinfection: Boil socks of heavily infected individuals to prevent reinfection. Place shoes in a box and subject to formaldehyde vapor for several hours; follow by airing to prevent irritation of skin from residual formalin.
        4) Quarantine: None.
        5) Immunization of contacts: None.
        6) Investigation of contacts and source of infection: None.
        7) Specific treatment: Topical fungicides. Expose feet to air by wearing sandals; use dusting powders. Griseoful-

vin by mouth may be indicated in severe, protracted disease.

C. *Epidemic measures:* Thorough cleaning and washing down floors of gymnasiums, showers and similar sources of infection. Education of the public concerning the mode of spread.

D. *International measures:* None.

D. RINGWORM OF THE NAILS
(Tinea unguium)

1. **Identification**— A chronic infectious disease involving one or more nails of the hands or feet. The nail gradually thickens, becomes discolored and brittle, and an accumulation of caseous-appearing material forms beneath the nail, or the nail becomes chalky and disintegrates.

Diagnosis by microscopic examination of potassium hydroxide preparations of the nail and of detritus beneath the nail should be confirmed by culture.

2. **Occurrence**— Common.

3. **Infectious agents**— Various species of *Trichophyton;* also *Epidermophyton floccosum,* and *Candida albicans.*

4. **Reservoir**— Man.

5. **Mode of transmission**— Presumably by direct extension from skin or nail lesions of infected persons, possibly from contaminated floors and shower stalls. Usually no transmission, even to close family associates.

6. **Incubation period**— Unknown.

7. **Period of communicability**— Possibly as long as an infected lesion is present.

8. **Susceptibility and resistance**— Injury to nail predisposes to infection. Reinfection is frequent.

9. **Methods of control**—

A. *Preventive measures:* Those for tinea corporis.

B. *Control of patient, contacts, and the immediate environment:*
   1) *Report to local health authority:* Official report not ordinarily justifiable, Class 5 (see Preface).
   2), 3), 4), 5), and 6): See Section C, above (Tinea pedis).
   7) *Specific treatment:* Griseofulvin by mouth is the treat-

ment of choice; should be given until nails grow out (about 6 months for fingernails, 18 for toenails).

C. *Epidemic measures:* Not applicable.

D. *International measures:* None.

∞

DIARRHEA, ACUTE UNDIFFERENTIATED

Acute diarrheal disease, an ubiquitous clinical syndrome of diverse and frequently unidentifiable etiology, presents with loose stools and often fever as the most common manifestations. While it may include specific infectious diseases such as cholera, shigellosis, salmonellosis, amebiasis, enteropathogenic *Escherichia coli* infections, or acute viral gastroenteritis (q.v.), it also may be caused by other viruses or helminths or protozoa. A variety of other organisms of low pathogenicity also may be etiologically associated when present in large numbers, especially if there are modifying conditions such as poor nutrition, metabolic abnormalities, concurrent disease, or unaccustomed environmental stresses. Abnormally frequent and liquid stools often result from chemical, nutritional, metabolic or psychogenic stimuli.

Recognition of specific entities may rest entirely upon clinical and epidemiological grounds because of the difficulty in identifying specific infectious agents, especially in developing areas where undifferentiated diarrheal disease is most prevalent, where multiple infections and concurrent disease are more common, and where facilities for clinical and laboratory differentiation are limited. Identification of the causative infectious agent(s) should be attempted whenever possible. Within the group of the undifferentiated diarrheas two entities require brief elaboration; they are (1) the diarrhea of early childhood (weanling diarrhea) of developing countries, and (2) traveler's diarrhea or "turista."

Diarrhea of Early Childhood

Diarrhea of early childhood is characterized by acute onset, frequent liquid or semi-liquid stools and rapid progression. Approximately one-third of cases have blood and/or mucus in the stools and pus may be present; fever is absent or low and there may be malaise, toxemia, intestinal cramps and tenesmus. Usually after an acute clinical course of four to five days, a low grade indisposition, accompanied by irregular loose stools, a deteriorating nutritional state, and occasional recurrent acute episodes frequently follow for 1-3 months. Affects children before and after weaning, but is most prevalent after weaning, usually around four to thirty months of age; common in areas of poor sanitation and prevailing malnutrition. Protein-calorie malnutrition is commonly associated and acute diarrheal episodes may precipitate kwashiorkor. The case fatality rate in the first two years of life is 1 to 5%. In developing areas the incidence may be as high as 115 cases per 100 children per year for breast fed infants under 5 months of age; by weanling age may reach 275 attacks per 100 children per year. Mortality rates of over 50 per 1000 per year may be observed in pre-school children. Highest incidence tends to parallel hot, dry periods. A specific pathogenic agent is infrequently recovered; in some localities infections with *Shigella*, enteropathogenic *E. coli*, *Salmonella*, *Entamoeba histolytica*, *Giardia lamblia*, other parasites or viruses are found in 10-40% of cases, either alone or as mixed infections, without necessarily being the cause of the diarrhea. Control includes provision of a nutritious diet, both as a supplement to breast feeding and after weaning, and improvement of personal hygiene and environmental and food sanitation. Cases are treated by correction of fluid and electrolyte abnormalities and nutritional deficiencies; antibiotics are of questionable value.

Traveler's Diarrhea (Turista)

Traveler's diarrhea is a clinical syndrome common among newly arrived or departing travelers, especially in tropical areas, and is characterized by diarrhea, often accompanied by abdominal pain, nausea and vomiting, and sometimes fever. It lasts 1-3 days and occasionally longer; thought to be infectious. Viral agents such as those isolated in winter-vomiting disease (see Gastroenteritis, Acute Viral) or pathogenic or enterotoxic strains of *Escherichia coli* may be important etiologically. The disease primarily affects adults sporadically, but families or groups of travelers of all ages may be affected in apparent common source outbreaks, which may originate from infections acquired in transit. Despite the popularity of a variety of commonly used medicines and nonmedicinal precautions employed prophylactically as well as therapeutically, there is no convincing evidence that the syndrome can be either prevented or treated effectively. With good reason, some have seriously questioned the role of antibiotics, and of drugs which inhibit intestinal motility, such as paregoric, for either prevention or treatment. Symptomatic treatment should include the liberal use of safe, clear fluids and juices to prevent dehydration and electrolyte disturbances, especially in the aged, in infants, and in those with underlying diseases. Kaolin or bismuth preparations may be helpful.

∞

DIARRHEA, ENTEROPATHOGENIC *ESCHERICHIA COLI*

1. **Identification:** Enteropathogenic *Escherichia coli* are of 2 types, invasive and enterotoxic (toxin producing). Invasive strains behave much like shigella in causing disease primarily localized in the colon, and manifested by fever and mucoid and occasionally bloody diarrhea; pathologic changes in the colon resemble those seen with shigellosis. On the other hand, enterotoxic strains behave more like cholera in producing a profuse watery diarrhea without blood or mucus; abdominal cramping, acidosis, prostration, and dehydration are common; fever may or may not be present; few if any histopathologic changes occur. Both invasive and enterotoxic strains may cause epidemic and sporadic disease; newborns are most susceptible and fatality rates may range from 0 to 40%; older children and adults may also be affected.

Specific diagnosis is by isolation of pathogenic strains of *E. coli* from stools of affected persons. Invasiveness can be demonstrated by the development of keratoconjunctivitis after instillation in the guinea pig eye (Sereny test); toxigenicity may be demonstrated by an assay system for enterotoxin. Serotypes which have been frequently associated with infantile diarrhea in the past can be identified serologically with commercially available antisera; however, these strains are not always pathogenic and may be found in healthy persons.

2. **Occurrence**—Outbreaks occur in nurseries and institutions and as food or waterborne outbreaks in the community. In areas with poor sanitation endemic diarrhea may be due to pathogenic *E. coli*, especially in persons under 2 years of age. Some cases of "traveler's diarrhea" (turista) (see p. 97) may be due to *E. coli*.

3. **Infectious agents**—Several serogroups are more commonly encountered in association with diarrheal illness, e.g., 026:B6, 055:B5,

086:B7, 0111:B4, 0112:B11, 0119:B14, 0124:B17, 0125:B15, 0126:B16, 0127:B8, 0128:B12, and 0142:K86. However, pathogenicity is not always established by serotyping; tests for toxigenicity or invasiveness may be necessary, especially in sporadic cases.

4. **Reservoir** — Infected persons; often may be asymptomatic.

5. **Mode of transmission** — Fecal contamination of food, water or fomites. Spread from mother to infant may occur during delivery, or by the fecal-oral route, or by fomites such as weighing scales or tables. Infants with diarrhea are particularly infectious because they excrete extraordinarily large numbers of organisms. Uninfected hospital personnel whose hands are contaminated following care of colonized infants may transmit organisms to other infants. Poor handwashing after patient contact, faulty personal toilet hygiene of adult carriers, and poor environmental sanitation contribute to perpetuation of epidemics. Airborne (dust) transmission may occur, but its relative importance has not been established.

6. **Incubation period** — 12-72 hours.

7. **Period of communicability** — Not known; presumably for the duration of fecal colonization, which may be a month or longer.

8. **Susceptiblity and resistance** — Infants are most susceptible, particularly prematures. Breast-feeding may confer some protection. Immunity to enterotoxin has been demonstrated but its duration is unknown.

9. **Methods of control** —

   A. *Preventive Measures:*
      1) For general measures for prevention of disease by fecal-oral spread, see Typhoid Fever 9A (p. 351).
      2) Prevention of hospital nursery outbreaks depends primarily on adequate handwashing practices, a scrupulously clean nursery and proper culturing and isolation of patients with diarrhea.
         a) Prepare feeding formulas aseptically; bottle, apply nipple, cover with a cap, sterilize, and refrigerate with nipple and caps on bottles until feeding time. Evaluate sterility by periodic bacteriological sampling of locally prepared formulas; sampling commercially prepared formulae is not necessary except in epidemiologic investigations.
         b) Provide a nursery for the newborn and premature infants not connecting directly with other nurseries, and with separate isolation facilities for those ill or suspect. Provide each infant with individual equip-

ment kept at the bassinet; use no common bathing or dressing tables and no bassinet stands for holding or transporting more than one infant at a time.

c) Keep no normal newborn infant in the same nursery with sick infants or older children. Admit to the nursery no infant born outside the hospital or to a mother with diarrheal or respiratory illness until after quarantine for at least six days, preferably after bacteriological examination of stools. Control visitors to minimize spread of infection. Monitor laundry procedures to assure absence of pathogens from the finished product as returned to the nursery.

d) Keep systematic daily record for each infant of number and consistency of stools.

e) Spread of disease (even in the absence of an outbreak) can be limited by the practice of keeping in one area the entire cohort of infants born during one time period. They should not be mixed with infants of other cohorts from birth to the time of discharge. Personnel should not care for infants from more than one cohort.

B. *Control of patient, contacts, and the immediate environment:*

1) *Report to local health authority:* Obligatory report of epidemics; no individual case report, Class 4 (see Preface). Two or more concurrent cases in a nursery are to be interpreted as an epdiemic.

2) *Isolation:* Of infected infants, also suspects.

3) *Concurrent disinfection:* Of all discharges and articles soiled therewith. Thorough terminal cleaning.

4) *Quarantine:* Use of isolation and cohort methods. (9A2e above.)

5) *Immunization of contacts:* None.

6) *Investigation of contacts and source of infection:* (see 9C2 below).

7) *Specific treatment:* In the enterotoxic form of the disease fluid and electrolyte fluid therapy (oral or IV) may be the most important measure (see Par 9 B7, cholera p. 74). In cases of infant diarrhea, an oral, non absorbable antibiotic to which the strain is sensitive is usually indicated.

C. *Epidemic measures:* For nursery epidemics, the following—

1) Admit no more babies to the contaminated nursery; suspend maternity service unless a clean nursery is avail

able with separate personnel and facilities; promptly discharge infected infants when medically possible. For the babies exposed in the contaminated nursery, provide separate medical and nursing personnel skilled in the care of communicable disease. Observe contacts for at least two weeks after the last case leaves the nursery; promptly remove each new case to isolation. Maternity service may be resumed after discharge of all contact babies and mothers, and thorough cleaning and terminal disinfection. Put into practice recommendations of 9A above so far as feasible in the emergency.

2) Epidemiologic investigation:

a) Conduct an investigation into the distribution of cases by time, place, and person and exposure to risk factors to determine how transmission is occurring.

b) Assure adequate treatment of missed cases by follow-up examination of all infants discharged from hospital during the two weeks preceding first recognized case.

c) Examine mothers and maternity service personnel for early signs of illness.

d) Bacteriologic surveys of ill and well infants is an important means of defining high risk areas and discovering reservoirs; also finding the suspect serotype in higher frequency among ill persons than among well ones helps establish its pathogenicity.

e) Survey hospital for unsanitary conditions.

f) Investigation of preparation of feeding formulas.

g) Inquire into techniques of aseptic nursing of infants and changing diapers and other clothing. Chemoprophylaxis for contacts should be approached with caution but may have some value.

D. International measures: WHO Collaborating Centres (see Preface).

∞

DIPHTHERIA

1. Identification—An acute infectious disease of tonsils, pharynx, larynx or nose, occasionally of other mucous membranes or skin. Lesion is marked by a patch or patches of grayish membrane with a surrounding dull red inflammatory zone. The throat is moderately sore in faucial diphtheria, with cervical lymph nodes somewhat enlarged and tender; in severe cases, there is marked swelling and edema of the neck. Laryngeal diphtheria is serious in infants and young children, while nasal diphtheria is mild, often chronic and marked by one-sided nasal discharge and excoriations. Inapparent infections outnumber recognized cases. The lesions of cutaneous diphtheria are variable and may be indistinguishable from impetigo. Late effects of absorption of toxin include cranial and peripheral motor and sensory nerve palsies and myocarditis, often severe. Case fatality of 5 to 10% has changed little in 50 years.

Diagnosis is confirmed by bacteriologic examination of lesions. Failure to demonstrate the bacillus in suspected diphtheria is not a valid reason for withholding specific treatment.

Diphtheria should be suspected in differential diagnosis of bacterial and viral pharyngitis, Vincent's angina, infectious mononucleosis, syphilis, and candidiasis, especially following antibiotics. Administration of antibiotics for all sore throats, on the assumption that most are streptococcal, may delay diagnosis and therapy of diphtheria with fatal result.

2. **Occurrence** — A disease of colder months in temperate zones, primarily involving unimmunized children under 15 years of age; often found also among adults in population groups whose immunization was neglected. In the tropics infection is more often inapparent and cutaneous diphtheria is more common.

3. **Infectious agent** — *Corynebacterium diphtheriae.* Toxigenic strains cause severe and fatal cases.

4. **Reservoir** — Man.

5. **Mode of transmission** — Contact with a patient or carrier or rarely with articles soiled with discharges from lesions of infected persons. Raw milk has served as a vehicle.

6. **Incubation period** — Usually 2 to 5 days, occasionally longer.

7. **Period of communicability** — Variable, until virulent bacilli have disappeared from discharges and lesions; usually 2 weeks or less but seldom more than 4 weeks. Carriers may shed organisms for 6 months or more.

8. **Susceptibility and resistance** — Infants born of immune mothers are relatively immune; protection is passive and usually lost before the 6th month. Recovery from clinical attack is not always followed by lasting immunity. Immunity is often acquired through inapparent infection. Passive temporary immunity of from 15 days to 3 weeks follows administration of antitoxin; prolonged

active immunity can be induced by giving toxoid. Antitoxic immunity does not protect against infection of the mucous membranes and the carrier state.

9. Methods of control —

A. *Preventive measures:*

1) The only effective control is by active immunization with diphtheria toxoid on a population basis, including an adequate program to maintain immunity. When protection has been neglected in infancy, immunization should be started as soon as the opportunity arises. Alternative procedures are: (a) Multiple antigens — At 2 or 3 months of age, diphtheria toxoid combined with tetanus toxoid containing an aluminum adjuvant and pertussis vaccine (DTP); give 3 intramuscular injections of 0.5 ml each at intervals of at least 4 weeks and a fourth dose approximately one year after the 3rd injection. A booster dose of DTP should be given to children 3 through 6 years of age when they start kindergarten or elementary school. After 6 years of age (8 years in Australia) use Tetanus and Diphtheria Toxoids, (Adult Type) (Td), which contains only 2 Lf of diphtheria toxoid. For primary immunization it is given in two doses 4-6 weeks apart, followed by a reinforcing dose 1 year later. Booster doses of Td should be given every 10 years. (b) Single antigens — Only used when there is a definite contraindication to a component in the combined antigens. Primary immunization follows the same schedule; booster dose schedule as above.

2) Adults subject to unusual risk, such as physicians, teachers, nurses, other hospital personnel, and staff and patients of institutions for the mentally handicapped, should be immunized and should receive a booster dose every 10 years.

3) Educational measures to inform the public and particularly the parents of young children of the hazards of diphtheria and the necessity and advantages of active immunization.

B. *Control of patient, contacts and the immediate environment:*

1) *Report to local health authority* — Case report is obligatory in most states and countries. Class 2A (see Preface).

2) *Isolation* — Until 2 cultures, taken not less than 24 hours

apart, and not less than 24 hours after cessation of antimicrobial therapy, from throat and nose, fail to show diphtheria bacilli. Where culture is impractical, isolation may be ended after 14 days with a fair degree of safety.

3) *Concurrent disinfection* — Of all articles in contact with patient, and all articles soiled by discharges of patient. Terminal cleaning.

4) *Quarantine* — All intimate contacts should be placed under modified quarantine until nose and throat cultures are negative. All carriers should be treated (9B7 below). Adult contacts whose occupation involves handling of food or close association with children should be excluded from those occupations until bacteriological examination proves them not to be carriers.

5) *Immunization of contacts* — Contacts intimately exposed and not previously immunized with toxoid should be given the first dose of toxoid and an appropriate antibiotic if culture is positive. Daily examination by a physician is advised for older children and adults, with such further active immunization as may be indicated; persons previously immunized should have a booster dose of toxoid. Groups of older persons, as in institutions, barracks, or other congested quarters, may be given routine immunization with Td.

6) *Investigation of contacts* — Search for carriers and unreported and atypical cases among intimate contacts; restrict and treat.

7) *Specific treatment* — If diphtheria is suspected, antitoxin should be given without awaiting bacteriological confirmation. After completion of tests to rule out anaphylactic reactions, give a single dose of 20,000 to 100,000 units, depending upon the duration of symptoms, area of involvement and severity of the disease. Intramuscular administration usually suffices; in severe infections antitoxin, both intravenously and intramuscularly, may be indicated. Sulfonamides are of no value; both penicillin and erythromycin are effective and one should be used after cultures are taken, in conjunction with but not as a substitute for antitoxin.

If a carrier state is demonstrated, give 600,000 to 2,000,000 units of aqueous procaine penicillin intramuscularly daily for 10 days, or erythromycin 1.0 gm orally for 7 days. If antibiotic treatment fails, tonsillectomy may be performed but not before 3 months after onset of disease leading to the carrier state.

C. Epidemic measures

1) Immediate intensification of efforts to immunize the largest possible number of the population group involved, with emphasis on protection of infants and pre-school children. Sample immunization surveys define levels of immunity and set priorities for selected area immunization.

2) In areas with good health facilities, carry out a prompt field investigation of reported cases to verify diagnosis, determine subtype of *C. diphtheriae*, identify contacts, trace sources of infection and define population groups at special risk.

D. International measures — Active immunization of susceptible infants and young children traveling to or through countries where diphtheria is a common disease; a booster dose of toxoid for those previously inoculated.

DIPHYLLOBOTHRIASIS

(Broad or Fish tapeworm disease)

1. Identification — A nonfatal intestinal tapeworm disease of long duration. Symptoms commonly are trivial or absent. A few patients develop vitamin B-12 deficiency anemia; massive infections may be associated with toxic symptoms.

Diagnosis is confirmed by identification of eggs or proglottids (segments) of the worm in feces.

2. Occurrence — Endemic worldwide in temperate zones. Where eating raw or only partly cooked fish is popular, 1 to 3% of some populations are infected. Prevalence increases with age. Persons in U.S.A. become infected through eating uncooked, infected fish from midwestern or Canadian lakes.

3. Infectious agent — *Diphyllobothrium latum*, a cestode; also several other species.

4. Reservoir — Mainly an infected person discharging eggs in feces; other hosts include dogs, bears and other fish-eating mammals.

5. Mode of transmission—Man acquires the infection by eating raw or inadequately cooked fish. Larvae developing in the flesh of freshwater fish (pike, perch, burbots) infect definitive hosts, i.e. man or animals. Eggs from segments of worm are discharged into bodies of fresh water in which they mature, hatch, and produce infection in first intermediate hosts (copepods). Susceptible species of freshwater fish ingest infected copepods and become second intermediate hosts in which the worms transform into the plerocercoid stage which is infective for man.

6. Incubation period—From 3 to 6 weeks.

7. Period of communicability—Not directly transmitted from man to man. Man and other definitive hosts continue to disseminate eggs in the environment as long as worms remain in the intestine, sometimes for many years.

8. Susceptibility and resistance—Man is universally susceptible. No apparent resistance follows infection.

9. Methods of control—

　A. Preventive measures:
　　1) Thorough heating (56° C for 5 minutes) of freshwater fish or freezing for 24 hours at -10° C insures protection.

　B. Control of patient, contacts, and the immediate environment:
　　1) Report to local health authority: Official report not ordinarily justifiable, Class 5 (see Preface).
　　2) Isolation: None.
　　3) Concurrent disinfection: None; sanitary disposal of feces.
　　4) Quarantine: None.
　　5) Immunization of contacts: None.
　　6) Investigation of contacts: Not usually justified.
　　7) Specific treatment: Niclosamide (Yomesan), available from the Center for Disease Control, Atlanta, GA (see Preface), or quinacrine hydrochloride (Atabrine) are the drugs of choice.

　C. Epidemic measures: None.

　D. International measures: None.

ANISAKIASIS is a newly recognized disease of the gastrointestinal tract characterized by intestinal colic, fever and eosinophilic abscesses caused by ingestion of raw or inadequately cooked herring and other salt water fish containing the larval stages of a nematode (*Anisakis marina*). The exact life cycle of this parasite has not been fully worked out but probably involves sea mammals, with man as an incidental host. First reported in Holland during the mid-1950's after human ingestion of slightly salted raw herring. The distribution of anisakiasis may be worldwide; many cases are reported from Japan where the ingestion of fresh and raw salt water fish is common. The parasite, found in a variety of salt water fish, is rapidly destroyed by heat and is killed by freezing.

DRACONTIASIS
(Guinea worm disease, Dracunculiasis)

1. Identification — An infection of the subcutaneous and deeper tissues with a large nematode. A blister appears, usually on a lower extremity, especially the foot, as the gravid, meter-long female prepares to discharge the larvae. Burning and itching of the skin in the area of the lesion and frequently fever, nausea, vomiting, diarrhea, dyspnea, generalized urticaria, and eosinophilia may precede vesicle formation. When the vesicle ruptures the worm discharges larvae whenever the infected part is immersed in water. The prognosis is good unless there are multiple worms or unless a bacterial infection occurs which may produce severe crippling sequelae.

Diagnosis is by microscopic identification of larvae or recognition of the adult worm.

2. Occurrence — In India, Africa, Middle East, West Indies, and northeastern South America. Local prevalence varies greatly; in some localities nearly all inhabitants are infected, in others few, mainly young adults. Worms morphologically similar to *Dracunculus medinensis*, occur in dogs, mink, otter, foxes and raccoons in North America but no authentic indigenous case has been reported in man.

3. Infectious agent — *Dracunculus medinensis*, a nematode worm.

4. Reservoir — An infected person.

5. Mode of transmission — Larvae discharged into fresh water are swallowed by crustacea of the genus *Cyclops* and in about 2 weeks develop into the infective stage. Man swallows the infected copepods by drinking water from contaminated step-wells and ponds; larvae are liberated in the stomach or duodenum, migrate through the viscera, become adults, and reach the subcutaneous tissues.

6. **Incubation period**—About 12 months.

7. **Period of communicability**—Until larvae have been completely evacuated from the uterus of the gravid worm, usually 15 to 20 days. Larvae may survive in water up to 3 weeks. Not directly transmitted from man to man.

8. **Susceptibility and resistance**—Susceptibility is universal; no acquired immunity; multiple and repeated infections may occur in the same person.

9. **Methods of control**--

A. *Preventive measures:*

1) Provision of potable water. Abolition of step-wells and other measures to prevent contamination of drinking water by infected persons through immersion of affected parts.
2) Boiling of drinking water or filtration through fine mesh cloth to remove copepods.
3) Chemical treatment of water with chlorine or copper sulfate may destroy copepods.
4) Education of the public to drink only boiled or filtered water. Instruction of infected persons in mode of spread of the infection and the danger in contaminating wells or other water supplies.

B. *Control of patients, contacts, and the immediate environment:*

1) *Report to local health authority:* Official report not ordinarily justifiable, Class 5 (see Preface).
2) *Isolation:* None.
3) *Concurrent disinfection:* None.
4) *Quarantine:* None.
5) *Immunization of contacts:* None.
6) *Investigation of contacts and source of infection:* Obtain information as to source of drinking water at probable time of infection. Search for other cases.
7) *Specific treatment:* Metronidazole or niridazole or thiabendazole.

C. *Epidemic measures:* In hyperendemic situations, field survey to determine prevalence, to discover sources of infection and to guide control measures as described in 9A.

D. *International measures:* None.

ENTEROBIASIS
(Pinworm disease, Oxyuriasis)

1. **Identification**—Generally a benign intestinal disease with mild or nonspecific symptoms. If severe, it may cause anal itching with disturbed sleep, irritability, and local irritation due to scratching. A variety of severe manifestations including appendicitis, salpingitis and pelvic granuloma have been described, but these complications occur only rarely. Most infections are usually asymptomatic.

Diagnosis is by applying transparent adhesive tape to the perianal region and examining it microscopically for eggs; the material is best obtained in the morning before bathing or defecation.

2. **Occurrence**—Distribution is worldwide and infection rates are quite high in some areas. The most common helminth infection in the United States, it is variously estimated that 5-15% of the general population of the United States harbors the worm. Prevalence is highest in children of school age, next highest in those of preschool age, and lowest in adults except for mothers of infected children. Infection is usually familial. Crowding is an important factor; prevalence is often high in institutions and is lower in the tropics than in colder climates.

3. **Infectious agent**—*Enterobius vermicularis,* an intestinal round worm infecting only man.

4. **Reservoir**—Man. Pinworms of animal hosts are not transmissible to man.

5. **Mode of transmission**—Direct transfer of infective eggs by hand from anus to mouth of the same or new host, or indirectly through clothing, bedding, food, or other articles contaminated with eggs of the parasite. Dustborne infection by inhalation is possible in heavily contaminated households. Eggs are infective within a few hours after leaving the gastrointestinal tract; they survive only a few days. They hatch in the small intestine; young worms mature in the lower small intestine, cecum, and upper portions of the colon. Gravid worms migrate to the rectum to discharge eggs on perianal skin; may migrate up the genital tract of females and enter the peritoneal cavity. Retro-infection occurs when eggs hatch in the perianal region and the larvae migrate into the large intestine through the anus.

6. **Incubation period**—The life cycle requires 3 to 6 weeks. The worm burden ordinarily builds up from successive reinfections and may not be recognized for months.

7. Period of communicability—As long as gravid females are present in the intestine. Individual worms survive only about 2 months but reinfection from self or other infected members of the family or institution is usual.

8. Susceptibility and resistance—Susceptibility is universal. Differences in frequency and intensity of infection are due to differences in exposure or to an acquired resistance.

9. Methods of control—

A. Preventive measures:

1) Daily bathing, with showers preferred to tub baths.
2) Frequent change to clean underclothing, night clothes, and bed sheets, preferably after bathing.
3) Education in personal hygiene, particularly the washing of hands after defecation, and always before eating or preparing food; also to discourage habits of nail-biting and scratching bare anal area.
4) Reduction of overcrowding in living accommodations.
5) Adequate provision of toilets and privies with handwashing facilities; and maintenance of cleanliness in these facilities.
6) Removal of sources of infection by treatment of cases.

B. Control of patient, contacts, and the immediate environment:

1) Report to local health authority: Official report not ordinarily justifiable, Class 5 (see Preface). Advise school authorities of school outbreaks.
2) Isolation: None.
3) Concurrent disinfection: Sanitary disposal of feces. Change bed linen and underwear of infected person daily with care to avoid dispersing eggs into the air. Eggs on discarded linen are killed by exposure to temperatures of 55°C (132°F) for a few seconds; either boiling or use of a properly functioning household washing machine is therefore effective.
4) Quarantine: None.
5) Immunization of contacts: None.
6) Investigation of contacts: Examine all members of an affected family or institution.
7) Specific treatment: Pyrantel, pyrvinium pamoate (Povan), thiabendazole or piperazine citrate (Antepar). All infected members of a household or institution should be treated simultaneously.

C. Epidemic measures: Outbreaks in schools and institutions require strict hygienic measures and cleanliness. Toilet seats should be washed daily with disinfectants. Adequate treatment facilities should be provided.

D. International measures: None.

FASCIOLOPSIASIS

1. **Identification**—A trematode disease of the small intestine, particularly the duodenum. Symptoms result from local inflammation and ulceration of the intestinal wall, obstruction of the lumen and systemic toxic effects. Diarrhea usually alternates with constipation; vomiting and anorexia are frequent. Large numbers of worms may produce acute intestinal obstruction. Patients may show edema of the face, abdominal wall, and legs within 20 days after massive infection; ascites is common, eosinophilia is usual, secondary anemia is occasional, and death is rare.

Diagnosis is by finding the large flukes or characteristic eggs in feces; worms are occasionally vomited.

2. **Occurrence**—Widely distributed in the Orient, especially central and south China. Prevalence is often extremely high.

3. **Infectious agent**—*Fasciolopsis buski,* a large trematode or fluke.

4. **Reservoir**—Man, pig and dog are definitive hosts of adult flukes.

5. **Mode of transmission**—Eggs passed in feces develop in water within 3 to 7 weeks under favorable conditions; miracidia hatch, and penetrate planorbid snails as intermediate hosts; cercariae develop, are liberated and encyst on aquatic plants. Man becomes infected by eating these plants uncooked. In China the chief sources of infection are the nuts of the red water-caltrop grown in enclosed ponds, and tubers of the so-called "water chestnut"; infection frequently results when the hull or skin is peeled off with teeth and lips. Period of development from infection of snail to development of encysted infective metacercariae is 7 to 8 weeks.

6. **Incubation period**—About 7 weeks from ingestion of infective larvae. Eggs appear in the stool a month after infection (prepatent period).

7. Period of communicability—As long as viable eggs are discharged by patient; without treatment probably for many years. Not directly transmitted from man to man.

8. Susceptibility and resistance—Susceptibility is universal. In malnourished individuals the ill effects are pronounced; the number of worms influences severity of disease.

9. Methods of control—

A. *Preventive measures:*
1) Education of the public in endemic areas on the mode of transmission and life cycle of the parasite.
2) Drying of suspected plants, or if eaten fresh, dipping into boiling water for a few seconds; both methods kill metacercariae.

B. *Control of patient, contacts, and the immediate environment:*
1) *Report to local health authority:* In selected endemic areas; in most countries not a reportable disease, Class 3C (see Preface).
2) *Isolation:* None.
3) *Concurrent disinfection:* Sanitary disposal of feces.
4) *Quarantine:* None.
5) *Immunization of contacts:* None.
6) *Investigation of contacts and source of infection:* In the individual case, of little value. A community problem (see 9C below).
7) *Specific treatment:* Tetrachlorethylene or hexylresorcinol crystoids are effective.

C. *Epidemic measures:* Identify aquatic plants which are eaten fresh and harbor encysted metacercariae; identify infected snail species living in water with such plants; prevent contamination of water with human feces.

D. *International measures:* None.

FASCIOLIASIS in animals is caused by the fluke, *Fasciola hepatica,* which commonly infects the bile ducts of sheep, cattle and other ruminants throughout the world; hepatic infection has been reported in man in South America, the Caribbean area, Europe, and parts of the U.S.A.

FILARIASIS

(Wuchereriasis, Brugiasis)

1. Identification—

A. Bancroftian filariasis is an infection with the nematode worm *Wuchereria bancrofti;* man is the only vertebrate host. Early acute manifestations may include fever, lymphadenitis, lymphangitis of the extremities, orchitis, epididymitis, funiculitus and abscess. Prolonged and repeated infection with obstruction to lymph flow often leads to hydrocele or to elephantiasis of the limbs, genitalia or breasts, or to chyluria. Many infected persons show no clinical manifestations. Female worms give rise to embryos which, in the absence of lymphatic obstruction, reach the blood stream. Two forms occur: one form exhibits microfilariae in the peripheral blood at night (nocturnal periodicity) with greatest concentrations of larvae between 10:00 p.m. and 2:00 a.m. In the other form microfilariae are continuously present in the circulating blood (i.e., sub-periodic) although they often occur in greater concentration in the peripheral circulation in the daytime (diurnal sub-periodicity). The latter form is primarily endemic in the South Pacific, where the principal vectors are day-biting mosquitoes.

B. Malayan filariasis is caused by the nematode worm *Brugia malayi.* One nocturnally periodic form is transmitted by *Mansonia* mosquitoes, principally in rural populations throughout much of Asia. A nocturnally sub-periodic form, also transmitted by *Mansonia* species, occurs in a variety of wild and domestic animals, and is a true zoonosis in Malaysia. Clinical manifestations are similar to those of bancroftian filariasis, except that genital and inguinal lesions are less conspicuous.

Many perons with clinical manifestations do not have circulating microfilariae (occult filariasis). In some of these cases, infection is manifested by marked eosinophilia associated with pulmonary infiltrates (tropical eosinophilia or tropical pulmonary eosinophilia).

Microfilariae are best detected during optimum periods of microfilaremia, or after a provocative dose of diethylcarbamazine (in areas where there is no onchocerciasis or loiasis), by concentration techniques or, if not feasible, by direct examination of hemolyzed blood in a counting chamber or of stained thick blood films.

In its broadest connotation, filariasis means infection of humans with one of several species of filarial worms. In addition to *W. bancrofti* and *B. malayi*, these include *Onchocerca volvulus* and *Loa loa* which in man cause onchocerciasis and loiasis respectively (see pp. 216 and 182). Infection with *Dipetalonema perstans,* a worm parasite widely distributed in Africa, northern South America and some of the Caribbean Islands, is largely limited to the body cavities, especially the peritoneum and pleura, but is of doubtful pathogenicity. Symptoms occasionally have been attributed to its unsheathed microfilariae which appear in the peripheral blood, without a clear cycle of periodicity. *D. streptocerca* is apparently confined to the forested regions of West and Central Africa; the adult worm was only recently demonstrated in man; its microfilariae are found in the skin, the same as those of *Onchocerca* and it is suspected of causing cutaneous edema and elephantiasis. *Mansonella ozzardi* is limited to the New World, specifically from northern Argentina to the Yucatan and the West Indies. Adults live in the body cavities, but the unsheathed microfilariae they produce are found non-periodically in the peripheral blood. While generally asymptomatic and nonpathogenic, lymphadenopathy occasionally results from infection with *M. ozzardi. Culicoides* species are the vectors for both genera of worms; *Simulium* species have also been incriminated in the transmission of *M. ozzardi* in parts of Brazil. *Dirofilaria immitis* normally causes canine filariasis or heartworm in dogs of U.S.A. and subtropical and tropical areas. Rarely, when an infectious mosquito feeds on man, infective larvae gain entrance and develop into worms which though mature rarely produce microfilariae before they die. While often asymptomatic, coin lesions revealed by X-ray may be confused with other diseases. Biopsy reveals a worm in a pulmonary artery. Other species of *Dirofilaria,* commonly found in domestic or wild animals, e.g., *D. tenuis* which lives in the subcutaneous tissues of the raccoon, occasionally infect man but, like *D. immitis,* rarely produce microfilariae.

2. **Occurrence** — *Wuchereria bancrofti* is endemic in most of the warm regions of the world, including Latin America, Africa, Asia, and the Pacific Islands. *Brugia malayi* is endemic in Southeast Asia, India, Central China, South Korea, and all major islands of Indonesia, but no farther east than Ceram. Local foci of high prevalence are often surrounded by nonendemic areas. High prevalence depends upon a large reservoir of infection and abundant vector breeding; commonly a disease of heavily populated rural and urban areas with inadequate basic sanitation favoring vector breeding.

3. **Infectious agents** — *Wuchereria bancrofti* and *Brugia malayi,* nematode worms.

4. **Reservoir** — Man with microfilariae in the blood; in Malaysia occasionally other mammals infected with *B. malayi.*

5. **Mode of transmission** — By bite of a mosquito harboring infec-

tive larvae. *W. bancrofti* is transmitted in nature by many species, the most important being *Culex pipiens, C. fatigans, C. quinquefasciatus, Aedes polynesiensis, A. pseudoscutellaris,* and several species of *Anopheles,* some also vectors of malaria. *B. malayi* is transmitted by various species of *Mansonia, Anopheles,* and *Aedes.* Microfilariae, picked up by a mosquito while feeding on an infected person, penetrate the stomach wall of the mosquito, lodge in thoracic muscles, develop into infective larvae which migrate to the proboscis, and penetrate the new host as the mosquito bites.

6. Incubation period — While allergic inflammatory manifestations may appear as early as 3 months after infection, microfilariae do not appear in the blood until months later.

7. Period of communicability — Not directly transmitted from man to man. Man may infect mosquitoes as long as microfilariae are present in the blood. The mosquito is infective from about 10 days after a blood meal until all infective larvae are discharged.

8. Susceptibility and resistance — Universal susceptibility to infection, but considerable geographical differences in severity of lesions. Repeated infections apparently occur in endemic regions.

9. Methods of control —

   A. Preventive measures:
   1) Determine, by dissection, the vector or vectors; identify times and places of feeding and locate breeding places; if indoor night biters attack adults, spray buildings with an acceptable and effective residual insecticide, screen houses and use bed nets and insect repellents. Eliminate small breeding places such as old tires, coconut husks, etc. and treat others with biodegradable larvicides. Where *Mansonia* species are vectors, apply herbicides to plants which harbor their larvae.
   2) Education of the public concerning mode of transmission, and methods of mosquito control.

   B. Control of patient, contacts, and the immediate environment:
   1) *Report to local health authority:* In selected endemic regions; in most countries is not a reportable disease, Class 3C (see Preface). Reporting of cases with demonstrated microfilariae provides information on potential areas of transmission. Cases of elephantiasis without demonstrable microfilariae in the blood should not be reported as filariasis, but are usefully recorded in endemic

areas in estimating prevalence or in planning control
programs.

2) *Isolation:* Not practicable. So far as possible, patients
with microfilaremia should be protected from mos
quitoes to reduce transmission.

3) *Concurrent disinfection:* None.

4) *Quarantine:* None.

5) *Immunization of contacts:* None.

6) *Investigation of contacts and source of infection:* Only
as a part of a general community effort (see 9A and 9C).

7) *Specific treatment:* Diethylcarbamazine (Hetrazan
Banocide) results in rapid disapparence of most or al
microfilariae from the blood, but may not destroy the
adult female worm; microfilariae may again appear after
several months. Therefore, treatment must usually be
repeated at specified intervals. Low level microfilaremia
can only be detected by concentration techniques.

C. **Epidemic measures:** Vector control is the fundamenta
measure. In areas of high endemicity it is essential to ap
praise correctly the bionomics of mosquito vectors, preva
lence and incidence of disease, and environmental factors
responsible for transmission in each locality. Even partia
control by antimosquito measures may reduce incidence
and restrict the endemic focus. Measurable results are slow
because of the long incubation period. Mass treatment with
diethylcarbamazine (Hetrazan) often is an effective
measure.

D. **International measures:** None.
1) WHO Collaborating Centres (see Preface).

FOOD POISONING

Food poisoning is a generic term applied to illnesses acquired
through consumption of contaminated food or water. The term also
applies to intoxications caused by chemical contaminants (heavy
metals and others), toxins elaborated by bacterial growth
(staphylococci, botulinus), and a variety of organic substances that
may be present in natural foods such as certain mushrooms, mus
sels, eels, scombroid fish, and other seafood.

Acute salmonellosis is often classed with food poisoning, but since it is more an acute enteric infection than an intoxication it is presented elsewhere (p. 276). Food may also be the vehicle of transmission for many other infectious diseases. These include typhoid and paratyphoid fevers, shigellosis, streptococcal pharyngitis (septic sore throat), diphtheria, brucellosis, infectious hepatitis, amebiasis, cholera, and trichinosis and other helminthic infections. These, however, are not usually classified as forms of food poisoning. Epidemic nausea and vomiting of presumed viral origin can be confused with food poisoning.

Food-poisoning outbreaks are usually recognized by the sudden occurrence of illness within a short period of time among individuals who have consumed one or more foods in common. The diagnosis is generally indicated by epidemiologic findings. While single cases of food poisoning undoubtedly occur, they are difficult to identify unless, as in botulism, there is a distinctive clinical syndrome.

A. STAPHYLOCOCCAL FOOD POISONING

1. Identification—An intoxication (not an infection) of abrupt and sometimes violent onset, with severe nausea, cramps, vomiting, usually diarrhea, and prostration; sometimes with subnormal temperature and markedly lowered blood pressure. Deaths are rare; duration of illness is commonly not more than a day or two, but its intensity may result in surgical exploration in sporadic cases. Diagnosis is usually through recognition of a group of cases with the characteristic acute, predominantly upper gastrointestinal symptoms and the short interval between eating a common food item and the onset of symptoms.

Recovery of large numbers of enterotoxin-producing staphylococci on routine culture media from stomach contents, feces or a suspected food item supports the diagnosis. Phage typing and enterotoxin tests greatly aid epidemiologic investigation.

Differential diagnosis considers other recognized forms of food poisoning, and epidemic nausea, vomiting and diarrhea (winter vomiting disease).

2. Occurrence—Widespread and relatively frequent; one of the principal acute food poisonings in the U.S.A.

3. Toxic agent—Several enterotoxins of staphylococci are stable at boiling temperature. Staphylococci multiply in food, producing the toxin which causes poisoning.

4. Reservoir—Man in most instances; occasionally cows.

5. Mode of transmission—By ingestion of any of a wide variety of contaminated food products: pastries, custards, salads and salad dressings, sandwiches, sliced meats and meat products, in which toxin-producing staphylococci of human origin (from purulent discharges of an infected finger, infected eyes, abscesses, acneiform facial eruptions, nasal secretions, or the apparently normal skin of hands and forearms) or of bovine origin (contaminated milk or milk products) have multiplied in food allowed to stand for several hours before serving. Ham and bacon, pressed meat, milk from cows with infected udders, occasionally dried milk, cream, and butter, have been implicated in extensive outbreaks.

6. **Incubation period** — Interval between eating food and onset of symptoms is 1 to 6 hours, usually 2 to 4 hours.

7. **Period of communicability** — Not applicable.

8. **Susceptibility and resistance** — Most persons are susceptible, although individual reactions are variable.

9. **Methods of control** —

    A. Preventive measures:

        1) Prompt and thorough refrigeration of food (especially of sliced and chopped meats, custards and cream fillings) to avoid multiplication of staphylococci accidentally introduced. Immediate disposal or prompt refrigeration of left-over foods.

        2) Temporary exclusion from food handling of persons suffering from pyogenic skin, eye or respiratory infections.

        3) Education of food handlers in strict food protection, sanitation and cleanliness of kitchens, proper refrigeration, hand washing, cleaning of fingernails, and to the danger of working with a skin or eye infection.

    B. Control of patient, contacts, and the immediate environment:

        1) Report to local health authority: Report promptly. Obligatory report of epidemics of suspected or confirmed cases, Class 4 (see Preface).

        2), 3), 4), 5), 6), 7): Not pertinent. Control is of epidemics; single cases are rarely identified.

    C. Epidemic measures:

        1) By quick review of reported cases, determine time and place of exposure and the population at risk. A study of the prominent clinical features of the disease, coupled with an estimate of the incubation period, provides useful leads to the most probable etiological agent. Collect appropriate specimens of feces and vomitus for laboratory examination. Obtain a complete listing of the foods served. Interview an appropriate sample of the

patients and of those remaining well; in both groups identify those specific foods eaten and not eaten. Determine attack rates for each item of food. The rate for those eating the contaminated food will be higher than the rate for persons who did not eat the contaminated food.

2) Conduct a meticulous inquiry into the origin of the incriminated food and its manner of preparation and storage before serving. Look for possible sources of contamination and periods of inadequate refrigeration that would permit incubation of the etiological agent. Submit any remainder of the incriminated food for laboratory examination. Failure to isolate staphylococci does not exclude the presence of the heat-resistant enterotoxin.

3) Search for food handlers with skin infections, particularly of the hands. Culture all purulent lesions; culture nasal swabs of all food handlers. Antibiograms and phage-typing of representative strains of enterotoxin-producing staphylococci isolated from foods and food handlers and from vomitus or feces of patients are recommended.

D. *International measures:* WHO Collaborating Centres (see Preface).

B. CLOSTRIDIUM PERFRINGENS (C. welchii) FOOD POISONING

1. Identification—An intestinal disorder characterized by sudden onset of abdominal colic followed by diarrhea; nausea is common but vomiting is usually absent. Generally a mild disease of short duration, one day or less, and rarely fatal in healthy persons. Outbreaks of severe disease with a high fatality rate associated with a necrotizing enteritis have occurred in Germany and New Guinea.

Diagnosis is supported by semiquantitative bacteriological examination of food and patients' stools. Anaerobic techniques usually demonstrate the same serotype in both.

2. Occurrence—Widespread and relatively frequent in countries with cooking practices that favor multiplication of the *Clostridia*.

3. Infectious agent—Type A strains of *Clostridium perfringens (welchii)* cause typical food poisoning outbreaks; type C and F strains cause necrotizing enteritis.

4. Reservoir—Reservoir is soil, also the gastrointestinal tract of man and animals (cattle, pigs, poultry and vermin).

5. **Mode of transmission** — Ingestion of food contaminated by feces or soil in which conditions have permitted multiplication of the organism. Almost all outbreaks are associated with inadequately heated or reheated meats, usually stews, meat pies, or gravies made of beef, turkey or chicken. Spores survive normal cooking temperatures, germinate and multiply during cooling and rewarming. Outbreaks are usually traced to food catering firms, restaurants, cafeterias and schools which have inadequate cooking and refrigeration facilities for large-scale service. Heavy bacterial contamination is required for clinical disease.

6. **Incubation period** — From 8 to 22 hours, usually 10 to 12 hours.

7. **Period of communicability** — Not applicable.

8. **Susceptibility and resistance** — Most persons are probably susceptible. In volunteer studies, no resistance was observed to develop after repeated ingestion of filtrates or dead cells.

9. **Methods of control** —

   A. *Preventive measures:*
      1) Serve meat dishes hot, as soon as they are cooked, or cool them rapidly and refrigerate until serving time; reheating, if necessary, should be rapid. Do not partially cook meat and poultry one day and reheat the next. Stuffing or dressing placed inside fowl or meat cuts is frequently a source of food poisoning. Large cuts of meat should be adequately cooked; divide stews and similar dishes prepared in bulk into small lots for cooling and refrigeration.
      2) Educate food handlers in the risks inherent in large-scale cooking, especially of meat dishes.

   B. *Control of patient, contacts, and the immediate environment:* (See Staphylococcal Food Poisoning 9B1, p. 118).

   C. *Epidemic measures:* Identify contaminated food (See Staphylococcal Food Poisoning 9C1 and 2, pp. 118-119).

   D. *International measures:* None.

C. BOTULISM

1. **Identification** — A serious intoxication (not an infection) characterized by weakness, extreme dryness of the mouth, and oculomotor or other symmetrical motor cranial-nerve paralyses. Clinical manifestations relate primarily to the nervous system. Ptosis, visual difficulty (blurred or double vision), and sore throat are often the first complaints. Vomiting and diarrhea, occasionally

constipation, may be present initially. About one-third of patients die within 3 to 7 days, usually from respiratory failure or from superimposed infection.

Diagnosis is established by demonstration of the specific toxin in blood serum or stool or its presence in a suspected food item. Isolation of the organism from the suspected food or stool is helpful but not diagnostic.

2. Occurrence—Sporadic and family-grouped cases occur in most countries, always in relation to a food product so prepared or preserved as to permit toxin formation.

3. Toxic agent—Toxins produced by *Clostridium botulinum* (botulinus bacillus). Most outbreaks are due to type A, B, or E toxins of *C. botulinum*, a few to type F. Type E outbreaks are usually related to seafood, particularly fish. Toxin is produced in improperly processed foods, only under anaerobic conditions, and especially in low-acid foods. Toxin is destroyed by boiling; inactivation of spores requires higher temperatures. Ordinary refrigeration does not necessarily prevent toxin production.

4. Reservoir—Soil, water, and the intestinal tract of animals, including fish.

5. Mode of transmission—By ingestion of contaminated food, predominantly from jars or cans inadequately processed during canning and eaten without subsequent adequate cooking. Most poisonings in the U.S.A. are due to home-canned vegetables and fruits or to fish; meats are infrequent vehicles. In Europe, most cases are due to sausages and to smoked or preserved meats or fish. Cases of botulism secondary to wound infection have been reported.

6. Incubation period—Symptoms usually appear within 12 to 36 hours, sometimes several days after eating contaminated food. In general, the shorter the incubation period, the more severe the disease and the higher the case fatality rate.

7. Period of communicability—Not applicable.

8. Susceptibility and resistance—Susceptibility is general.

9. Methods of control—

    A. Preventive measures:

        1) Ensure effective control of processing and preparation of commercial canned and preserved foods.

        2) Education of housewives and others concerned with home canning and other processing of foods regarding the proper time, pressure and temperature required to destroy spores, and the need to boil home-canned vege-

tables at least 3 minutes with thorough stirring before serving.

3) While neither bulging cans nor a peculiar odor in commercially canned foods are indications of botulinum toxin, they do not exclude it; the contents of such cans should not be tasted but returned to the vendor.

B. *Control of patient, contacts, and the immediate environment:*

1) *Report to local health authority:* Case report of suspect and confirmed cases obligatory in most states and countries, Class 2A (see Preface); immediate telephone report indicated.

2) *Isolation:* None.

3) *Concurrent disinfection:* The contaminated food(s) should be sterilized before discarding or else buried deeply in soil. Contaminated utensils should be sterilized to inactivate any remaining toxin. Use of chlorine will assist in decontamination.

4) *Quarantine:* None.

5) *Management of contacts:* None for simple direct contacts. Those who are known to have eaten the specifically incriminated food should be purged with cathartics, given enemas, and kept under close medical observation. Presumptive treatment with polyvalent botulism antitoxin may be given or give monovalent antitoxin of the appropriate type, if known and available.

6) *Investigation of contacts and source of infection:* Search for contaminated food. Study the food habits and recent food history of those ill.

7) *Specific treatment:* Intravenous and intramuscular administration of botulinus antitoxin. Trivalent antitoxin (types A, B and E) and monovalent type E antitoxin may be obtained from the Center for Disease Control, Atlanta, GA (see Preface). Bivalent antitoxins (A and B) can be obtained from commercial sources (Lederle).

C. *Epidemic measures:* Suspicion or recognition of a case of botulism should immediately raise the question of a group outbreak involving a family or others who have shared a common meal. Home preserved foods should be the prime suspect until ruled out, although widely distributed commercially produced preserved foods are being frequently identified as sources of intoxication. When the latter is indicated by epidemiologic or laboratory findings, immediate recall of the product is necessary. Immediate search for persons who shared the suspected food and for any remaining food from the same source that may be similarly contaminated; such food, if found, to be submitted for laboratory examination. Blood from patients, and others exposed but not ill, should be obtained before administration of antitoxin and forwarded immediately to a reference laboratory.

D. International measures: None.

D. VIBRIO PARAHAEMOLYTICUS FOOD POISONING

1. Identification—An intestinal disorder characterized by watery diarrhea and abdominal cramps in the majority of cases, with nausea, vomiting, fever, and headache variably present. Occasionally a dysentery-like illness with bloody or mucoid stools, high fever, and high white blood count is observed. A disease of moderate severity with duration generally 1-7 days; systemic spread of infection and death rarely occur.

Diagnosis is confirmed by isolating Kanagawa positive strains of the organism from the patients' stool.

2. Occurrence—Sporadic cases and common source outbreaks have been reported from many parts of the world, particularly Japan, Southeast Asia, and the United States. Primarily occurs in warm months of the year.

3. Infectious agent—*Vibrio parahaemolyticus,* a halophilic vibrio. Eleven different "O" antigen groups and approximately 50 different "K" antigen types have been identified. Pathogenic strains are generally capable of producing a characteristic hemolytic reaction (the "Kanagawa phenomenon").

4. Reservoir—Marine coastal environs are the natural habitat. During the cold season, organisms are found in marine silt. During warm season, they are found free in coastal waters and are a natural contaminant of fish and shellfish.

5. Mode of transmission—Ingestion of raw seafood which has been inadequately cooked to destroy naturally contaminating vibrios or has been cross-contaminated due to handling in the same environment as raw seafood. A period of inadequate refrigeration is generally necessary to allow proliferation of contaminants to a level infectious for man (10^6 or greater). Person to person spread does not appear to occur.

6. Incubation period—Usually between 12 and 24 hours, with individual cases ranging from as little as 4 up to 96 hours.

7. Period of communicability — Non-communicable-man-to-man.

8. Susceptibility and resistance — Most persons are probably susceptible. No information is available regarding acquisition of immunity.

9. Method of control —

A. *Preventive measures:*
   1) Assure that cooked seafood reaches temperature adequate to kill the organism (may survive at 80°C for up to 15 minutes).
   2) Handle cooked seafood in an environment separated from that used for raw seafood to avoid cross-contamination.
   3) Keep all seafood, raw or cooked, adequately refrigerated prior to eating.
   4) Educate seafood handlers and processors with regard to the above preventive measures.

B. *Control of patient, contacts and immediate environment:*
   (See Staphylococcal Food Poisoning 9C, p. 118).

C. *Epidemic measures:* None.

D. *International measures:* None.

E. *BACILLUS CEREUS* FOOD POISONING

1. Identification — A gastrointestinal disorder characterized in some cases by sudden onset of nausea and vomiting and in others by intense abdominal colic and diarrhea. Generally persists no longer than 24 hours and is rarely fatal. Diagnosis is supported by identifying the causative organism in the suspect food and in feces of patients and by performing quantitative cultures with selective media to estimate the number of organisms present.

2. Occurrence — A well-recognized cause of foodborne disease in Europe; not commonly observed or reported in the U.S.A.

3. Infectious agent — *Bacillus cereus,* an anaerobic sporeformer; spores are heat resistant. A cell-associated enterotoxin may be responsible for symptoms.

4. Reservoir — An ubiquitous organism of soil.

5. Mode of transmission — Ingestion of food in which conditions have permitted multiplication of the organisms. Outbreaks have been most commonly associated with rice, vegetables, and meat dishes mishandled after cooking.

6. Incubation period — From 1 to 5 hours in cases where vomiting is the predominant symptom; from 6 to 16 hours where diarrhea is predominant.

7. **Period of communicability** — Unknown.

8. **Susceptibility and resistance** — Unknown.

9. **Methods of control** —

    A. Preventive measures: Foods which may be contaminated with *B. cereus*, such as grain and vegetable dishes, should not remain at ambient temperature after cooking. Spores can survive boiling, germinate, and multiply rapidly at room temperature. Leftover food should be refrigerated; reheating should be performed rapidly to avoid multiplication of microorganisms.

    B. Control of patient, contacts, and the immediate environment: (See Staphylococcal Food Poisoning 9B, p. 118).

    C. Epidemic measures: Identify contaminated food. (See Staphylococcal Food Poisoning 9C, p. 118).

    D. International measures: None.

GASTROENTERITIS, VIRAL

Viral gastroenteritis comprises at least two distinct entities with considerable clinical similarity, but distinct epidemiological differences. Epidemic viral gastroenteritis tends to occur in community-wide outbreaks; sporadic viral gastroenteritis principally affects children in limited outbreaks. They are presented separately.

A. EPIDEMIC VIRAL GASTROENTERITIS
(Norwalk type disease, Acute infectious non-bacterial gastroenteritis, Viral diarrhea, Epidemic diarrhea and vomiting, Winter vomiting disease, Epidemic collapse, Epidemic nausea and vomiting)

1. Identification — Epidemic viral gastroenteritis is usually a self-limited mild disease which often occurs in outbreaks and which is characterized by a spectrum of clinical symptoms which may include nausea, vomiting, diarrhea, abdominal pain, malaise, low grade fever or a combination thereof. Clinical features usually last 24-48 hours.

The virus may be identified in preparations made from stools of ill individuals by immune electron microscopy. Serologic evidence of infection also may be demonstrated by immune electron microscopy, using a particle-positive stool filtrate as antigen.

2. Occurrence—Probably world-wide; occurs in outbreaks most often but may also occur sporadically. Based on a long term family study in the United States, acute infectious nonbacterial gastroenteritis may be a common experience. Probably occurs in all age groups. Syndrome has a characteristic seasonal pattern, occurring most frequently from September to March.

3. Infectious agent—The 27 nm particle, a parvovirus-like agent, has recently been suggested as the etiologic agent of an outbreak in Norwalk, Ohio, on the basis of immune electron microscopy. At least one additional distinct serotype (the Hawaii agent) exists, and it is probable that there are other distinct serotypes, thus possibly accounting for the frequency of repeated episodes.

4. Reservoir—Man is the only known reservoir.

5. Mode of transmission—Unknown; possibly by fecal-oral route.

6. Incubation period—24-48 hours.

7. Period of communicability—During acute stage of disease and possibly shortly thereafter also.

8. Susceptibility and resistance—Susceptibility to disease is widespread since several, or possibly numerous, serotypes of 27 nm parvovirus-like agents exist. Rechallenge of volunteers with homologous infectious stool filtrate indicates that immunity to the specific agent occurs; however, the duration of such immunity is unknown.

9. Methods of control—

    A. Preventive measures:
        1) Undetermined. Until mode(s) of transmission can be definitively established, hygienic measures applicable to diseases transmitted via fecal-oral route (see Salmonellosis, p. 276).
        2) Prevent exposure of infants and young children to individuals with acute gastroenteritis.

    B. Control of patient, contacts, and the immediate environment:
        1) Report to local health authority: Obligatory report of epidemics; no individual case report, Class 4 (see Preface).

2) *Isolation:* Enteric precautions.

3) *Concurrent disinfection:* None.

4) *Quarantine:* None.

5) *Immunization of contacts:* None.

6) *Investigation of contacts and source of infection:* Individual sources of infection should be sought, especially in family and home, and possibly in food and/or water.

7) *Specific treatment:* Electrolyte and fluid replacement in severe cases.

C. *Epidemic measures:* Search for vehicles of transmission and source; determine course of outbreak to better define epidemiology.

D. *International measures:* None.

B. SPORADIC VIRAL GASTROENTERITIS
(Severe viral gastroenteritis of infants and children)

1. **Identification**—A sporadic severe gastroenteritis of infants and young children, characterized by diarrhea, with or without vomiting, patients usually febrile, has recently been associated with a reovirus-like 70 mm particle. Deaths from acute gastroenteritis associated with the reovirus-like agent in this young age group have been reported occasionally. Milder forms of gastroenteritis due to this agent probably also occur, but most studies have dealt with hospitalized infants and young children.

The virus is identified by electron microscopic examination of preparations made from stools from ill patients. Serologic evidence of infection can be demonstrated by the complement-fixation and/or indirect immunofluorescent techniques.

2. **Occurrence**—Probably world-wide; occurs sporadically, and also in outbreaks. During a 1 year period, in Melbourne, Australia, infection with the reovirus-like agent was the most common cause of sporadic acute gastroenteritis in infants and young children less than 5 years of age who required hospitalization. Infection has been observed most often in the winter months. In the Melbourne study it was the most common enteric pathogen in all but 2 months of the year; the 2 months when it was not were the hottest of the year. Virus has been detected in an infant as young as 10 days of age.

3. **Infectious agent**—The 70 nm reovirus-like agent (also designated orbivirus, rotavirus, and duovirus) has been shown to be the etiologic agent of a large percentage of severe diarrhea of infants and young children. This agent is related antigenically to the

Nebraska calf diarrhea virus, a neonatal calf diarrhea virus isolated in England, the virus of epizootic diarrhea of infant mice virus, and the simian agent (SA) 11 and "O" agent. It is not related antigenically to reovirus types 1, 2 or 3.

4. Reservoir—Probably humans; role of animals unknown.

5. Mode of transmission—Unknown; possibly fecal-oral or fecal-respiratory route(s).

6. Incubation period—Probably less than 48 hours.

7. Period of communicability—Maximum excretion of virus particles on 3rd or 4th day after onset of symptoms as determined by electron microscopy. The agent is rarely detectable after the 8th day.

8. Susceptibility and resistance—A study of the prevalence of serum antibody to the reovirus-like agent among infants and young children in the Washington, D.C. area revealed that there was a rapid acquisition of antibody at a very early age; by 3 years of age over 90% of those studied had acquired antibody. No information is available on the protective effect of antibody.

9. Methods of control—

   A. *Preventive measures:*
      1) Undetermined. Until mode(s) of transmission can be definitively established, hygienic measures applicable to diseases transmitted via fecal-oral route (see Salmonellosis, p. 276), or possibly fecal-respiratory route.
      2) Prevent exposure of infants and young children to individuals with acute gastroenteritis.

   B. *Control of patient, contacts, and the immediate environment:*
      1) Report to local health authority: Obligatory report of epidemics; no individual case report, Class 4 (see Preface).
      2) Isolation: Of infected infants and children, especially in hospitals. Enteric precautions.
      3) Concurrent disinfection: None.
      4) Quarantine: None.
      5) Immunization of contacts: None.
      6) Investigation of contacts and source of infection: Individual sources of infection should be sought, especially in family and home, and possibly in food and/or water.
      7) Specific treatment: Fluid and electrolyte replacement in severe cases.

C. *Epidemic measures:* Search for vehicles of transmission and source; determine course of the outbreak to better define epidemiology.

D. *International measures:* None.

GIARDIASIS
(Giardia enteritis, Lambliasis)

1. **Identification** — A protozoal infection of the small bowel; while often asymptomatic, may also be associated with a variety of intestinal symptoms, chronic diarrhea, steatorrhea, abdominal cramps, bloating, frequent loose and pale, greasy, or malodorous stools, fatigue and weight loss. Malabsorption of fats or of fat-soluble vitamins may occur. Symptomatic patients may harbor large numbers of organisms *(Giardia lamblia);* improvement occurs upon removal of the parasites by appropriate chemotherapy. There is no invasion beyond the bowel lumen; damage and inflammatory changes of duodenal and jejunal mucosal cells may occur in severe giardiasis.

Diagnosis is by identification of cysts or trophozoites in feces or of trophozoites in duodenal drainage; the latter is more reliable but rarely necessary. The presence of *G. lamblia* (in either stools or duodenal drainage) is not necessarily indicative of a causal relationship to symptoms; other intestinal pathogens or other causes of malabsorption should be ruled out.

2. **Occurrence** — Worldwide. Children are infected more frequently than adults. Prevalence is higher in areas of poor sanitation and in institutions. The carrier rate in different areas of the U.S.A. may range between 1.5 and 20%, depending on the community and age group surveyed. Present in Russia; of 27 tour groups traveling to Russia between 1970 and early 1974, 23% of 1419 persons became ill with giardiasis related epidemiologically to drinking tap water in Leningrad.

3. **Infectious agent** — *Giardia lamblia,* a flagellated protozoan.

4. **Reservoir** — Man; possibly domestic animals.

5. **Mode of transmission** — Fecal contamination of water and by

hand-to-mouth transfer of cysts from the feces of an infected individual. Localized outbreaks occur from contaminated water supplies.

Asymptomatic individuals are probably more important in transmission than persons with active disease, due to fragility of the trophozoite form. The effect of chlorination on *Giardia* cysts is unknown, but probably is not lethal in standard concentrations (similar to *Entamoeba histolytica*).

6. Incubation period—Variable. In experimental infections, incubation periods range from 6 to 22 days. In a waterborne epidemic in the United States, clinical illnesses occurred 1 to 4 weeks after exposure.

7. Period of communicability—Entire period of infection.

8. Susceptibility and resistance—Asymptomatic carrier rate is high; pathogenicity of *G. lamblia* for humans has been established by clinical studies, but its mechanism is not clear.

9. Methods of control—

A. Preventive measures:
1) Education in personal hygiene of families, and personnel and inmates of institutions.
2) Sanitary disposal of feces.
3) Protection of public water supplies against fecal contamination.

B. Control of patient, contacts, and the immediate environment:
1) *Report to local health authority:* Obligatory report of epidemics, Class 4 (see Preface).
2) *Isolation:* None.
3) *Concurrent disinfection:* Sanitary disposal of feces.
4) *Quarantine:* None.
5) *Investigation of contacts and source of infection:* Microscopic examination of feces of household members and other suspected contacts, supplemented by search for environmental contamination.
6) *Specific treatment:* Metronidazole (Flagyl) is the drug of choice; quinacrine hydrochloride (Atabrine) is also effective. Relapses may occur with either drug.

C. Epidemic measures: Epidemiological investigation of clustered cases in an area or institution to determine source of infection and mode of transmission; look for common vehicle, such as water; institute applicable preventive or control measures. Control of person to person transmission requires special emphasis on personal cleanliness and sanitary disposal of feces.

D. International measures: None.

❦

GONOCOCCAL DISEASE

Urethritis, salpingitis, proctitis, cervicitis, and pharyngitis of adults, vulvovaginitis of children and opthalmia of the newborn and adults are inflammatory conditions which are caused by *Neisseria gonorrhoeae*. All are maintained in a population by the continued presence of gonorrhea and together they constitute an epidemiologic entity. Similar principles of control apply to the group.

Clinically indistinguishable infections of the same anatomic structures may be caused by other infectious agents. This presentation relates specifically to gonococcal disease, but the final paragraph under identification of each of the 3 gonococcal conditions gives the general characteristics of these other infections. They occur frequently and methods of control are often ill-defined.

A. GONORRHEA (GONOCOCCAL URETHRITIS)
(Clap, Strain, Gleet, Dose, Jack)

1. Identification— An infectious disease of venereal origin, limited to columnar and transitional epithelium and accordingly differing between male and female in course, in seriousness and in ease of recognition. In males, a purulent discharge from the anterior urethra appears usually 2 to 9 days or later after an infecting exposure. The infection is often self-limited, but may extend to the posterior urethra where it may produce epididymitis and prostatitis, and result in a chronic carrier state. Asymptomatic urethral carriage also may occur. In females a few days after exposure, an initial urethritis or cervicitis occurs, often so mild as to pass unnoticed in the typical disease. In some there is pelvic invasion at the first, second, or later menstrual period, with mild or severe symptoms of salpingitis or pelvic peritonitis. Residual and often chronic infection is common. In both sexes, pharyngeal and anal infections are not uncommon. Septicemia may occur, with dermatitis, arthritis, endocarditis, and meningitis. Death is rare, but early and late manifestations, and especially complications, are frequent and may be seriously incapacitating.

Bacteriologic culture on special media (e.g., modified Thayer-Martin media) confirms diagnosis. In males, typical gram-negative intracellular diplococci can be considered diagnostic. In females, repeated cervical and rectal cultures may be necessary to detect residual infection. Fluorescent antibody-stained smears lack specificity, and are only an adjunct to cultures.

Widespread and frequent non-gonococcal urethritis, possibly also of sexual origin, seriously complicates the clinical diagnosis of gonorrhea. In some countries the incidence exceeds that of gonorrhea and the condition is reportable. It may be initiated by a number of infectious agents.

2. **Occurrence** — A common disease everywhere, affects both sexes and practically all ages, especially younger adult groups among whom sexual activity is greatest; is seriously under reported. In recent years, incidence has increased worldwide.

3. **Infectious agent** — *Neisseria gonorrhoeae*, the gonococcus.

4. **Reservoir** — Man is the only known reservoir.

5. **Mode of transmission** — By contact with exudates from mucous membranes of infected persons, almost wholly as a result of sexual activity. Even in children it is most frequently a result of sexual contact or molestation.

6. **Incubation period** — Usually 2 to 5 days, sometimes 9 days or longer.

7. **Period of communicability** — May extend for months or years if untreated, especially in females who frequently are asymptomatic. Specific therapy usually ends communicability within hours or days.

8. **Susceptibility and resistance** — Susceptibility is general. Although secretory antibody has been demonstrated, acquired immunity after attack is not evident.

9. **Methods of Control** —

   A. *Preventive measures:* Same as for syphilis (p. 316), except for measures applying specifically to gonorrhea, i.e. primarily the use of chemoprophylactic agents in the eyes of the newborn (in U.S.A.) (C9A1) and special attention (prophylactic treatment) to contacts of infectious patients (9B6).

   B. *Control of patient, contacts, and the immediate environment:*
      1) *Report to local health authority:* Case report is required in many states and countries, Class 2B (see Preface).

2) *Isolation:* None. Antibiotics in adequate dosage promptly render discharges non-infectious. Patients should refrain from sexual intercourse with untreated previous sexual partners to avoid reinfection.

3) *Concurrent disinfection:* Care in disposal of discharges from lesions and articles soiled therewith.

4) *Quarantine:* None.

5) *Immunization of contacts:* Not applicable (see 9B6).

6) *Investigation of contacts:* Interview of patients and tracing of contacts are fundamental elements of a program for control. Trained interviewers obtain the best results. All sexual contacts within 10 days of onset should be located and treated at once. Examine serologically for syphilis, initially and 4 months after starting treatment of gonorrhea. Orogastric and rectal cultures on all infants born to infected mothers.

7) *Specific treatment:* On clinical, laboratory or epidemiological grounds, aqueous procaine penicillin G intramuscularly in 2 injections (2.4 million units each) at one visit, immediately preceded by 1 gm. of oral probenecid. Repository preparations (benzathine penicillin G) are contraindicated. For patients sensitive to penicillin and for infections resistant to penicillin, use spectinomycin, tetracyclines or erythromycin. Concurrent syphilis must be ruled out. (see 9B6 above).

C. *Epidemic measures:* Intensification of routine procedures, especially therapy of contacts on epidemiologic grounds.

D. *International measures:* See Syphilis 9D (p. 318).

B. GONOCOCCAL VULVOVAGINITIS OF CHILDREN

1. Identification—An inflammatory reaction of the urogenital tract of prepubescent females, characterized by redness and swelling of the mucous membranes and a mucopurulent discharge that varies from case to case. In severe infections, excoriation of the labia and thighs and extension to the urethra and bladder may occur. A self-limited disease; more than three-fourths of patients recover spontaneously within 3 to 6 months; a carrier state sometimes persists.

Diagnosis is established by bacteriologic culture of exudates; stained smears are unreliable.

Gonococcal vulvovaginitis must be differentiated from acute vulvovaginitis due to a variety of other infectious agents. The several diseases are usually indistinguishable clinically; recognition is by bacteriological means.

2. **Occurrence** — Extent not known but presumably widespread, particularly in families of social and economic levels where standards of personal, sexual and general hygiene are low. Epidemics are most frequent in institutions for children.

3. **Infectious agent** — *Neisseria gonorrhoeae,* the gonococcus.

4. **Reservoir** — Man is the only known reservoir.

5. **Mode of transmission** — Intimate, direct contact with exudates from infected adult patients in the home; direct sexual contact; infrequently, contact with contaminated moist articles, or insertion of contaminated instruments and foreign bodies into the vagina and rectum, or indiscriminate use of rectal thermometers. The existence of transient inapparent gonococcal infection among children has been demonstrated.

6. **Incubation period** — Usually 3 to 9 days.

7. **Period of communicability** — While discharges persist, usually 3 to 6 months; may continue after clinical manifestations cease.

8. **Susceptibility and resistance** — Susceptibility is related to the type of epithelium lining the vagina; until puberty, the columnar or transitional epithelium is receptive to attack by gonococci; after puberty, the stratified squamous type is not attacked by gonococci. One attack does not protect against subsequent infection.

9. **Methods of control** —

   A. *Preventive measures:*
      1) Fundamentally dependent on control of gonorrhea (see above); general measures are those of syphilis (see p. 316).
      2) Proper supervision of institutions for children, with rigid enforcement of hygienic principles and early sex education.

   B. *Control of patient, contacts, and the immediate environment:*
      1) *Report to local health authority:* Case report is required in most states and countries, Class 2B (see Preface).
      2) *Isolation:* Until 24 hours after administration of antibiotics.
      3) *Concurrent disinfection:* Care in disposal of discharges from lesions and articles soiled therewith.
      4) *Quarantine:* None.
      5) *Immunization of contacts:* None; chemotherapy on suspicion of infection.

6) *Investigation of contacts:* The proved importance of sexual transmission among children calls for trained interviewers to elicit history of sexual contact among playmates, family members and older persons within the family group and outside. Histories are unreliable; actual search for gonorrhea among persons in the environment of the child is necessary.

7) *Specific treatment:* Aqueous procaine penicillin G intramuscularly in a single dose of 75,000-100,000 units/kg and 25 mg/kg oral probenecid.

C. *Epidemic measures:*

1) Prompt search for source of infection within the institution or group affected and introduction of measures to protect preadolescent girls.

2) Education of those in charge of children as to causes of outbreaks and the sources and development of the disease, with special emphasis upon personal hygiene of children. The importance of probable sexual transmission should be emphasized.

D. *International measures:* None.

C. GONOCOCCAL OPHTHALMIA NEONATORUM
(Gonorrheal ophthalmia, Acute conjunctivitis of the newborn)

1. **Identification**—Acute redness and swelling of the conjunctiva of one or both eyes, with mucopurulent or purulent discharge in which gonococci are identifiable by microscopic and cultural methods. Corneal ulcer, perforation and blindness may occur if specific treatment is not given promptly.

Gonococcal ophthalmia neonatorum is only one of a number of acute inflammatory conditions of the eye or the conjunctiva occurring within the first 3 weeks of life, and collectively known as ophthalmia neonatorum. Differentiation is bacteriological. The gonococcus is the most important, but not always the most frequent, infectious agent; may also include meningococci, hemophilic bacilli, chlamydia (inclusion conjunctivitis, p. 84) and others. All purulent inflammation of the conjunctiva should be regarded as gonococcal until proved otherwise.

2. **Occurrence**—Varies widely according to measures for prevention of infection of eyes of the newborn by attendants at delivery, but is infrequent where care is adequate. Globally, the disease continues to be an important cause of blindness.

3. **Infectious agent**—*Neisseria gonorrhoeae,* the gonococcus.

4. **Reservoir**—Man is the only known reservoir.

5. **Mode of transmission**—Contact with the infected maternal birth canal during childbirth.

6. **Incubation period**—Usually 36 to 48 hours.

7. **Period of communicability**—For 24 hours following specific treatment or in its absence until discharges from infected membranes have ceased.

8. **Susceptibility and resistance**—Susceptibility is general. Immunity to subsequent gonococcal disease does not follow attack.

9. **Methods of control**—

A. *Preventive measures:*
   1) Use of an established effective preparation for protection of the eyes of babies at birth; instillation of 1% silver nitrate solution stored in individual wax capsules remains the preferred prophylactic agent for general use.
   2) Depends fundamentally on the control of venereal disease (see syphilis, p. 316). Routine cervical and rectal culturing for gonococci during prenatal period, especially in third trimester.

B. *Control of patient, contacts, and the immediate environment:*
   1) *Report to local health authority:* Case report is required in most states and countries, Class 2B (see Preface).
   2) *Isolation:* For the first 24 hours after administration of an antibiotic.
   3) *Concurrent disinfection:* Care in disposal of conjunctival discharges and articles soiled therewith.
   4) *Quarantine:* None.
   5) *Immunization of contacts:* Not applicable; prompt treatment on recognition or clinical suspicion of infection.
   6) *Investigation of contacts:* Examination and treatment of mothers and their sexual partners.
   7) *Specific treatment:* Parenteral and local penicillin.

C. *Epidemic measures:* None; a sporadic disease.

D. *International measures:* None.

GRANULOMA INGUINALE
(Donovaniasis, Granuloma venereum)

1. Identification — A mildly communicable, nonfatal, chronic, and progressive autoinoculable disease of the skin and mucous membrane of external genitalia and anal region. A small nodule, vesicle or papule becomes a creeping, exuberant, ulcerative, or cicatricial process of the skin, frequently painless and extending peripherally with characteristic rolled edges and formation of fibrous tissue; in many cases the lesion is actively granulomatous. Lesions have predilection for warm and moist surfaces such as folds between scrotum and thighs or labia and vagina. If neglected, the process may result in extensive destruction of genital organs and spread to other parts of body. Not infrequently, this infection is associated with squamous cell carcinoma of the penis.

Laboratory diagnosis by demonstrating intracytoplasmic Donovan bodies in Giemsa stained spreads of granulation tissue or by punch biopsy tissue taken from lesions, and by histologic examination of biopsy specimens.

2. Occurrence — An infrequent disease of tropical, subtropical and temperate areas; apparently more frequent among males than females, and among persons of lower economic status; predominantly at ages 20 to 40 years. Rare in prostitutes and heterosexual partners of cases; patients are frequently homosexual.

3. Infectious agent — *Calymmatobacterium granulomatis (Donovania granulomatis).*

4. Reservoir — Man.

5. Mode of transmission — Presumably by direct contact with active lesions during sexual activity.

6. Incubation period — Unknown; presumably between 8 to 80 days.

7. Period of communicability — Unknown; probably for the duration of open lesions on the skin or mucous membranes.

8. Susceptibility and resistance — Susceptibility is variable; immunity apparently does not follow attack.

9. Methods of control —

   A. Preventive measures: Except for those measures applicable only to syphilis, preventive measures are those for syphilis, See Syphilis 9A. (p. 316).

   B. Control of patient, contacts, and the immediate environment:
      1) Report to local health authority: In selected endemic

areas (U.S.A., some states); not a reportable disease in most states and countries, Class 3B (see Preface).

2) *Isolation:* None; avoid close personal contact until lesions are healed.

3) *Concurrent disinfection:* Care in disposal of discharges from lesions and articles soiled therewith.

4) *Quarantine:* None.

5) *Immunization of contacts:* Not applicable; prompt treatment on recognition or clinical suspicion of infection.

6) *Investigation of contacts:* Examination of sexual contacts, especially homosexual contacts.

7) *Specific treatment:* Tetracyclines and erythromycin are effective; recurrence is not rare, but usually responds to a second course of therapy unless malignancy is present.

C. *Epidemic measures:* Not applicable.

D. *International measures:* See Syphilis 9D. (p. 318).

HEMORRHAGIC FEVERS OF ARGENTINIAN AND BOLIVIAN TYPES

1. Identification—Acute febrile illnesses, duration 7 to 15 days. Onset is gradual with malaise, headache, sustained fever and sweats, followed by prostration. Exanthem appears on thorax and flanks 3 to 5 days after onset; may later show petechiae. Enanthem with petechiae on the soft palate is frequent. Severe infections result in epistaxis, hematemesis, melena, hematuria, and gingival hemorrhage; encephalopathies with intention tremors are frequent. Bradycardia and hypotension with clinical shock are important findings, and leukopenia and thrombocytopenia are characteristic. Moderate albuminuria is present with many cellular and granular casts and vacuolated epithelial cells. Relapses occur.

Diagnosis is by isolation of virus from blood, spleen or throat washings, and serologically by complement fixation or neutralization test.

2. Occurrence—First described in Argentina in 1955, in rural areas among laborers in corn fields. Occurs from March to October (autumn and winter) with peak in May or June; mainly at ages 15 to 44 years; 5 times as frequently in males as females. Estimated fatality rate varies from 5% to 30%, greatest among older patients. A similar disease was subsequently described in a series of epidemics in urban areas (small villages) of Bolivia.

3. Infectious agent — The Junin virus of the Tacaribe group of arenaviruses for the Argentinian disease, and the closely related Machupo virus for the Bolivian.

4. Reservoir — In Argentina, wild rodents of corn fields are vertebrate hosts; domestic rodents, particularly *Calomys callosus*, in Bolivia.

5. Mode of transmission — Saliva and excreta of infected rodents contain the virus. Possibly food-borne. Laboratory infections occur. There is no proof of arthropod transmission.

6. Incubation period — Commonly 10 to 14 days.

7. Period of communicability — Probably not often directly transmitted from man to man although this has occurred for the Bolivian disease.

8. Susceptibility and resistance — All ages appear susceptible but immunity of unknown duration follows infection.

9. Methods of control — Specific rodent control where the reservoir host has been identified. Use of specific immunoglobulins is under consideration.

❧

HEMORRHAGIC FEVER WITH RENAL SYNDROME
(Hemorrhagic nephrosonephritis, Epidemic hemorrhage fever)

1. Identification — An acute infectious disease characterized by fever of 3 to 6 days duration, conjunctival injection, prostration, anorexia, vomiting, hemorrhagic manifestations which begin about the third day, proteinuria about the fourth day, and hypotension about the fifth; renal abnormalities, varying from mild to acute renal failure, continue for several weeks. About one-fourth of cases show an alarming hypotension and the majority of deaths (fatality about 6%) occur during shock; other deaths from renal shutdown. Convalescence is usually rapid during the third week.

Specific laboratory tests are not available; clinical laboratory findings such as proteinuria, leukocytosis, thrombocytopenia, and elevated blood urea nitrogen assist in establishing the diagnosis.

2. **Occurrence** — In Korea in the vicinity of the 38th parallel among civilians and United Nations troops since 1951. Earlier Japanese and Russian reports of experience in Manchuria and in Siberia along the Amur River indicate that women and children acquire the malady as well as men. Recently recognized in European USSR in the Yaroslav region north of Moscow and suspected elsewhere. A few cases occur throughout the year, but in Korea there are two seasonal outbreaks, one in May-June and one in October-November. The majority of cases are isolated events but outbreaks have involved 5 to 20 persons within a small area, all infections apparently acquired at the same time and place; a rural disease presently occuring among civilians in other areas of Korea.

3. **Infectious agent** — Unknown; Berkefeld and Seitz filtrates of human materials induce hemorrhagic fever in experimentally inoculated volunteers. The agent has not been established in laboratory animals although experimentally inoculated tissue cultures have been reported to be positive by fluorescent antibody tests in the USSR.

4. **Reservoir** — Assumed to be maintained in nature by rodents, with man only an accidental host.

5. **Mode of transmission** — Unknown; epidemiologic observations in Korea suggested an analogy to scrub typhus and implicated a nonflying arthropod vector of limited mobility; trombiculid mites were suspected. Presently, transmission from rodent excreta is suspected.

6. **Incubation period** — Usually 12 to 16 days, but varying from 9 to 35.

7. **Period of communicability** — Apparently not directly transmitted from man to man.

8. **Susceptibility and resistance** — Newcomers to endemic areas are uniformly susceptible; indigenous populations probably have some acquired resistance. Mild or inapparent infections are suspected but unproved. Second attacks have not been observed.

9. Methods of control —

   A. Preventive measures: Without adequate information on etiologic agent and mode of transmission, preventive measures employed are those of a disease with field rodent host.

   B. Control of patient, contacts, and the immediate environment:
   1) Report to local health authority: In selected endemic

areas; in most countries not a reportable disease, Class 3A (see Preface).

2) *Isolation:* None.

3) *Concurrent disinfection:* None.

4) *Quarantine:* None.

5) *Immunization of contacts:* None.

6) *Investigation of contacts:* None.

7) *Specific treatment:* None. Appropriate treatment for shock and/or for renal shutdown.

C. *Epidemic measures:* Rodent control.

D. *International measures:* None.

HEPATITIDES, VIRAL

Two distinct diseases are grouped as the viral hepatitides; they are similar in many ways but differ in etiology and in some epidemiological, immunological, clinical and pathological characteristics. Their prevention and control vary greatly. Each will therefore be presented in a separate section.

A. HEPATITIS A

(Epidemic hepatitis, Epidemic jaundice, Infectious hepatitis, Catarrhal jaundice, Viral Hepatitis type A)

1. **Identification**—Onset is usually abrupt with fever, malaise, anorexia, nausea and abdominal discomfort, followed within a few days by jaundice. Multiple organs may be involved. Varies from a mild illness lasting 1 to 2 weeks, to a severely disabling disease lasting several months. Convalescence usually is prolonged. In general, severity increases with age, but complete recovery without sequelae or recurrences is the rule. Many cases are mild and without jaundice, especially in children, and recognizable only by liver function or serum enzyme tests.

Antigen has been demonstrated by electron microscopic techniques; specific serological tests have been developed but are not available for general use as yet. Differential diagnosis usually depends on clinical laboratory and epidemiologic evidence for the exclusion of other causes of febrile jaundice.

2. **Occurrence**—Worldwide, sporadic and epidemic, with a tendency to cyclic recurrences. Outbreaks are common in institutions, in low-cost housing projects, in rural areas, and in military forces, particularly during wars. Epidemics often evolve slowly, involve wide geographic areas and last many months. Most common among school-age children and young adults. In most temperate zone countries incidence is 10 to 20% higher during autumn and winter compared to spring and summer.

3. **Infectious agent**—Particles measuring 27 nm with characteristics of an enterovirus or a parvovirus have been visualized in infective feces of human subjects.

4. **Reservoir**—Man, chimpanzees and, less frequently, certain other nonhuman primates.

5. **Mode of transmission**—Person-to-person contact, presumably in the majority of cases by the fecal-oral route. The infectious agent may be found in feces, blood and urine. Common-vehicle outbreaks have been related to contaminated water and food, including milk, sliced meats, salads, raw or undercooked clams and oysters, and bakery products. The infectious agent is present in circulating blood prior to the onset of jaundice and for a few days later. Spread by ingestion or by parenteral inoculation of infected blood or blood products occurs.

6. **Incubation period**—Dose related; from 15 to 50 days, average 28-30 days.

7. **Period of communicability**—Studies of transmission in humans and epidemiological evidence indicate maximum infectivity during the latter half of the incubation period, continuing for a few days after onset of jaundice (or during peak transaminase activity in anicteric cases).

8. **Susceptibility and resistance**—Susceptibility is general. Low incidence in infants and preschool children suggests that mild and anicteric infections are common. Degree and duration of homologous immunity after attack are unknown but presumed to be long lasting.

9. **Methods of control**—

   A. *Preventive measures:*
   1) Education of the public directed toward good sanitation and personal hygiene, with special emphasis on sanitary disposal of feces.
   2) Proper sterilization of syringes and needles and other equipment used for parenteral injections (see Hepatitis B, 9A, p. 146) or use disposable units.

3) Travelers to highly endemic areas, including North and tropical Africa, the Middle East, Asia, and parts of South America, may be given prophylactic doses of immune serum globulin (ISG). For expected exposures up to 2 months, a single dose of 0.02 ml per kg of body weight is recommended; for more prolonged exposures, 0.06 ml per kg should be repeated at intervals of 4 to 6 months.

Staff, attendants and newly admitted patients in mental institutions, notably homes for retarded children, who experience intensive prolonged exposure may be given ISG in doses of 0.04 to 0.1 ml per kg of body weight, repeated one time after a 4 to 6 month interval.

B. *Control of patient, contacts, and the immediate environment:*
   1) *Report to local health authority:* Reporting obligatory in all states of the U.S.A., although not now required in many countries; Class 2A (see Preface).
   2) *Isolation:* Enteric precautions during first 2 weeks of illness and at least 1 week after onset of jaundice.
   3) *Concurrent disinfection:* Sanitary disposal of feces, urine, and blood.
   4) *Quarantine:* None.
   5) *Immunization of contacts:* No vaccine for active immunization exists. Passive immunization with ISG, 0.02 ml per kg of body weight, should be given intramuscularly as soon as possible after exposure. Recommended for all household contacts regardless of age.
   6) *Investigation of contacts:* Search for missed cases and maintain surveillance of contacts.
   7) *Specific treatment:* None.

C. *Epidemic measures:*
   1) Epidemiologic investigation to determine mode of transmission, whether from person to person or by common vehicle, and to identify the population exposed to increased risk of infection. Search for suspicious illnesses among food handlers. Eliminate any common sources of infection. Provide ISG for exposed contacts.
   2) Special efforts to improve sanitary and hygienic practices, to reduce fecal contamination of foods and water, and to prevent careless disposal of urine.
   3) Focal outbreaks of disease in institutions may warrant mass prophylaxis with ISG.

D. *International measures:* None.

B. HEPATITIS B

(Homologous serum jaundice, Serum hepatitis, Australia
antigen hepatitis, Viral hepatitis type B).

1. Identification—Onset is usually insidious, with anorexia,
vague abdominal discomfort, nausea and vomiting, sometimes
anthralgias, often progressing to jaundice. Fever may be absent or
mild. Severity ranges from inapparent cases detectable only by bio-
chemical tests of liver function to fulminating, fatal cases of acute
hepatic necrosis. The fatality rate also varies widely in different
situations, i.e., from 1% or less (as after use of yellow fever vaccine
containing human plasma in World War II), to 40% or greater following common exposure to a particular lot of human serum. The
fatality rate associated with post transfusion hepatitis commonly
ranges from 6 to 12%.

Prolonged hepatitis B antigenemia, without overt signs of
disease, is found in 1-5 per 1,000 persons in western countries. There
may or may not be a history of clinical acute hepatitis. Sometimes
there is an associated transaminase increase, while biopsy findings
range from normal to an active hepatitis, with or without cirrhosis.
In terms of liver disease, the prognosis for such individuals is
unknown.

In patients manifesting persistant hepatitis, chronic active hepatitis, and cryptogenic cirrhosis, various studies have shown antigenemia in about one-third. In contrast, patients with biliary
cirrhosis or alcohol associated liver disease rarely show
antigenemia. Circulating auto-antibodies rarely are encountered in
those with antigenemia but are not infrequent in patients without
antigenemia. Claims have been advanced associating antigenemia
with various signs of immuno-deficiency but these have not been
confirmed. Finally, hepatomas may be associated with antigenemia
in up to 60% of the cases.

The hepatitis B surface antigen (HBsAg), previously termed
hepatitis-associated antigen (HAA) or Australia or SH antigen,
and HBcAg, the core antigen, constitute hepatitis B virus (HBV).
They can be demonstrated in the blood at some stage in the large
majority of cases by a variety of techniques, the most sensitive of
which is radioimmunoassay. It is associated with the capability of
such blood to be infectious. It is also found in saliva, semen and
urine. Electron microscopy of serum from patents with HBsAg
shows at least three different sized particles, the largest of which
(the Dane particle) is probably the complete virus. HBsAg is antigenically heterogenous; in addition to a common antigenic deter-

minant, designated a, there are mutually exclusive determinants y and d, and mutually exclusive determinants w and r. Thus, there are four possible subtypes: *adw, ayw, adr, ayr*. A new determinant, *e*, separate from the HB_s Ag, has recently been defined. An additional determinant, x, may be specified by the genotype of the host. Individuals from the same area of the world tend to have the same subtype, as do families, and individuals in single source epidemics.

Viral infection in man results in production of specific antibodies which can be demonstrated by passive hemagglutination and radioimmunoassay. In addition to antibody directed against the surface antigens of the virus (anti-HB_s), an antibody directed against the internal core component of the Dane particle (anti-HB_c) has been described.

2. Occurrence—Worldwide; endemic with little seasonal variation. Although widespread infection in childhood may occur in areas of Africa and Asia, in North America it is most common in adults. While endemic in the U.S.A. and Canada the infection has not yet become widely distributed; serologic evidence of previous infection varies from less than 5% in children to 6 to 30% in the general adult population. Presently recognized among recipients of blood or blood products, and among individuals heavily exposed to these products such as patients and employees in renal dialysis centers. Incidence is high among narcotic addicts. Serious outbreaks have originated in clinics and physicians' offices among patients who have received parenteral inoculations from contaminated and inadequately sterilized syringes and needles. Cases also have been traced to tattoo parlors.

3. Infectious agent—A virus of probable DNA nucleic acid content capable of expressing several non-infective morphological forms in addition to an infectious virion.

4. Reservoir—Man, and possibly chimpanzees.

5. Mode of transmission—By parenteral (intravenous, intramuscular or subcutaneous) inoculation of human blood, plasma, serum, thrombin, fibrinogen, packed red cells, cryoprecipitate, and other blood products from an infected person. Immune serum globulin, heat-treated albumin, and fibrinolysin have not been shown to transmit illness. Contaminated needles, syringes and other intravenous equipment also are important vehicles of spread. The infection may be spread through contamination of wounds or lacerations (track finder's hepatitis). It may also be transmitted by ingestion of infective blood; this route probably is an important source of transmission in occupations related to the handling of blood and blood products. Fecal-oral transmission has not been convincingly demonstrated. May also be transmitted in the course of close personal contact. Transmission through interrupted feedings of mosquitoes has been suspected in Africa.

6. **Incubation period**—Usually 45 to 160 days, average 60-90 days; variation may in part be related to size of inoculum.

7. **Period of communicability**—Blood from experimentally inoculated volunteers has been shown to be infective many weeks before the onset of first symptoms. Blood remains infective through the acute clinical course of the disease and during the chronic carrier state, the latter of which may persist for years. Many, *but not all*, carriers have demonstrable HB$_s$Ag or anti-HB$_c$ or both. Many persons may be carriers without having experienced a clinically recognized attack.

8. **Susceptibility and resistance**—Susceptibility is general. Usually, the disease is milder in children. It is not known whether transmission occurs across the placenta, or whether it may occur during parturition or in the neonatal period. Chronic antigenemia is common in individuals infected in infancy.

9. **Methods of Control**—

   A. *Preventive measures:*
      1) Limit administration of unscreened whole blood or potentially hazardous blood products to those patients in clear and immediate need of such therapeutic measures.
      2) Enforce strict discipline in blood banks; reject as donors all individuals who have a history of viral hepatitis, show evidence of drug addiction, have received a blood transfusion within the preceding 6 months, or have HB$_s$ Ag or anti-HB$_c$ in their blood. Use professional donors only in emergencies.
      3) Maintain surveillance of all cases of post-transfusion hepatitis, including a register of all persons who donated blood for each case. Notify blood banks of these potential carriers so that future donations may be promptly identified.
      4) Adequately sterilize all syringes and needles and stylets for finger puncture. A fresh sterile syringe and needle is essential for each individual receiving skin tests, other parenteral inoculations or venipuncture. Use disposable equipment whenever possible. Discourage tattooing.
      5) Most lots of immune serum globulin have too little hepatitus B antibody (anti-HB$_s$) to be of value.

B. Control of patient, contacts, and the immediate environment:

1) *Report to local health authority:* Official report is obligatory in the U.S.A., although not now required in many countries; Class 2A (see Preface).

2) *Isolation:* Enteric precautions for duration of stay for hospitalized patients.

3) *Concurrent disinfection:* Of equipment contaminated with blood.

4) *Quarantine:* None.

5) *Immunization of contacts:* None. Experimental studies suggest promise in the use of passive immunization with gamma globulin containing a high titer of anti-HB_s.

6) *Investigation of contacts:* See 9C below.

7) *Specific treatment:* None.

C. Epidemic measures: When two or more cases occur in association with some common exposure, conduct extensive search for additional cases among personal associates such as drug addicts, or among patients who have attended a particular clinic in common, or who have been admitted to a particular hospital ward where parenteral inoculations have been given. Institute strict aseptic techniques. If a blood product such as pooled plasma, thrombin or fibrinogen is implicated, trace all recipients of the same lot in a search for additional cases. Recall all outstanding vials of any infective lots.

D. International measures: None.

∞

HERPANGINA, VESICULAR STOMATITIS WITH EXANTHEM AND ACUTE LYMPHONODULAR PHARYNGITIS

(Hand, Foot, and Mouth Disease)

1. Identification — Herpangina is an acute viral disease characterized by sudden onset, fever and small (1-2 mm) discrete, grayish papulo-vesicular pharyngeal lesions on an erythematous base, which gradually progress to slightly larger ulcers. These lesions, usually on the anterior pillars of the tonsillar fauces, soft palate, uvula, and tonsils, may be present for 4 to 6 days after the onset of illness. No fatalities reported. In one series febrile convulsions occurred in 5% of cases.

Vesicular Stomatitis with Exanthem (Hand, Foot, and Mouth Disease) differs from herpangina in that oral lesions are more diffuse and may occur on the buccal surfaces of the cheeks and gums and on the sides of the tongue. Papulo-vesicular lesions which may persist from 7 to 10 days, also occur commonly on hands, feet, and legs; occasionally maculopapular lesions appear on the buttocks.

Acute Lymphonodular Pharyngitis also differs from herpangina lesions are firm raised, discrete, whitish to yellowish nodules surrounded by a 3 to 6mm zone of erythema. They occur predominantly on the uvula, anterior tonsillar pillars and posterior pharynx, with no exanthem.

Clinical diagnosis of these similar but specific syndromes is facilitated by epidemic occurrence. Virus may be isolated in suckling mice from lesions and stool specimens. Serologic and virologic diagnostic procedures are not routinely available.

These diseases are not to be confused with vesicular stomatitis caused by the virus found in cattle and horses, which in man usually occurs in dairy workers, animal husbandrymen and veterinarians. Foot-and-mouth disease of cattle, sheep and swine rarely affects man except for laboratory workers handling the virus; however man can be a mechanical carrier of the virus and the source of animal outbreaks.

Stomatitis due to herpes virus requires differentiation; it has larger, deeper, more painful lesions commonly located in the front of the mouth.

2. **Occurrence** — Probably throughout the world for herpangina and vesicular stomatitis with exanthem, both sporadically and in epidemics; greatest incidence is in summer and early autumn; occurs mainly in children under 10 years, but adult cases are relatively frequent. Single outbreaks of acute lymphonodular pharyngitis, predominantly in children, may occur in summer and early fall.

3. **Infectious agents** — Coxsackievirus, group A: types 2, 3, 4, 5, 6, 10 and 22 for herpangina; type 16 predominantly and types 5 and 10 less often, for vesicular stomatitis with exanthem, and type 10 for acute lymphonodular pharyngitis.

4. **Reservoir** — Man.

5. **Mode of transmission** — Direct contact with nose and throat discharges and feces of infected persons (who may be asympto

matic) and by droplet spread, but no reliable evidence of spread by insects, water, food or sewage.

6. Incubation period — Usually 3 to 5 days for herpangina and vesicular stomatits with exanthem; 5 days for acute lymphonodular pharyngitis.

7. Period of communicability — During the acute stage of illness and perhaps longer, since these viruses persist in stools for several weeks.

8. Susceptibility and resistance — Susceptibility to infection is general. Immunity is acquired by infection, either clinical or inapparent; duration unknown.

Second attacks may occur with group A coxsackievirus of a different immunological type.

9. Methods of control —

A. *Preventive measures:* Reduce person-to-person contact where practicable by measures such as ventilation and crowd reduction.

B. *Control of patient, contacts, and the immediate environment:*
1) *Report to local health authority:* Obligatory report of epidemics; no case report, Class 4 (see Preface).
2) *Isolation:* None.
3) *Concurrent disinfection:* Of nose and throat discharges, feces and articles soiled therewith.
4) *Quarantine:* None.
5) *Immunization of contacts:* None.
6) *Investigation of contacts and source of infection:* Of no practical value.
7) *Specific treatment:* None.

C. *Epidemic measures:* General notice to physicians of increased incidence of the disease, together with a description of onset and clinical characteristics. Isolation of diagnosed cases and all children with fever, pending diagnosis.

D. *International measures:* WHO Collaborating Centres (see Preface).

∞

HERPES SIMPLEX

1. **Identification**—Herpes simplex is a viral infection marked by latency and repeated, recurrent localized lesions. The primary infection usually is asymptomatic and occurs in early childhood. In perhaps 10% of primary infections, overt disease may appear as a mild or severe illness marked by fever and malaise lasting a week or more; may be associated with a gingivostomatitis accompanied by vesicular lesions in the oropharynx, a severe keratoconjunctivitis, a vulvovaginitis, a generalized cutaneous eruption complicating chronic eczema (Kaposi's varicelliform eruption), a meningoencephalitis, or a fatal generalized infection as seen in newborn infants.

Reactivation of latent infection commonly results in herpes labialis (fever blisters or cold sores) manifested by superficial clear vesicles on an erythematous base, involving the face and lips, which crust and heal within a few days. Reactivation is precipitated by various forms of trauma, physiological changes, or intercurrent disease such as pneumococcal pneumonia, bacterial meningitis, and malaria. Reactivation may also involve other body tissues, particularly ectodermal tissues. It occurs in the presence of circulating antibodies which may not be elevated by reactivation.

Central nervous system involvement occurs usually as a primary infection but may appear in a recrudescence. Serological studies indicate that many cases of meningoencephalitis are due to this virus. Fever, headache, leucocytosis, signs of meningeal irritation, drowsiness, confusion, stupor, coma, and lateralizing signs usually referable to one or the other temporal region may occur. The condition can be confused with a variety of other intracranial lesions and requires differentiation from brain abscess and tuberculous meningitis.

A distinct clinical entity of genital herpes is found in adults and is venereally transmitted. Primary and recurrent disease occur as in the non-genital primary reservoir; may be precursor to cancer of the cervix. In males, lesions usually appear on the glans penis or prepuce, but in both sexes may be found in other genital or perineal sites. In most cases genital herpes is caused by herpes simplex virus type 2 (HSV type 2), biologically and antigenically differentiable from HSV type 1 recovered from most non-genital infections. HSV type 2 also has been associated with aseptic meningitis.

Diagnosis is suggested by characteristic cytologic changes (intranuclear inclusions), but is confirmed by isolation of the virus from lesions, from the spinal fluid or surgical tissue in CNS cases, from oral or genital mucous membranes and from semen. Diagnosis also can be confirmed by a rise in specific neutralizing antibodies.

2. **Occurrence** — Worldwide in distribution; 70 to 90% of adults possess circulating antibodies. Infection with HSV type 1 is most prevalent before the fifth year of life. HSV type 2 is rare before adolescence; type 2 antibody is found in about 20% of adults. The prevalence is greater (to 60%) in lower socioeconomic groups and with increasing promiscuity.

3. **Infectious agent** — Herpes simplex virus. Herpes simplex virus types 1 and 2 can be separated by their characteristics in tissue culture, embryonated eggs and experimental animals in addition to their antigenic differentiation. Such differentiation is less distinct than serotypic differentiation in many other viruses, but has been found to be clinically useful.

4. **Reservoir** — Man.

5. **Mode of transmission** — Direct contact with virus in saliva of carriers is probably the most important mode of spread. Direct inoculation of the hands of attendants handling infants with the eczematoid disease occurs; preexisting lesions in the recipient may play a significant role. Transmission of HSV type 2 to nonimmune adults is often by some form of sexual contact. The cervix is a prime reservoir in females; semen may constitute the principal reservoir in males.

6. **Incubation period** — Up to 2 weeks.

7. **Period of communicability** — Secretion of virus in the saliva for as long as 7 weeks after recovery from stomatitis has been reported; virus can be isolated from the saliva of asymptomatic adults.

8. **Susceptibility and resistance** — Probably man is universally susceptible.

9. **Methods of control** —

  A. *Preventive measures:*
    1) Personal hygiene and health education directed toward minimizing the transfer of infectious material.
    2) Particular care to avoid contaminating the skin of eczematous patients with infectious material.
    3) Genital herpes in late pregnancy is serious because of the risk of neonatal herpes which may be highly fatal. Cesarean section is often indicated before membranes rupture.

  B. *Control of patient, contacts, and the immediate environment:*
    1) *Report to local health authority:* Official case report ordinarily not justifiable, Class 5 (see Preface).

    2) Isolation: Patients with herpetic lesions should be kept away from newborns, children with eczema or burns, or from immuno-suppressed patients.

    3) Concurrent disinfection: None.

    4) Quarantine: None.

    5) Immunization of contacts: None.

    6) Investigation of contacts: Seldom of practical value.

    7) Specific treatment: None, except that topical 5-iodo-2' deoxyuridine (Idoxuridine) may modify the acute manifestation of herpetic keratitis and early dendritic ulcers. Corticosteroids should never be used for ocular involvement unless administered under the control of a skilled ophthalmologist. The value of Idoxuridine, cytosine, arabinoside and adenine arabinoside intravenously are under evaluation for treatment in encephalitic and generalized infections, particularly in immuno-suppressed individuals.

C. Epidemic measures: Not applicable.

D. International measures: None.

B-VIRUS INFECTION

B-Virus Infection, or Herpesvirus simiae encephalomyelitis—caused by *Herpesvirus simiae,* a closely related virus—is an ascending encephalomyelitis occurring in veterinarians, laboratory workers and other individuals having close contact with monkeys or monkey cell cultures. After an incubation period of up to 3 weeks, there is an acute febrile onset, with headache, lymphocytic pleocytosis, and a variable neurological pattern, usually ending in death 1 day to 3 weeks after onset of symptoms. An occasional recovery has been associated with considerable residual disability. The virus causes a natural infection of monkeys analogous to *Herpes simplex* virus (HSV) infection in man. Human disease is acquired by the bite of apparently normal monkeys, or by exposure of naked skin to infected saliva or to monkey tissue cultures. There is no treatment. Prevention depends on use of proper protective gauntlets and care to minimize exposure to monkeys. If there has been exposure to monkey saliva, wash thoroughly with soap and water.

HISTOPLASMOSIS

Two clinically different mycoses have been designated as histoplasmosis because the pathogens that cause them, when growing on culture media as molds, cannot be distinguished morphologically. Detailed information will be given for the infection caused by *Histoplasma capsulatum*, followed by a brief resume of histoplasmosis caused by *H. capsulatum var. duboisii*.

1. **Identification** — A systemic mycosis of varying severity, with the primary lesion usually in the lungs. While infection is common, overt clinical disease is not. Five clinical forms are recognized: (a) *Asymptomatic:* Detectable only by acquired hypersensitivity to histoplasmin. Calcification of primary lung lesion may occur. (b) *Acute benign respiratory:* Probably common in endemic areas and easily overlooked; varies from mild respiratory illness to temporary incapacity with general malaise, weakness, fever, chest pains, and dry or productive cough. Erythema multiforme and erythema nodosum may occur. Recovery is slow and spontaneous, with or without multiple, small scattered calcifications in the lung, hilar lymph nodes and spleen. (c) *Acute disseminated:* Varying degrees of hepatosplenomegaly, accompanied by septic-type fever, prostration, and a rapid course are characteristic. It often resembles miliary tuberculosis, is most frequent in infants and young children and, without therapy, is usually fatal. (d) *Chronic disseminated:* Symptoms are variable, depending on organs infected. May present as unexplained fever, anemia, patchy pneumonia, hepatitis, endocarditis, meningitis, or mucosal ulcers of mouth, larynx, stomach or bowel. Adrenal infection is common but usually asymptomatic. More common in the adult male. Cytotoxic or corticosteroid therapies may predispose to dissemination. Course is usually subacute, with variable progression over weeks up to a few years; outcome usually fatal unless treated. (3) *Chronic pulmonary:* Clinically and radiologically resembles chronic pulmonary tuberculosis; more common in males over 40 years old. The disease progresses over months or years, with periods of quiescence and sometimes spontaneous cure. Death may result from respiratory insufficiency or cor pulmonale.

Clinical diagnosis is most rapid if the fungus can be seen in Giemsa's or Wright's stained smears of ulcer exudates, bone marrow, sputum or blood. Special stains are necessary to demonstrate the fungus in biopsies of ulcers, liver, lymph nodes, or lung. Several serologic tests for serum anti-*Histoplasma* antibody are available. Rising titers in paired sera are strong evidence for active disease, although recent positive skin tests with histoplasmin can raise the titer and the serological tests can cross react with other mycoses.

2. **Occurrence** — Foci of infection are common over wide areas of the Americas, Europe, Africa and eastern Asia and Australia; clinical disease is far less frequent and severe progressive disease is rare. Histoplasmin hypersensitivity, sometimes in as much as 80% of a population and indicating antecedent infection, is prevalent in parts of eastern and central U.S.A. Prevalence increases from childhood to 30 years of age; differences by sex are usually not observed except that the chronic disseminated form is more common in males. Outbreaks have occurred in families or in groups of workmen with common exposure to bird or bat droppings; airborne epidemics may occur in areas where contaminated soil has recently been disturbed. Histoplasmosis also occurs in dogs, cats, rats, skunks, opossums, foxes and other animals.

3. **Infectious agents** — *Histoplasma capsulatum (Emmonsiella capsulatum)*, a dimorphic fungus growing as a mold in soil and as a yeast in animal and human hosts.

4. **Reservoir** — Soil around old chicken houses, in caves harboring bats and around starling roosts; also around houses sheltering the common brown bat, and in other soils with high organic content.

5. **Mode of transmission** — Inhalation of airborne spores in dust.

6. **Incubation period** — In reported epidemics, symptoms appear within 5 to 18 days after exposure, commonly 10 days.

7. **Period of communicability** — Not usually transmitted from man to man.

8. **Susceptibility and resistance** — Susceptibility is general. Inapparent infections are extremely common in endemic areas and usually result in increased resistance to infection.

9. **Methods of control** —

    A. *Preventive measures:* Minimize unavoidable exposure to a contaminated and enclosed environment such as chicken coops and their surrounding soil, by spraying with water to reduce dust; masks may be worn. Infectious foci can be decontaminated with 3% formalin.

    B. *Control of patient, contacts, and the immediate environment:*

        1) *Report to local health authority:* In selected endemic areas (U.S.A.); in many countries not a reportable disease, Class 3B (see Preface).

        2) *Isolation:* None.

        3) *Concurrent disinfection:* Of discharges from skin lesions, sputum and articles soiled therewith. Terminal cleaning.

    4) Quarantine: None.

    5) Immunization of contacts: None.

    6) Investigation of contacts: Household contacts for evidence of infection from a common environmental source.

    7) Specific treatment: For disseminated or chronic pulmonary cases, amphotericin B (Fungizone) is the drug of choice; side effects require that it be used with caution.

C. Epidemic measures: Occurrence of grouped cases of acute pulmonary disease in or outside of an endemic area, particularly with history of exposure to dust within a closed space, should arouse suspicion of histoplasmosis. Suspected sites such as chicken houses, barns, silos, caves, starling roosts, or basements should be investigated.

D. International measures: None.

AFRICAN HISTOPLASMOSIS—Usually presents as a subacute granuloma of the skin or bone. Infection, though usually localized in skin or bone, may be disseminated in the skin, subcutaneous tissue, lymph nodes, bones and joints, lungs and abdominal viscera. Disease is more common in males and may occur at any age, but especially in the second decade of life. Thus far, the disease has been recognized only in Africa. Diagnosis is made by culture and by demonstrating in smear or biopsy the yeast cells of *Histoplasma capsulatum var. duboisii.* These cells are much larger than the yeast cells of *H. capsulatum.* The true prevalence of African histoplasmosis, its reservoir, mode of transmission and incubation period are unknown. It is not communicable from man to man. Amphotericin B (Fungizone) is an effective therapeutic agent.

HYDATIDOSIS

(Hydatid disease, Echinococcosis)

    This disease is producted by the presence of cysts of varying size which are the larval stage of *Echinococcus.* The adult worms are found in *Canidae* hosts. There are two different but closely related species causing different clinical manifestations: (1) unilocular echinococcosis or hydatid disease, and (2) multilocular or alveolar hydatid disease.

Microscopic examination for hooklets, protoscolices (scolices) and cyst membranes in sputum, vomitus, urine or feces after rupture of cysts, or in discharges from a sinus, aids in the diagnosis. Immunoelectrophoresis, indirect hemagglutination, latex flocculation and intradermal tests are helpful. Confirmation is by examination of tissues obtained surgically or at necropsy.

A. Infection by *Echinococcus granulosus*

(Unilocular Echinococcosis)

1. Identification — The well encapsulated cysts of *E. granulosus* are found in the liver and lungs and less commonly in the kidney, heart, bone, central nervous system and thyroid. No tissue or organ of the body is exempt from infection. Symptoms are variable and depend upon the location of the slowly growing cysts, which may attain great size. In the liver and the lungs, as well as in other tissues, cysts may give no symptoms throughout life and calcified cysts may be found incidentally during x-ray examination or at autopsy. In vital organs they may cause severe symptoms and death.

2. Occurrence — This parasite is common in countries where dogs are used to herd grazing animals and also have intimate contact with humans. The Middle East, Greece, Cyprus, Italy, North Africa, Asia, Australia, New Zealand, Argentina, Ecuador, Uruguay, southern Brazil and Chile are enzootic areas. Infections acquired in continental U.S.A. are relatively rare.

3. Infectious agent — *Echinococcus granulosus*, a tapeworm of the dog.

4. Reservoir — Definitive hosts are the dog, wolf, dingo and other *Canidae*, infected with adult worms. The usual intermediate hosts are herbivores.

5. Mode of transmission — By ingestion of infective eggs in food and water contaminated with feces of infected animals, by hand-to-mouth transfer of dog feces and through objects soiled with dog feces. Eggs may survive for several months in pastures, gardens and around households. Ingested eggs hatch in the intestine, and larvae migrate to various organs and produce cysts. The dog-sheep-dog cycle is important in most areas where *E. granulosus* is endemic. In other regions it is the dog-cattle or dog-pig cycle. In northwest Canada, the disease is maintained in a moose-wolf-moose sylvan cycle from which sled dogs may bring the parasite to man. A dog-kangaroo-dog cycle is found in Australia.

6. Incubation period — Variable, from months to years, depending upon the number and location of cysts and how rapidly they grow.

7. Period of communicability—Not directly transmitted from man to man or from one intermediate host to another. Dogs begin to pass eggs of the parasite approximately 7 weeks after infection. Adult worms may survive for 2-3 years.

8. Susceptibility and resistance—Children are more likely to be infected and have less natural resistance to infection with the larval stage than adults. Man does not harbor the adult worm.

9. Methods of control—

A. Preventive measures:
1) Rigid control of slaughtering of herbivorous animals so that dogs have no access to uncooked viscera. Dogs become infected by eating hydatid cysts, principally those present in food mammals, but also in wild animals.
2) Licensing and treatment of systematic dogs; reducing their numbers in endemic areas so far as may be compatible with occupational requirements for dogs.
3) Education of school children and of the general public in endemic areas to the dangers of close association with dogs and of the need for controlled slaughtering of animals.
4) Incineration or deep burial of dead, potentially infected intermediate hosts.

B. Control of patient, contacts, and the immediate environment:
1) *Report to local health authority:* In selected endemic areas; not a reportable disease in most states and countries, Class 3B (see Preface).
2) *Isolation:* None.
3) *Concurrent disinfection:* None.
4) *Quarantine:* None.
5) *Immunization of contacts:* None.
6) *Investigation of contacts and source of infection:* Examination of familial associates for suspicious tumors. Search for source of infection in dogs kept in and about houses.
7) *Specific treatment:* None. Surgical removal of isolated cysts is sometimes curative.

C. Epidemic measures: In highly endemic areas, destruction of wild and stray dogs, wolves, coyotes, and foxes. Mass anthelmintic treatment of dogs. Bunamidine HCl is drug of choice; Yomesan has varied effectiveness and must be repeated periodically. Detection and treatment of infected dogs has been more successful.

D. International measures: Coordinated programs by neighboring countries where the disease is endemic, to control infection in animals and movement of dogs from known enzootic areas.

B. Infection by *Echinococcus multilocularis*
(Alveolar Hydatid Disease)

1. Identification—This disease, primarily of the liver, is due to the poorly circumscribed cysts of *Echinococcus multilocularis.* The cysts may be found also in the lungs and other organs. The development of the cysts is not restricted by a strong and intact laminated membrane so that they are invasive in the liver and may disseminate by metastasis. The clinical effects of the infection depend upon the size and location of the cyst or cysts; the prognosis is grave because of the invasive and metastatic potentials.

2. Occurrence—In Central Europe, Siberia, Northern Japan, Alaska, Southern Canada and U.S.A. In the United States it has been reported in North and South Dakota, Iowa, Montana and Minnesota.

3. Infectious agent—*Echinococcus multilocularis.*

4. Reservoir—*E. multilocularis* is commonly maintained in nature in Alaska in a normal fox-vole-fox cycle. The adult tapeworms are found in foxes, wolves, dogs and cats; the intermediate hosts are rodents.

5. Mode of transmission—By ingestion of infective eggs passed in the feces of infected *Canidae* and *Felidae.* Fecally soiled dog fur, harnesses and environmental fomites serve as vehicles of infection.

6. Incubation period, 7. Period of communicability, 8. Susceptibility and resistance and 9. Methods of control—As in Section A., *Echinococcus granulosus,* preceding, except that surgical removal is seldom successful.

∞

INFLUENZA

1. **Identification** — An acute infectious disease of the respiratory tract characterized by abrupt onset of fever, chills, headache, myalgia, and sometimes prostration. Coryza and sore throat are common, especially in later stages of the disease. Cough is almost universal, often severe and protracted. Usually a self-limited disease, with recovery in 2 to 7 days. Recognition is commonly by epidemiologic characteristics; sporadic cases can be identified only by laboratory procedures.

Influenza derives its importance from the rapidity with which epidemics evolve, the height of the attack rates, and the seriousness of complications, notably bacterial pneumonia. Severe disease and deaths normally occur among the elderly and those debilitated by chronic cardiac, pulmonary, renal or metabolic disease. However, in the 1918 epidemic the highest fatality rates were among young adults. Whether this was an attribute of the strain or of the particular epidemiologic conditions is not known. While fatality generally is low, epidemics are associated with a general mortality much in excess of nonepidemic expectancy; approximately 62,000 excess deaths occurred in the U.S.A. during the pandemic of influenza, type A, in 1957-58 and 27,900 excess deaths were estimated during the 1968-69 epidemic due to the Hong Kong strain of type A.

Laboratory confirmation is by recovery of influenza viruses from pharyngeal or nasal secretions during the early febrile stage of disease in embryonated hen's eggs or tissue culture and by demonstration of a specific serologic response in acute and convalescent sera.

2. **Occurrence** — In pandemics, epidemics, localized outbreaks, and as sporadic cases. During the past 75 years, pandemics began in 1889, 1918, 1957, and 1968. Attack rates during epidemics range from less than 15% to 25% in large communities to 40% or higher in closed populations. Major epidemics tend to be periodic: epidemics of influenza type A have appeared in the U.S.A. at intervals of 2 to 3 years; influenza type B usually not less than 4 to 6 years. A major exception in the U.S.A. occurred in 1968 when the pandemic of influenza, type A (Hong Kong strain), followed one year after a major type A epidemic. In temperate zones, epidemics tend to occur in winter; in the tropics often without reference to season.

Influenzal viral infections also occur in swine, horses, and other animals in many parts of the world, but transmission from animals to man has not been demonstrated.

3. Infectious agent—Three types of influenza virus are recognized: A, B and C. Types A and B have long been associated with epidemics; type C thus far has appeared only in sporadic cases and in minor localized outbreaks. Identification of the broad types of influenza virus, A, B and C, is determined by complement fixation with group-specific antisera. A revised system of nomenclature for strains of virus type A was adopted on 1/1/72 by the World Health Organization. Strains are now described by geographic origin, strain number and year of isolation as well as by an index identifying the character of the haemagglutinin (H) and the neuraminidase (N). Strains from species other than man are in addition identified by the species of host from which they were isolated, i.e., swine (sw), equine (eq), avian (av). For subtypes of influenza virus type A isolated from man the prototype strains by the new nomenclature are A/PR/8/34 (HON1), A/FM/1/47 (H1N1), A/Japan/305/57 (H2N2) and A/Hong Kong/1/68 (H3N2). In the A/Japan/57 strain both the haemagglutinin and the neuraminidase were unrelated to those of the A/FM/47 strain and the A/Japan/57 strain was designated as a new subtype. However, because the A/Japan/57 and A/Hong Kong/68 strains had identical neuraminidase components, the A/Hong Kong/68 strain was not considered to be a separate subtype from A/Japan/57. Completely new subtypes appear at irregular intervals. They are responsible for the pandemics. Lesser antigenic changes in the strains are, at least in part, responsible for the interpandemic epidemics. Strains of influenza virus type B also show antigenic variation but, due to complex interrelationships, subtypes have not been designated.

4. Reservoir—Man is the reservoir of human infections, although mammalian reservoirs, such as swine and horses, and avian species are suspected as sources of new human strains, e.g., by recombination with human strains.

5. Mode of transmission—By direct contact, through droplet infection, or by articles freshly soiled with discharges of the nose and throat of infected persons; probably airborne among crowded populations in enclosed spaces such as barracks, ships or school buses.

6. Incubation period—Short, usually 24 to 72 hours.

7. Period of communicability—Probably limited to 3 days from clinical onset.

8. Susceptibility and resistance—Susceptibility is universal. Infection produces immunity to the specific infecting virus. Infections with related viruses broaden the base of immunity. Immunization produces serologic responses specific for the subtypes present in the vaccine, and booster responses to related strains with which the individual has had prior experience.

Age-specific attack rates during an epidemic reflect existing immunity from past experience with strains related to the epidemic subtype. Attack rates are also markedly influenced by the degree of exposure. In general, incidence is highest in school-age children. Rates decrease progressively among adults as age increases, though exceptions occur: In the 1962-63 epidemic in the U.S.A., the third major recurrence of type A2 influenza, incidence was rather uniform for all ages. Normally, severe disease and deaths occur among the elderly and those with pre-existing disease (see par. 1).

9. **Methods of control—**

A. *Preventive measures:*
   1) Active immunization is effective when vaccine is potent and contains antigens which closely match the prevailing strain of virus. Because of the uncertainty that epidemic influenza will occur in any given year and that vaccines will be effective, immunization programs should be directed at persons with greatest risk of serious complication or death (see par. 1).

   During years when widespread epidemics of influenza type A are anticipated, immunization may also be considered for those engaged in essential community services if sufficient vaccine is available. Immunization should be accomplished before influenza is expected.
   2) Amantidine hydrochloride, 100 mg twice daily, is effective in the chemoprophylaxis of influenza type A, but not type B. The degree of protection approximates that of an effective vaccine. Its use should be considered in persons at high risk to complications who are not immunized or when an appropriate vaccine is not available.
   3) Education of the public in basic personal hygiene.

B. *Control of patient, contacts, and the immediate environment:*
   1) *Report to local health authority:* Obligatory reporting since January 1, 1971, as a Class 1 Disease under Surveillance by WHO, and as Class 4 in other jurisdictions. Report identity of infectious agent as determined by laboratory examination, if possible.
   2) *Isolation:* Generally, none recommended; it may be desirable to attempt isolation of highly susceptible individuals from acutely ill patients.
   3) *Concurrent disinfection:* None.
   4) *Quarantine:* None.

5) *Protection of contacts:* Too late for immunization to be effective. As a public health measure a limited role for antiviral chemoprophylaxis against type A strains has been shown (see 9A 2).

6) *Investigation of contacts:* Of no practical value.

7) *Specific treatment:* None. Sulfonamides and antibiotics have no beneficial effect on the uncomplicated disease; their administration may be considered if bacterial complications occur.

C. *Epidemic measures:*

1) The severe and often disrupting effects of epidemic influenza on community activities may be mitigated in part by effective health planning and education, particularly at the local level. Continued community surveillance by local health authorities of the extent and progress of outbreaks within areas of their jurisdiction is essential, followed by prompt report to state and national health agencies of the prevailing epidemic pattern. An economical and effective index of the progress, extent and severity of epidemic influenza in large population groups is current measurement of excess mortality from pneumonia, influenza, bronchitis and other respiratory diseases. Such reports permit evaluation of the epidemic as a whole and are useful to health officers and others responsible for the control of influenza.

2) Closing of schools is not an effective control measure, but may be unavoidable because of extensive pupil or teacher absenteeism.

3) Hospital administrators should anticipate the increased demand for beds and staff during epidemic periods; curtailment of visiting privileges may be warranted. Elective admissions, as well as unnecessary hospitalization of mild uncomplicated influenza, should be discouraged during these periods.

D. *International measures:* In accordance with a resolution of the 22nd World Health Assembly, influenza is now a Disease under Surveillance by WHO. The following measures are recommended:

1) Prompt report to WHO of epidemics within a country, with complete description of epidemiologic characteristics.

2) Prompt identification of the causative virus in individual epidemics, with immediate report and submission

of prototype strains to WHO. Throat washings and blood samples may be sent to any one of the 92 WHO national influenza reference centers, located in 61 countries throughout the world.

3) Continuing epidemiologic studies and prompt identification of viruses by national health agencies; exchange of information with WHO to increase understanding of the basic epidemiology of influenza, to establish the broad movements of an epidemic, and to aid in early recognition of outbreaks in previously uninvolved areas.

4) Continuing effort to ensure enough commercial and/or governmental facilities to provide for rapid production of sufficient quantities of vaccine should epidemic influenza, due to a major antigenic variant of the virus, appear anywhere in the world.

KERATOCONJUNCTIVITIS, EPIDEMIC (EKC)

(Shipyard conjunctivitis, Shipyard eye, Infectious punctate keratitis)

1. **Identification**—An acute infectious disease of the eye with unilateral or bilateral inflammation of conjunctivae and edema of the lids and periorbital tissues. Onset is sudden, with pain, photophobia, blurred vision, and occasionally low-grade fever, headache, malaise and tender preauricular lymphadenopathy. Approximately 7 days after onset in about half of the cases, the cornea exhibits petechial hemorrhages and/or round subepithelial infiltrates, the latter of which may form punctate ulcers that stain with fluorescein. Duration of acute conjunctivitis is about 2 weeks, although the keratitis may continue to evolve, leaving discrete subepithelial opacities which may interfere with vision. In severe cases conjunctival membranes develop and are frequently followed by conjunctival scarring.

Diagnosis is confirmed by recovery of virus from appropriate cell cultures inoculated with eye swabs or conjunctival scrapings and by serum neutralization or hemagglutination-inhibition tests.

2. **Occurrence**—Presumably worldwide. Both sporadic cases and large outbreaks have occurred in the Far East, Hawaii, North America and Europe. Outbreaks in industrial environments in temperate climates are usually centered around the dispensary

where eye-to-eye transmission takes place. Similarly, outbreaks occur in eye hospitals and the offices of physicians.

3. **Infectious agent** — Type 8 adenovirus, occasionally other types.

4. **Reservoir** — Man.

5. **Mode of transmission** — Direct contact with eye secretions of an infected person or with contaminated instruments or solutions. In industrial plants epidemics are centered in first aid stations or dispensaries where treatment is frequently administered for minor trauma to the eye; transmission then occurs through fingers, instruments or solutions contaminated by other cases. Similar outbreaks have originated in eye clinics and offices of physicians. When dispensary professional staff and/or other dispensary and clinic personnel acquire the disease they may act as sources of infection. In the Orient, family spread is common, with children implicated in introducing the infection.

6. **Incubation period** — Probably 5 to 12 days.

7. **Period of communicability** — From late in the incubation period to 14 days after onset.

8. **Susceptibility and resistance** — There is usually complete immunity after adenovirus 8 infection. Similar conjunctivitis with minor keratitis may occur with other adenoviruses. Trauma and eye manipulation increase the risk of infection.

9. **Methods of control** —

   A. *Preventive measures:*
   1) Avoidance of communal eye medicaments.
   2) Asepsis in ophthalmologic procedures in industrial dispensaries and ophthalmic clinics and offices should include vigorous hand washing before examining each patient and the systematic sterilization of instruments after being used. Medical personnel with overt conjunctivitis should be kept out of contact with patients.
   3) Use of safety measures such as goggles in industrial plants.
   4) Education as to personal cleanliness and the danger in using common towels and toilet articles.

   B. *Control of patient, contacts, and the immediate environment:*
   1) *Report to local health authority:* Obligatory report of epidemics; no individual case report, Class 4 (see Preface).
   2) *Isolation:* Patients should use separate towels and linen

during the acute stage of the disease. Infected medical personnel should not come in contact with patients.

3) *Concurrent disinfection:* Of conjunctival and nasal discharges and articles soiled therewith. Terminal cleaning.

4) *Quarantine:* None.

5) *Immunization of contacts:* None.

6) *Investigation of contacts and source of infection:* In outbreaks the source of infection should be identified and precautions taken to prevent further transmission.

7) *Specific treatment:* None during the acute phase. If the residual opacities interfere with the patient's ability to work these may be treated with topical corticosteroids.

C. *Epidemic measures:*

1) Education medical personnel to wash hands and sterilize instruments carefully prior to and following eye examinations.

2) Organize convenient facilities for prompt diagnosis and treatment.

D. *International measures:* WHO Collaborating Centres (see Preface).

LARVA MIGRANS

A. VISCERAL LARVA MIGRANS

1. Identification — A chronic and usually mild disease of young children due to migration of certain nematode larvae in the organs and tissues. It is characterized by eosinophilia of variable duration, hepatomegaly, hyperglobulinemia and fever. In severe cases the white cell count may reach 80,000/cu mm or more, with 80-90% eosinophils. Symptoms may persist for as long as a year or two. Endophthalmitis, caused by larvae entering the eye, occurs with some frequency in older children; pneumonitis or neurological disturbances may occur. Rarely a fatal disease.

Demonstration of larvae of *Toxocara* by liver biopsy confirms the clinical diagnosis. Sero-diagnostic tests are of some value and are increasingly available.

Aberrant larvae of *Strongyloides stercordalis* are found occasionally in tissues, including some ectopic sites, but they do not persist or migrate in the tissues for long periods as do the larvae of *Toxocara,* the usual causative agents of visceral larva migrans.

2. **Occurrence**—Probably worldwide. Has had most attention in U.S.A. and Britain, but prevalence is probably no greater in them than in most countries. The severe form occurs sporadically as isolated cases in a family, mainly affecting children aged 14 to 40 months, but also occurs at older ages especially among mentally retarded children. The next older or younger sibling often shows eosinophilia or other evidence of light or residual infection. Adults infrequently infected; gardeners and others working with soil are particularly at risk.

3. **Infectious agents**—Larvae of *Toxocara canis* and *Toxocara cati.*

4. **Reservoir**—Dog and cat respectively.

5. **Mode of transmission**—By direct or indirect transmission of infective *Toxocara* eggs from contaminated soil to the mouth; directly related to eating of dirt by young children. Eggs reach the soil in feces from infected cats and dogs. They then require several weeks incubation to become infective, but remain viable and infective in soil for many months; they are adversely affected by low moisture content of soil and by freezing. After ingestion, embryonated eggs hatch in the intestine, larvae penetrate the wall and migrate to the liver and lungs by the lymphatic and circulatory systems. From the lungs, larvae spread to various organs, causing damage by their wanderings and through formation of granulomatous lesions.

6. **Incubation period**—Probably weeks or months, depending upon intensity of infection, reinfection and sensitivity of the patient.

7. **Period of communicability**—Not directly transmitted from man to man.

8. **Susceptibility and resistance**—The lower incidence in older children and adults probably relates to less exposure. Dogs usually acquire infection as puppies; infection in the female dog may end or become dormant with sexual maturity; with pregnancy, however, *T. canis* frequently becomes active and infects her fetuses. Sex and age differences are less marked for cats; older animals are somewhat less susceptible than young.

9. **Methods of control**—
   A. *Preventive measures:*
      1) Prevent contamination of soil by feces of dogs and cats

in areas immediately adjacent to houses and play areas of children especially in multiple housing projects.

2) Bury deeply, or otherwise dispose of stools of dogs and cats passed in play areas. Children's sand boxes offer an attractive site for defecating cats; cover when not in use.

3) Deworm dogs and cats less than 6 months old and there-after as indicated. Destroy worms and feces passed as a result of treatment.

4) Educate the family as to source and origin of the in-fection, particularly the danger of eating dirt.

5) Hands should always be washed after handling soil and before eating.

B. Control of patient, contacts, and the immediate environment:

1) Report to local health authority: Official report not ordinarily justifiable, Class 5 (see Preface).

2) Isolation: None.

3) Concurrent disinfection: None.

4) Quarantine: None.

5) Immunization of contacts: None.

6) Investigation of contacts and source of infection: (See 9A3). Observed dirt-eating at area of known fecal contamination by dogs is a presumptive evidence in support of the diagnosis. Disinfection of soil is not feasible.

7) Specific treatment: Diethylcarbamazine; thiabendazole is of less value.

C. Epidemic measures: Not applicable.

D. International measures: None.

B. CUTANEOUS LARVA MIGRANS

Infective larvae of cat and dog hookworm (*Ancylostoma brasiliense* and *Ancylostoma caninum*) cause a dermatitis in man, called "creeping eruption." This is a disease of utility men, gardeners, children, seabathers and others who come in contact with sandy soil contaminated with cat and dog feces; in the U.S.A., most prevalent in the Southeast. The larvae, which enter the skin, migrate intracutaneously for long periods, but eventually penetrate to deeper tissues. Each larva causes a serpiginous track, advancing several mm to a few cm a day. The disease is self-limited, with spon-taneous cure after several weeks or months. Individual larva can be killed by freezing the area with ethyl chloride spray; thiabendazole systemically or as a topical ointment is effective. In the Orient a form of creeping eruption is caused by *Gnathostoma spinigerum*, a parasite of cats and dogs. Man is infected by eating raw fish containing third stage larvae.

Differentiate from "swimmers itch" caused by intracutaneous invasion by cercariae of bird or mammalian schistosomes, which reaches maximal intensity in 2-3 days and heals in a week or more.

LASSA FEVER

1. **Identification**—An acute febrile illness with a duration of 7 to 31 days. Onset is gradual with malaise, headache, sore throat, cough, vomiting, myalgia, diarrhea, chest and abdominal pain; fever is persistent or intermittent-spiking. Oropharyngeal ulcers, lymphadenopathy, conjunctivitis and swelling of the face or neck are commonly observed. In severe cases shock, pleural effusion, cardiac and renal failure, and encephalopathy are noted. Hemorrhagic manifestations occur rarely. Leukopenia, albuminuria, and hemoconcentration are common findings. Relapses occur. Alopecia and deafness are infrequent sequellae.

Diagnosis is by isolation of virus from blood, pleural fluid, or throat washings and serologically by complement-fixation or neutralization test. Handling specimens may be dangerous.

2. **Occurrence**—First described in Nigeria in 1969; nosocomial outbreaks occurred in Nigeria and Liberia in 1970 and 1972. Naturally occurring epidemic disease in all age groups was seen in Sierra Leone over the 2-year period 1970-1972. Fatality rates from 30% to 50%. Inapparent infections, diagnosed serologically, are common.

3. **Infectious agent**—One or more closely related arenaviruses, distantly sero-related to LCM, Machupo, and Junin viruses.

4. **Reservoir**—Probably wild rodents; in Sierra Leone, the multimammate rat *Mastomys natalensis* is implicated.

5. **Mode of transmission**—Probably from saliva and urine of infected rodents and man. Person-to-person and laboratory infections occur.

6. **Incubation period**—Commonly 7 to 14 days.

7. **Period of communicability**—Nosocomial infections occur dur-

ing the acute febrile phase when virus is present in the throat. Virus excreted in urine of patients for 3 weeks or longer.

8. **Susceptibility and resistance** — All ages are susceptible; immunity of unknown duration follows infection.

9. **Methods of control** —

    A. Preventive measures: Specific rodent control.

    B. Control of patient, contacts, and the immediate environment:

        1) Report to local health authority: Individual cases should be reported, Class 2A (see Preface).

        2) Isolation: Until virus free, or three weeks, strictly enforced.

        3) Concurrent disinfection: Patient's urine, sputum, blood and all objects with which the patients had contact, with formalin or active chlorine disinfection. Terminal disinfection.

        4) Quarantine: Three weeks.

        5) Immunization of contacts: None.

        6) Investigation of contacts and source of infection: Place of residence of patient during two weeks prior to onset. Search for unreported or undiagnosed cases.

        7) Specific treatment: None. Perfusion of one or two units of convalescent plasma (proved free of Lassa virus) tried on a few occasions with presumed beneficial effect.

    C. Epidemic measures: Not determined.

    D. International measures: None.

MARBURG VIRUS DISEASE

Marburg virus disease is a systemic febrile illness which occurs rarely; it is characterized by sudden onset with prostration, fever, pains in the limbs and headache, followed by vomiting, diarrhea, a maculo-papular rash, an enanthem and a hemorrhagic diathesis. Laboratory findings indicate multiple system involvement, including liver, CNS, kidney, pancreas and heart. Leucopenia and transaminase elevation are characteristic. Of 31 persons infected by exposure to African green monkeys in 1967 in Germany and Yugoslavia, seven died. In three cases in Southern Africa in 1975, one died. Diagnosis is by isolation of the virus in tissue culture, guinea pigs, or monkeys, visualization by electron microscope, or by serologic tests. The virion measures 665 by 75 nm and is filamentous and often curled; it is not related to other known infectious agents. The reservoir is unknown. Transmission occurs by direct contact with infected blood, organs or semen and possibly by aerosol. The incubation period is 5 to 7 days. Transmission through semen has occurred after 7 weeks postinfection. Control measures in 9B, C and D in Lassa Fever apply, plus restriction of intercourse until semen is free of virus.

∞

LEISHMANIASIS, CUTANEOUS

(Aleppo, Baghdad or Delhi boil, Oriental sore; in the Americas, Espundia Uta, Chiclero or Bauru ulcer.)

1. **Identification** — A polymorphic disease of skin and mucous membranes characterized by ulcerating, indolent lesions which are single and self-limiting (simple cutaneous form), or multiple nodular (diffuse type), or muco-cutaneous lesions that involve the nasopharyngeal membranes after an initial skin infection. The later form can be fatal.

Diagnosis is by microscopic identification of Leishman-Donovan bodies in stained smears of scrapings from edges of lesions; also by culture on suitable media such as Novy, MacNeal and Nicolle's (NNN). An intradermal test (Montenegro's test) using material derived from leptomonads generally becomes positive early in the disease and remains so thereafter; no serological test is of practical value.

2. **Occurrence** — Northwest India and Pakistan, the Middle East, Southern Russia, the Mediterranean littoral, North, West, East and Central Africa; in the Americas, endemic in Mexico (especially Yucatan), most of Central America, and every country of South America except Chile. In some areas the population at risk may be large, including young children, while in other areas the disease is restricted to occupational groups such as those involved in work in forested areas. Generally more common in rural than urban areas.

3. **Infectious agents** — Old World, *Leishmania tropica;* New World, *L. brasiliensis* and *L. mexicana* — flagellate protozoa.

4. **Reservoir** — Unknown in some areas, but certain animals, such as rodents or domestic animals, mainly dogs, are proven reservoirs in other areas.

5. Mode of transmission—Commonly through bite of infective female phlebotomines (sandflies); possibly by direct contact of abraded skin with a lesion of another person; or questionably through mechanical transmission by other flies.

6. Incubation period—From a few days to many months.

7. Period of communicability—As long as parasites remain in lesions; in untreated cases a year or more. Spontaneous healing is the rule except for the muco-cutaneous and diffuse forms. Duration of infectivity of vector unknown.

8. Susceptibility and resistance—Susceptibility is probably general. Immunity is usual after lesions heal.

9. Methods of control—

A. Preventive measures:

1) There is much variation from area to area, depending on the habits of the vector phlebotomines and mammalian hosts. Where these habits are known, applicable control measures may be carried out. These measures include:

a. Periodic application of insecticides with residual action. Phlebotomine flies have a flight range of under 200 meters and are highly susceptible to control by systematic spraying with residual insecticides. Spraying should cover exterior and interior of doorways and other openings if infection occurs in dwellings, as well as possible breeding places, such as stone walls, animal houses and rubbish heaps.

b. Elimination of rubbish heaps and other breeding places.

c. Destruction of animals implicated locally as reservoirs.

d. Avoidance of sandfly-infested areas after sundown; use of insect repellents and protective clothing if exposure to sandflies is unavoidable.

2) Education of the public concerning modes of transmission and methods of controlling phlebotomines.

B. Control of patient, contacts, and the immediate environment:

1) *Report to local health authority:* Official report ordinarily not justifiable, Class 5 (see Preface).

2) *Isolation:* None. Protect patient from phlebotomines by fine mesh screen (10-12 holes to the linear centimeter or 25-30 to the linear inch; aperture size not more than 0.89 mm. or 0.035 inches) and by spraying quarters with

insecticide having residual action, and by use of repellents.

3) *Concurrent disinfection:* None.

4) *Quarantine:* None.

5) *Immunization of contacts:* None.

6) *Investigation of contacts and source of infection:* Determine local transmission cycle and interrupt it in most practical fashion.

7) *Specific treatment:* A variety of agents, including pentavalent antimonials, pyrimethamine (Daraprim), quinacrine hydrochloride, amphotericin B and cycloguanil pamoate (Camolar) may be effective; response varies by geographic area. Antimony sodium gluconate (Pentostam), the recommended drug, is available in the U.S.A. from the Center for Disease Control, (CDC), Atlanta, GA, (see Preface) on an investigational basis. In the Americas, a combination of pyrimethamine and cycloguanil pamoate has given good results. Pentamidine isethionate, available from CDC, is the drug of choice for the diffuse cutaneous form. While spontaneous healing of lesions is the rule, infections with *L brasiliensis* should always be treated.

C. *Epidemic measures:* In areas of high incidence, intensive efforts to control the disease by provision of diagnostic facilities, by mass treatment campaigns and by appropriate measures against phlebotomine flies and the mammalian reservoir hosts.

D. *International measures:* WHO Collaborating Centres (see Preface).

LEISHMANIASIS, VISCERAL

(Kala azar)

1. Identification—A chronic systemic infectious disease characterized by fever, hepatosplenomegaly, lymphadenopathy, anemia with leucopenia, and progressive emaciation and weakness. Untreated, a highly fatal disease. Fever is of gradual or sudden onset, long continued and irregular, often with 2 daily peaks; alternating

periods of apyrexia and low-grade fever follow. Chemotherapy may lead to post-Kala azar leishmanoid dermal lesions.

Diagnosis is by demonstrating Leishman-Donovan bodies in stained smears from bone marrow, spleen, liver, lymph node or blood; by recovery of the parasite, by culture of these materials on appropriate media such as Novy, MacNeal and Nicolle's (NNN), or after injection into hamsters and by indirect fluorescent antibody and other serological tests.

2. **Occurrence** — A rural disease of most tropical and subtropical areas of the world: Asia, the Middle East, Africa, South and Central America. In Europe: Southern Russia, the Caspian littoral, Portugal and Mediterranean islands. In many affected areas, a relatively common disease, mainly scattered cases among infants, children and adolescents, but occasionally in epidemic waves. Incidence is modified by the use of antimalarial insecticides.

3. **Infectious agent** — *Leishmania donovani;* a flagellated protozoan.

4. **Reservoir** — Known or presumed reservoirs include man, dogs and other canines, cats and wild rodents. The relative importance of one or the other of these animals is strikingly different from one geographic area to another.

5. **Mode of transmission** — Through bite of infective sandflies of the genus *Phlebotomus*. The fly is infected by ingesting parasites present in skin or peripheral blood of an infected reservoir host.

6. **Incubation period** — Generally 2 to 4 months; as short as 10 days or as long as 2 years.

7. **Period of communicability** — As long as parasites persist in the circulating blood or skin of the mammalian reservoir host. If man is the reservoir host, infectivity for phlebotomines may extend beyond treatment and clinical recovery. Direct transmission from man to man, and transmission by blood transfusion, through sexual contact or bite of infected laboratory animals have been reported.

8. **Susceptibility and resistance** — Susceptibility is general. Kala azar induces apparent lasting immunity, but recovery from cutaneous leishmaniasis does not confer immunity against kala azar or vice versa.

9. **Methods of control** —

   A. *Preventive measures:* Prevention of the disease is accomplished by eliminating transmission of infection to man. Methods will vary according to the local ecology and resources. Anti-phlebotomine measures such as applications of residual insecticide to the area of sandfly-man contact are generally the most practical. (see Cutaneous Leishmaniasis 9A, p. 171).

B. *Control of patient, contacts, and the immediate environment:*

1) *Report to local health authority:* In selected endemic areas; in many countries not a reportable disease, Class 3B (see Preface).

2) *Isolation:* None. (see 9B, 2, Leishmaniasis, Cutaneous, p. 171).

3) *Concurrent disinfection:* None.

4) *Quarantine:* None.

5) *Immunization:* None.

6) *Investigation of contacts and source of infection:* Ordinarily none.

7) *Specific treatment:* Antimony sodium gluconate (Pentostam), available from Center for Disease Control (CDC), Atlanta, GA (see Preface) is effective. Antimony-resistant and antimony-sensitive cases may be treated by diamidine compounds such as stilbamidine, or pentamidine isethionate. These are not used routinely because of their toxicity. In Mediterranean areas and the Sudan the parasite is more resistant than in India.

C. *Epidemic measures:* Epidemic measures must include a study of the local life cycle, followed by selection of measures that will affect mammalian and phlebotomine hosts so as to stop transmission. No method suitable for mass application will detect the infected individual in the absence of overt disease.

D. *International measures:* Coordinated programs of control among neighboring countries where the disease is endemic. WHO Collaborating Centres (see Preface).

LEPROSY

(Hansen's Disease)

1. Identification—A chronic communicable disease characterized by lesions of the skin (infiltration, macules, plaques, papules and nodules), by involvement and often palpable enlargement of peripheral nerves with consequent anesthesia, muscle weakness and paralysis, and by trophic changes in skin, muscle and bone. Two distinct major types occur: lepromatous and tuberculoid; infections of intermediate character are described as borderline; also an indeterminate form corresponds to earliest manifestations of the disease. In lepromatous leprosy there are diffuse skin lesions and invasion of mucous membranes of the upper respiratory tract as well as of the lymphoid system and some viscera; skin lesions may ulcerate, iritis and keratitis are common. The tuberculoid form is usually localized, with discretely demarcated skin lesions, relatively early nerve involvement, and frequently spontaneous healing in 1-3 years. Residual paralysis and anesthesia leading to trophic ulcers and other complications may result from either major form of leprosy. Progress of the disease is slow; death is usually due to other causes.

Diagnosis is supported by the demonstration of acid-fast bacilli in suspected lesions. Large numbers of bacilli are characteristically present in lepromatous and borderline lesions; these patients are therefore potentially infectious. Bacilli are sparse and occasionally not demonstrable in tuberculoid lesions which are nearly always anesthetic. Diagnosis of leprosy is best confirmed by biopsy of a suspected skin lesion with evaluation by a knowledgeable pathologist.

2. **Occurrence** — Mostly in the tropics and subtropics. Prevalence rates of 5 per 1000 or higher are found only in the tropics; however, socioeconomic conditions are probably more important than climate. Estimated world total is 11 million or more cases. A few countries with temperate climates have estimated rates of 1 per 1000; high rates are found throughout the Far East. In Europe, low endemicity is found in Greece, Portugal and Spain, while in several other countries, residual foci only. Reported rates in the Americas range from less than 0.1/1000 to 4.63/1000. Two to three thousand known cases live in the U.S.A., mostly representing infections acquired in endemic areas elsewhere. Newly recognized cases are more frequently diagnosed in California, Texas, Hawaii, Florida, Puerto Rico and New York City.

3. **Infectious agent** — *Mycobacterium leprae*, the leprosy (Hansen's) bacillus. Other than in man it has multiplied in the footpads of mice, in the tissues of immunosuppressed rodents, and in the armadillo.

4. **Reservoir** — Man is the only known reservoir.

5. **Mode of transmission** — Not established; bacilli from nasal discharges of infectious patients gain entrance presumably through the skin or respiratory tract. Household contact is important.

6. **Incubation period** — Shortest known is 7 months; probably the average is 3 to 5 years, although many years may elapse before recognition.

7. **Period of communicability** — If morphologically normal bacilli are demonstrable, and especially if the patient is untreated, infectiousness should be considered possible. Some clinical, laboratory, and epidemiologic evidence suggests that in previously untreated patients infectiousness is lost in most instances within 3 months of continuous therapy with dapsone (DDS), but these findings require support on a much wider scale.

8. **Susceptibility and resistance** — No proven racial immunity. Most adults appear to be non-susceptible when exposed, although subclinical infections may be the rule. Clinically diagnosable leprosy may arise in response to massive or repeated challenge; its form depends on the presence or absence of the capacity of the individual to mount a cell-mediated immunity. The lepromin (Mitsuda) test (4 weeks reading) is of no value in diagnosis, but is useful in confirming the classification (and hence the prognosis); it is completely negative in lepromatous leprosy and variably positive in tuberculoid. Positivity increases with age, urban residence, tuberculous infection, and exposure to opportunist mycobacteria.

9. **Methods of control** —

   A. *Preventive measures:*
   1) The effectiveness of DDS in suppressing infectiousness and the ease of treatment of early cases have shifted the emphasis in leprosy control from isolation to early detection and ambulatory treatment of infectious cases and surveillance of household and other close contacts for disease. Hospital facilities are valuable for initiating treatment, management of reactions and for surgical correction of deformities.
   2) Health education stressing the availability of effective therapy and the absence of infectivity of patients under continuous and effective treatment.
   3) In large controlled studies in Uganda and New Guinea prophylactic BCG apparently effected a considerable reduction in the incidence of tuberculoid leprosy among child contacts. A controlled study in Burma is showing little protection, but results of these 3 important studies are not yet final. Prophylactic DDS therapy also appeared to confer good protection to child contacts in a smaller study in Madras in India and to those under 25

in a study in Andhra Pradesh. Prophylactic acedapsone (DADDS) has given good protection in a study in Micronesia. Unpublished reports from WHO supported chemoprophylactic studies in the Philippines and India suggest that approximately 50% protection with DDS in therapeutic doses can be achieved; however, this protection appears to be of a temporary nature only.

B. *Control of patient, contacts, and the immediate environment:*
   1) *Report to local health authority:* Case reporting obligatory in most states and countries and desirable in all (Class 2B, see Preface).
   2) *Isolation:* Hospitalization is indicated only for the medical reasons listed in 9A1. No special procedures are required when cases are hospitalized. No restrictions in employment and attendance at school are indicated from the public health standpoint for patients whose disease is regarded as noninfectious.
   3) *Concurrent disinfection:* Of nasal discharges and discharges from lesions. Terminal cleaning.
   4) *Quarantine:* None.
   5) *Immunization of contacts:* BCG vaccine, or DADDS or DDS preventive therapy of household contacts of infectious cases may be used for partial protection. (see 9A3 above).
   6) *Control of contacts:* Periodic examination of household and other close contacts at 6 to 12 month intervals for at least 5 years after last contact with an infectious case.
   7) *Specific treatment:* The standard treatment is oral DDS 6-10 mg per kg body weight per week for both adults and children. In lepromatous leprosy continue therapy for at least 10 years following the disappearance of signs of disease activity, and in tuberculoid disease for at least 1-1/2 years following the disappearance of activity. Studies indicated rifampicin is more rapidly bacteriocidal than DDS, but is an expensive drug. Acedapsone (DADDS), an injectable repository sulfone, is being studied and may be useful in overcoming the irregularities inherent in daily oral DDS medication, but if used in the treatment of lepromatous leprosy, a few months of daily rifampicin should probably be added. Patients whose bacilli have become sulfone resistant are best treated with rifampicin or B663 (clofazimine). To avoid bacterial drug resistance, some recommend daily

rifampicin for the first three months of DADDS therapy.

C. *Epidemic measures:* Not applicable.

D. *International measures:* International controls should be limited to untreated infectious cases only. WHO Collaborating Centres (see Preface).

LEPTOSPIROSIS
(Weil's disease, Canicola fever, Hemorrhagic jaundice, Mud fever, Swineherd's disease.)

1. Identification — A group of diseases with protean manifestations, including fever, headache, chills, severe malaise, vomiting, muscular aches and conjunctivitis; occasionally meningitis, infrequently jaundice, renal insufficiency, hemolytic anemia and hemorrhage in skin and mucous membranes. Rash occurs occasionally. Clinical illness lasts from a few days to 3 weeks; relapses may occur. Infections may be asymptomatic. Fatality is low, but increases with advancing age and may reach 20% or more in patients with jaundice and kidney damage.

Diagnosis is confirmed by agglutination and complement-fixation tests on sera and isolation of leptospires from blood during the acute illness or from urine after the first week in special media such as Fletcher's, or bovine albumin polysorbate, or by inoculation of young guinea pigs (200 gm.), hamsters or gerbils.

2. Occurrence — Outbreaks occur among swimmers exposed to water contaminated by urine of domestic or wild animals. An occupational hazard to rice workers, sugarcane field workers, farmers, sewer workers, miners, veterinarians, animal husbandmen, abattoir workers, fish workers and military troops; a recreational hazard to bathers, campers and sportsmen in infected areas. Distribution of reservoirs of infection and of one or another serotype of leptospira is worldwide, in urban and rural, developed and primitive areas.

3. Infectious agents — Many serotypes of leptospira, such as icterohaemorrhagiae, pomona, canicola and autumnalis, have been recovered from human cases in U.S.A.; and probably others. At present 18 serogroups and more than 170 serotypes are recognized from various parts of the world.

4. **Reservoir**—Farm and pet animals, including cattle, dogs, horses and swine. Rats and other rodents are frequently infected; wild animals, including deer, squirrels, foxes, skunks, raccoons, opossums and even reptiles and amphibians (frogs) may be infected. In Europe, field mice, voles, shrews and hedgehogs are common reservoir hosts.

5. **Mode of transmission**—Contact with water, moist soil, or vegetation contaminated with urine of infected animals, as in swimming or accidental or occupational immersion; direct contact with infected animals. Infection presumably results from penetration of abraded skin or mucous membrane, or possibly through ingestion of food contaminated with urine of infected rats.

6. **Incubation period**—4 to 19 days, usually 10 days.

7. **Period of communicability**—Direct transmission from man to man is negligible.

8. **Susceptibility and resistance**—Susceptibility of man is general, varying with serotype.

9. **Methods of control**—

A. *Preventive measures:*
   1) Protection of workers in hazardous occupations by provision of boots and gloves.
   2) Identification of potentially contaminated waters.
   3) Education of the public on modes of transmission, avoidance of swimming or wading in potentially contaminated waters, and need for proper protection when work requires such exposure.
   4) Rodent control in human habitations, especially rural and recreational. Firing of cane fields before harvest.
   5) Segregation of domestic animals, and the prevention of contamination of living, working and recreational areas of man by urine of infected animals.
   6) Immunization of farm and pet animals prevents disease but not necessarily infection and renal shedding. The vaccine must represent the dominant local strains.

B. *Control of patient, contacts, and the immediate environment:*
   1) *Report to local health authority:* Obligatory case report in many states and countries, Class 2B (see Preface).
   2) *Isolation:* None.
   3) *Concurrent disinfection:* None.
   4) *Quarantine:* None.
   5) *Immunization of contacts:* None.

6) *Investigation of contacts:* Search for exposure to infected animals or history of swimming in contaminated waters.

7) *Specific treatment:* Penicillin, streptomycin, tetracycline antibiotics, and erythromycin are leptospirocidal; may be of value in the treatment of human disease when given early and in high dosage. Peritoneal or renal dialysis may be required in case of renal failure.

C. *Epidemic measures:* Search for source of infection, such as a pond used for swimming; eliminate contamination or prohibit use. Investigate industrial or occupational sources, including direct animal contact.

D. *International measures:* WHO Collaborating Centres (see Preface).

LISTERIOSIS

1. **Identification**—Usually manifested as an acute meningo-encephalitis with or without associated septicemia; less frequently, septicemia only. Onset of meningo-encephalitis is usually sudden, with fever, intense headache, nausea, vomiting and signs of meningeal irritation; delirium and coma often appear early; occasionally collapse and shock. Abortion, endocarditis, granulomatous lesions in liver and other organs, localized internal or external abscesses, and pustular or papular cutaneous lesions may occur. Septicemic listeriosis is an acute, mild, febrile illness, sometimes with influenza-like symptoms, which in pregnant women usually results in infection of the fetus and interrupted pregnancy. Infants may be stillborn, born with a massive septicemia, or develop meningitis in the neonatal period. The postpartum course of the mother is usually uneventful, but case fatality is 50% in newborn infants; approaches 100% when onset occurs in the first 4 days.

Diagnosis is confirmed by isolation of the infectious agent from spinal fluid, blood or lesions. Bacteriological methods are exacting and care must be taken to distinguish *Listeria monocytogenes* from other gram positive rods, particularly "diphtheroids." Microscopic examination of spinal fluid or meconium permits presumptive diagnosis. Fluorescent antibody tests may be useful in the examination of tissues and spinal fluid. Serologic tests are unreliable.

2. **Occurrence**—An uncommon infection. Typically sporadic, rarely in small epidemics. Occurs in all seasons, slightly more often in males than females. About 40% of clinical cases occur within the first 3 weeks of life; in adults it occurs mainly after age 40. Inapparent infections occur at all ages although they are of consequence only during pregnancy. Abortion occurs as early as the 2nd month of pregnancy but mainly in the 5th or 6th month; perinatal infection, during last trimester. Incidence unknown; in U.S.A. estimated as approximately 1 case per million population per year. European studies have disclosed large numbers of human carriers.

3. **Infectious agent**—*Listeria monocytogenes*, a bacterium.

4. **Reservoir**—Infected domestic and wild mammals, fowl and man. Asymptomatic fecal carriers have been observed in man and animals. The organism is frequently found free-living in water and mud. The seasonal use of silage as fodder is frequently followed by an increased incidence in animals.

5. **Mode of transmission**—Largely neonatal; infection is transmitted from mother to unborn infant in utero, or during its passage through infected birth canal. Papular lesions on hands and arms may occur from direct contact with infectious material, probably soils contaminated with infected animal feces. Person to person transmission through venereal contact is probable; infection from ingestion of contaminated food or inhalation is strongly suspected.

6. **Incubation period**—Unknown; probably 4 days to 3 weeks. Fetus is usually infected within several days after maternal disease.

7. **Period of communicability**—Mothers of infected newborn infants may shed infectious agent in vaginal discharges or urine for 7 to 10 days after delivery, rarely longer. Period of person to person communicability unknown.

8. **Susceptibility and resistance**—Unborn and newborn infants are highly susceptible. Children and young adults are generally resistant, adults less so after age 40. Disease is frequently superimposed on other debilitating illnesses, especially in patients receiving steroids or other immuno-suppressive agents. Little evidence of acquired immunity, even after prolonged severe infection.

9. **Methods of control**—

    A. Preventive measures:

        1) Education of pregnant women to avoid contact with infective materials on farms where the disease is endemic among livestock, and with known infected persons.

2) Proper precautions by veterinarians and farmers in handling aborted fetuses.

B. Control of patient, contacts, and the immediate environment:

1) *Report to local health authority:* Official report not ordinarily justifiable, Class 5 (see Preface).

2) *Isolation:* Of infected infants and their mothers until infectious agents are no longer present in bodily discharges.

3) *Concurrent disinfection:* Of discharges from the vagina of mothers, of discharges from eyes, nose and mouth of infants, of meconium, and of articles soiled therewith. Terminal cleaning.

4) *Quarantine:* None.

5) *Immunization of contacts:* None.

6) *Investigation of contacts and source of infection:* Of no practical value.

7) *Specific treatment:* Penicillin or ampicillin together with kanamycin, ampicillin alone, the tetracyclines, and chloramphenicol are effective. Ampicillin is preferred for maternal-fetal listeriosis; the tetracyclines are contraindicated for children under 7 years of age.

C. Epidemic measures: Not applicable; usually a sporadic disease.

D. International measures: None.

LOIASIS

1. **Identification** — A chronic filarial disease characterized by migration of the adult worm through subcutaneous or deeper tissues of the body, causing transient fugitive or calabar swellings of the trunk and extremities. Migration under the bulbar conjunctivae may be accompanied by pain and edema. Allergic reactions with giant urticaria and fever may occur occasionally, particularly in Caucasian hosts.

Female worms produce larvae (microfilariae) present in peripheral blood during the daytime, best demonstrated in stained thick blood smears or stained sediment of laked blood. The intradermal test with *Dirofilaria* antigen is diagnostically useful although nonspecific; eosinophilia is frequent.

Infection with other filariae such as *Wuchereria bancrofti, Brugia malayi, Onchocerca volvulus,* or *Dipetalonema perstans* requires differentiation in endemic areas.

2. Occurrence — Widely distributed in tropical West and Central Africa. In the Congo River basin up to 90% of indigenous inhabitants of some villages are infected.

3. Infectious agent — *Loa loa,* a nematode worm.

4. Reservoir — An infected person harboring microfilariae in the blood.

5. Mode of transmission — Transmitted by a "mangrove fly" of the genus *Chrysops. Chrysops dimidiata, C. silacea* and other species ingest blood and microfilariae. The larvae develop within 10 to 20 days in the fat body of the fly. The developed larvae migrate to the proboscis and are transferred to a human host by the bite of the infective flies.

6. Incubation period — Symptoms usually do not appear until several years after infection but may occur as early as 4 months. Microfilariae may appear in the peripheral blood 5 to 6 months after infection.

7. Period of communicability — The adult worms may live in man as long as 17 years and microfilariae may be present in the blood during this time; in the fly, communicability is from 10 to 20 days after its infection and until all infective larvae have migrated or until the fly dies.

8. Susceptibility and resistance — Susceptibility is universal; repeated infections occur and immunity, if present, has not been demonstrated.

9. Methods of control —

   A. Preventive measures:

     1) Measures directed against the aquatic fly larvae have not proved practical or effective, as breeding areas are usually extensive.

     2) Diethyltoluamide (DEET), dimethylphthalate or detamide (DET) applied to exposed skin are effective repellants.

   B. Control of patient, contacts, and the immediate environment:

     1) Report to local health department: Official report ordinarily not justifiable, Class 5 (see Preface).

     2) Isolation: Not practicable. So far as possible, patients with microfilariae in the blood should be protected from

Chrysops bites as a means of reducing transmission.

3) *Concurrent disinfection:* None

4) *Quarantine:* None.

5) *Immunization of contacts:* None.

6) *Investigation of contacts:* None; a community problem.

7) *Specific treatment:* Diethylcarbamazine (Hetrazan) causes disappearance of microfilariae and may kill the adult worm with resulting cure; however, hypersensitivity reactions commonly occur during therapy. Surgical removal of adult worm for relief of acute bulbar conjunctivitis is indicated.

C. *Epidemic measures:* Not applicable.

D. *International measures:* WHO Collaborating Centres (see Preface).

∞

LYMPHOCYTIC CHORIOMENINGITIS (LCM)

1. **Identification**—A viral disease of animals, especially mice, transmissible to man, with a marked diversity of clinical manifestations. Occasionally begins with an influenza-like attack and terminates by recovery; more frequently, after a few days of remission, meningeal symptoms suddenly appear. Attacks sometimes begin with meningeal or meningoencephalomyelitic symptoms. In most severe cases the primary pathologic findings are hemorrhagic meningoencephalitis with the specific symptoms depending solely on the area involved and the severity of the particular lesion. The course is usually short; it is very rarely fatal, and even with extremely severe disease (e.g. coma with meningoencephalitis) prognosis for recovery without sequelae is relatively good. The cerebrospinal fluid varies from entirely normal to pleocytotic depending on the severity of the pathologic changes.

Laboratory diagnostic methods include isolation of virus from blood, urine, nasopharynx, or spinal fluid early in the attack by intracerebral inoculation of guinea pigs or LCM-free mice or in tissue cultures, and rising titers of antibodies demonstrated by indirect immunofluorescence, complement fixation, or neutralization testing of paired sera. Requires differentiation from other aseptic meningitides.

2. **Occurrence** — Uncommon. Foci of infection often persist within limits of a city block for months or years, resulting in sporadic clinical disease. Outbreaks have occurred in USA and in Germany from Syrian hamsters sold as pets or laboratory animals.

3. **Infectious agent** — The virus of lymphocytic choriomeningitis, an arenavirus.

4. **Reservoir** — The infected house mouse, *Mus musculus;* naturally infected guinea pigs, hamsters, monkeys, dogs and swine have been implicated.

5. **Mode of transmission** — Virus is excreted in urine, saliva and feces of infected animals, usually mice. Transmission to man is probably through contaminated food or dust, possibly by arthropods; no evidence of man-to-man spread by ordinary contact. Biological products of animal origin have been found contaminated.

6. **Incubation period** — Probably 8 to 13 days; 15 to 21 days to meningeal symptoms.

7. **Period of communicability** — Not known to be directly transmitted from man to man. Naturally infected mice may carry and excrete the virus through life; the infected female transmits virus to offspring.

8. **Susceptibility and resistance** — Unknown. Sera of persons recovered from the disease neutralize virus, as occasionally do the sera of persons without a history of recognized attack.

9. **Methods of control** —

   A. *Preventive measures:* Cleanliness of home and place of work; elimination of mice and disposal of other diseased animals. Virologic surveillance of rodent breeding establishments, especially those producing hamsters and mice.

   B. *Control of patient, contacts, and the immediate environment:*
      1) *Report to local health authority:* Official report not ordinarily justifiable, Class 5 (see Preface).
      2) *Isolation:* None.
      3) *Concurrent disinfection:* Of discharges from the nose and throat, of urine and feces, and of articles soiled therewith.
      4) *Quarantine:* None.
      5) *Immunization of contacts:* None.
      6) *Investigation of contacts and source of infection:* Home and place of employment for presence of house mice or rodent pets.

7) *Specific treatment:* None.

C. *Epidemic measures:* Not applicable.

D. *International measures:* None.

LYMPHOGRANULOMA VENEREUM
(Lymphogranuloma inguinale, Lymphopathia venereum, Climatic bubo)

1. Identification — A venereally acquired systemic infectious disease of lymph channels and lymph nodes, possibly culminating in bubo formation, ulceration, elephantiasis of genitalia, and rectal stricture. May begin with a small, painless evanescent erosion, papule, nodule or herpetiform lesion, usually on the penis or in the vulva, rectum or urethra, followed shortly by acute, subacute or chronic adenitis, commonly inguinal with adherence to skin as well as underlying tissues and usually with multiple foci of suppuration; a bubo, usually painless, may be the first manifestation. Fever, chills, headache, vague abdominal aches, joint pains, and anorexia often occur during lymphatic progression. Spontaneous regression of buboes does not indicate recovery; course often long, disability great, but generally not fatal.

Diagnosis is by culture of bubo aspirate, or by complement-fixation test. Skin tests with Frei antigen significant if positive; may be negative if infection is not by the same antigenic type.

2. Occurrence — More common than ordinarily believed; widespread throughout the world, especially in tropical and subtropical areas. Endemic in southern U.S.A., and in Asian and African countries, particularly among lower socioeconomic classes; age incidence is that of greatest sexual activity; most frequent among sexually promiscuous persons, including homosexuals; sex differences not pronounced; all races affected.

3. Infectious agent — *Chlamydia (Bedsonia) trachomatis* which includes several antigenic types (TRIC agents).

5. Mode of transmission — Direct contact with open lesions of infected persons during sexual intercourse; indirect contact with articles, including clothing contaminated by discharges; children commonly infected from bedfellows.

6. Incubation period — Five to 21 days to primary lesion, usually

7 to 12; if bubo is first manifestation, 10 to 30 days, sometimes several months.

7. **Period of communicability** — Variable, from weeks to years, during presence of active lesions.

8. **Susceptibility and resistance** — Susceptibility general; status of natural or acquired resistance unclear.

9. **Methods of control** —

A. *Preventive measures:* Except for measures which are specific for syphilis, preventive measures are those for venereal diseases. See Syphilis 9A (pp. 316-317) and Granuloma inguinale 9A (p. 137).

B. *Control of patient, contacts, and the immediate environment:*
1) *Report to local health authority:* In selected endemic areas (U.S.A., some states); in most states and countries not a reportable disease, Class 3C (see Preface).
2) *Isolation:* None. Refrain from sexual contact until all lesions are healed.
3) *Concurrent disinfection:* None; care in disposal of discharges from lesions and of articles soiled therewith.
4) *Quarantine:* None.
5) *Immunization of contacts:* Not applicable; prompt treatment or recognition or clinical suspicion of infection.
6) *Investigation of contacts:* Search for sexual contacts of patient before and after appeared disease.
7) *Specific treatment:* Tetracycline antibiotics are effective for all stages, including buboes and ulcerative lesions. Administer orally for 10 days or longer as indicated by clinical response. Do not incise bubo; drain by aspiration.

C. *Epidemic measures:* Not applicable.

D. *International measures:* See Syphilis 9D (p. 138).

MADUROMYCOSIS
(Madura foot, Mycetoma)

1. **Identification** — A clinical syndrome of diverse etiology characterized by swelling and suppuration of subcutaneous tissues, and formation of sinus tracts. Lesions usually are on the foot or lower leg, sometimes on the hand, over the shoulders and back in burden bearers, and rarely in other sites.

Isolation of the fungus in culture and study of the granules in fresh preparations or histopathologic slides are necessary for conclusive identification.

2. **Occurrence** — Rare in continental U.S.A.; common in Mexico, northern Africa, southern Asia and other tropical and subtropical areas, especially where people go barefoot.

3. **Infectious agents** — Actinomycetic mycetoma is caused by *Nocardia brasiliensis, N. asteroides, N. caviae, N. madurae, N. pelletieri* or *Streptomyces somaliensis.* Mycotic mycetoma is caused principally by *Madurella mycetomi, M. grisea, Monosporium apiospermum, (Allescheria boydii), Phialophora jeanselmei, Cephalosporium recifei, C. falciforme, Leptosphaeria senegalensis, Neotestudina rosatii,* and *Pyrenochaeta romeroi,* or several others. Mycetoma may be difficult to distinguish from chronic osteomyelitis due to a variety of bacteria and fungi.

4. **Reservoir** — Presumably soil and decaying vegetation.

5. **Mode of transmission** — Subcutaneous implantation of spores or hyphal elements from a saprophytic source by penetrating wounds (thorns, splinters).

6. **Incubation period** — Usually months.

7. **Period of communicability** — Not directly transmitted from man to man.

8. **Susceptibility and resistance** — Unknown.

9. **Methods of control** —

   A. *Preventive measures:* Protection against small puncture wounds, as by wearing shoes or protective clothing.

   B. *Control of patient, contacts, and the immediate environment:*
      1) *Report to local health authority:* Official report ordinarily not justifiable, Class 5 (see Preface).
      2) *Isolation:* None.
      3) *Concurrent disinfection:* Ordinary cleanliness.
      4) *Quarantine:* None
      5) *Immunization of contacts:* None.

6) Investigation of contacts and source of infection: Not profitable.

7) Specific treatment: None. Sulfones or long-acting sulfonamides benefit some cases of actinomycetic mycetoma. Penicillin and other antibiotics are not useful. Resection of small lesions may be helpful, while amputation of an extremity with advanced lesions may be required.

C. *Epidemic measures:* Not applicable, a sporadic disease.

D. *International measures:* WHO Collaborating Centres (see Preface).

MALARIA

1. Identification—The four diseases that constitute the human malarias can be sufficiently similar in their symptoms to be difficult to differentiate without laboratory studies. The most serious, falciparum or malignant tertian malaria, may present in a very varied clinical picture including fever (not characterized by classical recurrence), chills and sweating, headache, icterus, coagulation defects, shock, renal failure, acute encephalitis and coma. It should be considered as a possible cause of coma and other central nervous symptoms, such as disorientation and delirium, in any person recently returned from a tropical area. Even in apparently mild forms of disease, prompt treatment is essential since irreversible complications may appear suddenly; case fatality among untreated children and nonimmune adults exceeds 10%.

The other human malarias, vivax or benign tertian, quartan, and ovale, generally are not life threatening except in the very young or in patients with concurrent disease. They may begin with indefinite malaise followed by a shaking chill and rapidly rising temperature, usually accompanied by headache and nausea and ending with profuse sweating. After an interval free of fever, the cycle of chills, fever, and sweating is repeated, either daily, every other day or every 3rd day. Duration of untreated primary attack varies from a week to a month or longer. Relapses are common and may occur at irregular intervals for several years.

Individuals who have been taking prophylactic drugs may show a wide variation in the incubation period and an atypical clinical picture.

Laboratory confirmation should always be sought through demonstration of malaria parasites in blood films by microscopic examination. Repeated examinations may be necessary; the thick film method is most likely to reveal the parasite; parasites are often not demonstrable in films from patients recently or actively under treatment. Antibodies, demonstrable by fluorescent antibody or other test, appear after the first week of the infection and persist for many years.

2. **Occurrence** — Epidemic malaria no longer occurs in many temperate zone countries but is a major cause of ill health in many parts of the tropics and subtropics. Certain tropical countries with a long history of hyperendemic malaria have greatly reduced the incidence by modern control measures. In other tropical countries where malaria control programs have been interrupted, malaria rates have risen to epidemic proportions. *Plasmodium falciparum* strains, refractory to cure with the 4-aminoquinolines (and many other synthetic drugs), occur in some areas of both hemispheres. In Asia the known range is from West Irian and Assam to Burma; in the Americas the confirmed distribution covers most of tropical South America east of the Andes, both the Caribbean and Pacific sides of Colombia and Panama. Resistance to the 4-aminoquinolines has not been confirmed in Africa.

3. **Infectious agents** — *Plasmodium vivax* for vivax or benign tertian malaria, *P. malariae* for quartan malaria, *P. falciparum* for falciparum or malignant tertian malaria and *P. ovale* for the less common ovale malaria seen only in West Africa. Mixed infections not infrequently occur in endemic areas.

4. **Reservoir** — Man is the only important reservoir of human malaria, although higher apes may harbor *P. malariae*. Monkeys are naturally infected by *P. knowlesi, P. cynomolgi, P. brasilianum, P. inui* and *P. simium,* all of which can infect man.

5. **Mode of transmission** — Transmitted by an infective female anopheline mosquito. Certain species of *Anopheles* ingest human blood containing plasmodia in the gametocyte stage. The male and female gametocytes unite in the stomach and sporozoites develop in from 8 to 35 days, depending on species of parasite and the temperature to which the vector is exposed. Sporozoites concentrate in the salivary glands and are injected into man as the insect thereafter takes blood meals. In the susceptible host, gametocytes usually appear in the blood within 3 to 14 days after onset of symptoms, according to species of parasite. Malaria may also be transmitted by injection or transfusion of blood of infected persons or by use of contaminated hypodermic syringes, as by drug addicts. Congenital transmission may occur.

6. Incubation period—Average 12 days for *P. falciparum,* 14 days for *P. vivax* and *P. ovale,* and 30 days for *P. malariae.* With some strains of *P. vivax,* there may be a protracted incubation period of 8 to 10 months. With infection by blood transfusion, incubation is usually short, but varies with the number of parasites in the transfused blood.

7. Period of communicability—For mosquito infection, as long as infective gametocytes are present in the blood of patients; varies with species and strain of parasite and with response to therapy. In untreated or insufficiently treated cases, infective gametocytes may be found indefinitely in quartan malaria, from 1 to 3 years in vivax, and generally not more than 1 year in falciparum malaria. The mosquito remains infective for the rest of her life, a few days to a month or more.

8. Susceptibility and resistance—Susceptibility is universal, but the degree sometimes is lessened by previous infection. Tolerance to infection is present in adults in highly endemic communities where exposure to infective anophelines is continuous over many years. Some African ethnic groups show a partial resistance to infection with *P. vivax.*

9. Methods of control—

   A. Preventive measures:

      1) Regular use of suppressive drugs in malarious areas.* For suppression or prophylaxis of nonimmune American civilians temporarily residing in or traveling through endemic areas, chloroquine (Aralen) 300 mg base (400 mg chloroquine phosphate), or amodiaquine (Camoquin) 400 mg base (520 mg amodiaquine dihydrochloride) once weekly. Alternative regimens would be: pyrimethamine (Daraprim), 25 mg once weekly; or proguanil monohydrochloride (chlorguanide) (Paludrine), 100 mg daily. For persons who have been on suppressive drugs and are leaving an endemic area, primaquine base, 15 mg (26.3 mg primaquine phosphate), may be given daily for 14 days concurrently with the suppressive chloroquine. Alternately, primaquine, 45 mg base, may be administered once a week for 8 weeks. In either case the suppressive drug is continued on the original schedule. All doses noted above are for adults of average weight; for children they should be adjusted according to weight.

* See "Information on Malaria Risk for International Travelers," published periodically in the "WHO Weekly Epidemiological Report."

2) Effective treatment of acute and chronic cases is an important adjunct to malaria control and is essential in attempted eradication, along with case detection methods to locate those still infected.

3) Application of residual insecticide (chlorinated hydrocarbons such as DDT, benzene hexachloride or dieldrin) in suitable formulae and dosage on the inside walls of dwellings and on other surfaces upon which vector anophelines habitually rest will generally result in effective malaria control, except where vector resistance to these insecticides has developed. When the latter occurs, the chlorinated hydrocarbons can be replaced by carbamate compounds (such as propoxur) or organophosphates (such as malathion or fenitrothion). These are effective in residual application, but may be more toxic to man in certain formulations. Entire communities should be treated in spraying projects, to be carried forward year after year until malaria ceases to be endemic. Afterward surveillance activities may be used to eliminate residual parasites in man. Countrywide effort over at least 4 consecutive years, followed by adequate surveillance, has eradicated malaria in some localized regions.

4) Where residual insecticide is not available, nightly spraying of living and sleeping quarters with a liquid or an aerosol preparation of pyrethrum or other space sprays is useful.

5) In endemic areas, install screens in living and sleeping quarters or use bed nets.

6) Insect repellents such as diethyltoluamide, dimethylphthalate, or 2-ethylhexane-diol, 1,3, (Rutgers 612) applied to uncovered skin and impregnated in the clothing of persons exposed to bites of vector anophelines, are useful, but need to be repeatedly reapplied for continued effectiveness.

7) Sanitary improvements, such as filling and draining which result in permanent elimination or reduction of anopheline breeding habitats should be encouraged. Larvicides (such as oil and Paris green) are not now commonly used where residual spraying is effective, but may be useful under special conditions. The chlorinated hydrocarbons are not recommended as larvicides, but organo-phosphorus compounds such as temephos (Abate) or fenthion may be of value. Effectiveness of

antilarval methods varies with the particular vector species involved.

8) Blood donors should be questioned for a history of malaria or possible exposure to the disease; in U.S.A., blood donors may be used six months after return from an endemic area if they have not taken antimalarial drugs and have been free of symptoms; if they have been on antimalarial prophylaxis, or have had malaria, or have immigrated or are visiting from endemic areas, they may be accepted as donors three years after cessation of chemoprophylaxis or chemotherapy or departure from the endemic area if they have remained asymptomatic. If the migrant or visitor is from an area where quartan malaria is endemic, transfusion transmission or *P. malariae* infection may occur under these conditions.

B. *Control of patient, contacts, and the immediate environment:*

1) *Report to local health authority:* Obligatory case report as a *Disease under Surveillance by WHO,* Class 1 (see Preface), in nonendemic areas, desirably limited to authenticated cases (U.S.A.); Class 3C (see Preface), is the more practical procedure in endemic areas.

2) *Isolation:* None. Patients should be in mosquito proof areas at night.

3) *Concurrent disinfection:* A single concurrent residual spraying of the neighborhood may be useful if a primary or relapsing case occurs in an area not under control but previously free from the disease and where potential vectors are active.

4) *Quarantine:* None.

5) *Immunization of contacts:* Not applicable.

6) *Investigation of contacts:* Determine history of previous infection among household members or of exposure to anophelines. In advanced stages of eradication, attempt to determine source of infection in every detected case by mass blood survey in the neighborhood; treat persons with fever by "presumptive" single-dose therapy even before result of blood examination is known. If a history of needle-sharing in illicit drug use is obtained from the patient, investigate and appropriately treat all persons who shared the injection equipment.

7) *Specific treatment for all forms of malaria in adults:*

a) For acute cases in nonimmune subjects, except *P. falciparum* infections acquired in South America or

Southeast Asia, chloroquine base orally over 3 to 5 days in dosages of 600 mg base initially, 300 mg base 6 hours later, and 300 mg on each of the next 2 to 5 days (total dose 1500 to 2400 mg); or amodiaquine base orally over 3 days in dosages of 600 mg base initially, and 400 mg base on each of the next 2 days (total dose 1400 mg); or quinine sulfate or dihydrochloride, 650 mg every 8 hours for 3 days, then every 12 hours for the next 7 days, or a total of 15,000 mg orally over a 10 day period.

b) For acute cases, emergency treatment of grave infections, or for persons unable to retain orally administered medication, chloroquine hydrochloride,* 300 mg base, intramuscularly, repeated if needed in 6 hours, but not more than 900 mg base per 24 hours; or quinine dihydrochloride* 650 mg (10 grains) diluted in a liter of normal saline, glucose or plasma administered intravenously and slowly, repeated if needed in 6 hours but not more than 3 injections per 24 hours. Intravenous chloroquine administration is seldom required, since intramuscular chloroquine produces a rapid response. If there is evidence of renal failure, quinine dosages should be reduced. All parenteral drugs should be discontinued as soon as oral drug administration can be initiated.

c) For *P. falciparum* infections acquired in South America or Southeast Asia: many of these infections respond poorly or not at all to the synthetic 4-aminoquinolines, pyrimethamine and/or chlorguanide. For such persons or any patient developing clinical malaria while on chloroquine prophylaxis, quinine orally (or parenterally if required) should be used in the dosage and on the schedules noted in the previous paragraphs. Concurrently, for the first 3 days of treatment, pyrimethamine may be administered in a dose of 25 mg twice daily by mouth for a total of 150 mg. In instances of repeated reappearance of clinical illness despite therapy as indicated above, or when quinine is not tolerated, good results may be obtained with combinations of sulfonamides or sulfones and pyrimethamine given over a 3-5 day period. (Promising new drugs, such as

---

* Available in U.S.A. from Center for Disease Control, Atlanta, Georgia, if not available locally (see Preface).

phenanthrene- and the quinoline-methanol compounds, effective against these refractory strains, are under active study).

d) For prevention of relapses in *P. vivax, P. malariae* and *P. ovale* infections acquired by mosquito bites, and treated as in 9B7a or 9B7b: the oral administration of primaquine, 15 mg base, daily for 14 days, usually is adequate to eradicate the secondary tissue forms of the parasite, but in some areas, e.g., New Guinea, it has been increased to 22.5 mg daily in relapsing infections. Primaquine may be administered concurrently with the other drug or following completion of the primary therapy. Certain individuals, particularly those originating from the eastern Mediterranean and African areas, may develop hemolysis from this dosage of primaquine.

All doses in this paragraph are for adults of average weight. Doses of antimalarial drugs for children should be adjusted according to age and especially weight.

C. Epidemic measures: A field survey to determine the nature and extent of the epidemic situation is the point of departure. Intensify residual spraying, directed against adult and larval stages, find and treat acute cases and use suppressive drugs. Sometimes the breeding places of anophelines responsible for an epidemic can be eliminated. Mass chemoprophylaxis must be considered.

D. International measures:

1) Disinsection of aircraft, ships or other vehicles on arrival in an area free from malaria or any of its vectors, if the health authority at the place of arrival has reason to suspect importation of malaria vectors.

2) Disinsection of aircraft before departure or in transit from an area where vectors have become resistant to a particular insecticide or insecticides, using an insecticide of a type to which the vectors are still susceptible.

3) Strong effort to maintain rigid antimosquito sanitation within the mosquito flight range of all ports and airports.

4) In special circumstances, administration of antimalarial drugs to migrants, seasonal workers or persons taking part in periodic mass movement into an area or country where malaria has been eliminated. Primaquine, 45 mg base, given as a single dose on a weekly basis renders the

gametocytes of the human malarias (including all *P. falciparum* drug-refractory strains tested) noninfectious for mosquitoes.

5) WHO is supporting a worldwide antimalarial eradication program; WHO Collaborating Centres (see Preface).

6) In accordance with the Resolution of the 22nd World Health Assembly, malaria is now a *Disease under Surveillance by WHO,* and procedures for the collection and distribution of information on an international basis have been developed.

BABESIOSIS

Several species of *Babesia,* a tick-transmitted hematogenous protozoan related to malaria parasites, are a common cause of febrile illness in domestic animals, but rarely in man. Five human cases have been reported, three in the United States, two of which were on Nantucket Island; all were caused by *Babesia microti,* a rodent parasite. Three of the five cases had had prior splenectomy; two of the three died. The survivors all received chloroquine. The diagnosis is based on the morphological appearance of the red cell parasite, easily mistaken for *Plasmodia* but atypical in shape, with no pigment production and without schizont or gametocyte forms.

MEASLES

(Morbilli, Hard measles, Rubeola, Red measles)

1. Identification—An acute, highly communicable viral disease with prodromal fever, conjunctivitis, coryza, bronchitis, and Koplik spots on the buccal mucosa. A characteristic dusky-red blotchy rash appears on the 3rd to 7th day, beginning on the face, becoming generalized, lasting 4 to 6 days and sometimes ending in bran-like desquamation. Leucopenia is usual. More severe in adults. In the U.S.A., death from uncomplicated measles is rare; such deaths as occur are from secondary pneumonia, mainly in children less than 2 years old; occasionally from postinfectious encephalitis. Measles is a severe disease among malnourished children of developing countries, with a fatality rate of 5 to 10% or more. It has been recently demonstrated that subacute sclerosing panencephalitis (SSPE) may develop in children 4-10 years following a natural measles infection.

Virus isolation from blood, conjunctivae and nasopharynx in tissue culture or demonstration of a rise in specific hemagglutination-inhibiting, hemolysis-inhibiting, or complement-fixing antibodies may be desirable, but the necessary laboratory facilities are often not readily available.

2. **Occurrence** — Common in childhood; in unimmunized populations probably 90% or more of persons surviving to age 20 years have had measles; few persons go through life without an attack. Endemic in large metropolitan communities, attaining epidemic proportions about every other year. In smaller communities and areas outbreaks tend to be more widely spaced and somewhat more severe. With long intervals between outbreaks, as in the Arctic and some island areas, measles often affects large portions of the population and the fatality rate may be higher. In temperate climates it is prevalent in all seasons, but primarily in late winter and early spring.

3. **Infectious agent** — Measles virus.

4. **Reservoir** — Man.

5. **Mode of transmission** — By droplet spread or direct contact with nasal or throat secretions or urine of infected persons; indirectly and less commonly airborne, or by articles freshly soiled with secretions of nose and throat. One of the most readily transmitted communicable diseases.

6. **Incubation period** — About 10 days, varying from 8 to 13 days, exposure to onset of fever; about 14 days until rash appears; uncommonly longer or shorter. Late measles immune serum globulin inoculation in attempted passive protection may extend incubation to 21 days.

7. **Period of communicability** — From the beginning of the prodromal period to 4 days after appearance of the rash.

8. **Susceptibility and resistance** — Practically all persons are susceptible; permanent acquired immunity is usual after attack. Infants born of mothers who have had the disease are ordinarily immune for approximately the first 6 months of life.

9. **Methods of control** —

    A. *Preventive measures:*

        1) Vaccination. Live attenuated measles virus vaccines have been widely used, while inactivated vaccines are much more limited in use and effectiveness.

a) Live attenuated vaccines: Several types are in use. A single injection induces active immunity in more than 95% of susceptible children for over 12 years, probably for life. The majority have mild or inapparent noncommunicable infection with minimal symptoms: 10-15% develop fever to 39.4°C (103°F) rectal on 4th to 10th day, lasting 2-5 days but with little disability; of these, 10-15% may have rash as fever subsides; a few have coryza, mild cough and Koplik spots. Concomitant measles immune globulin reduces these reactions but is not indicated with "further attenuated" vaccines. Uncommonly, mild seizures may occur without known sequelae as a febrile response to vaccine; rare reports of encephalitis (1 per million doses) may occur in normal children but its relation to vaccine is not established.

Indications for immunization: All children at 12 months of age or as soon thereafter as possible. In areas with high morbidity and mortality in children under 1 year of age, vaccine may be given between 6 and 12 months of age, but a booster dose must be given after a year of age (may be given simultaneoulsy with rubella and/or mumps vaccines). In the face of epidemic exposure, it may be desirable to vaccinate younger infants, recognizing an even greater need for the booster dose. Rarely indicated for adults as nearly all are immune; reactions approximate those of children. Recommended especially for institutionalized children and for those with cystic fibrosis, tuberculosis, heart disease, and asthma and other chronic pulmonary diseases.

Contraindications to the use of live vaccines are: Pregnancy, leukemia, lymphomas, other generalized neoplasms; resistance-depressing therapy, antimetabolites); severe illness; active tuberculosis not under treatment; severe egg sensitivity, and prior transfusion of whole blood or injection of immune serum globulin (human) in which case administration should be delayed 8-12 weeks to prevent neutralizing the vaccine.

b) Inactivated vaccine: Use not recommended in U.S.A. because of short-lived protection and because of unusual and severe reactions observed when individuals inoculated with inactivated vaccine develop natural measles infection later.

2) Education. Health departments and private physicians should encourage measles vaccine for all susceptible infants and children; those for whom vaccine is contraindicated and who are exposed to measles in families or institutions, should be protected by measles immune globulin (human).

B. Control of patient, contacts, and the immediate environment:

1) *Report to local health authority:* Obligatory case report in most states and in many countries, Class 2B (see Preface). Early report permits opportunity for better outbreak control.

2) *Isolation:* Impractical in the community at large; simply immunize siblings. In hospitals isolation from onset of catarrhal stage through 3rd day of rash reduces exposure of other children at high risk.

3) *Concurrent disinfection:* None.

4) *Quarantine:* Usually impractical and of no value. Quarantine of institutions, wards or dormitories for young children is of value; strict segregation of infants if measles occurs in an institution.

5) *Protection of contacts:* Live vaccine given before or on the day of exposure usually prevents natural measles; no known adverse effect if given later in incubation period. If vaccine is contraindicated, measles immune serum globulin given in the first 3 days after exposure will usually prevent disease; given later it will modify the attack.

6) *Investigation of contacts:* A search for and immunization of exposed susceptible children under 3 years of age is profitable. Carriers are unknown.

7) *Specific treatment:* None.

C. Epidemic measures:

1) Prompt reporting of suspected cases and comprehensive immunization programs to cover all potential susceptibles and limit spread.

2) In institutional outbreaks, protective doses of measles immune serum globulin (human), to all susceptibles for whom live vaccine is contraindicated. New admissions should be immunized, or passively protected.

3) In many less developed population groups and countries measles has a high fatality rate. If vaccine is available,

prompt use at the beginning of an epidemic is essential to limit spread; if vaccine supply is limited, priority should be given to young children for whom risk is greatest.

D. International measures: None.

MELIOIDOSIS

1. **Identification** — An uncommon disease, with a range of clinical manifestations from inapparent infection or asymptomatic pulmonary consolidation to a rapidly fatal septicemia. It may simulate typhoid fever or, more commonly, tuberculosis, including pulmonary cavitation, empyema, chronic abscesses, and osteomyelitis.

Diagnosis depends upon isolation of the causative agent, although acute and convalescent agglutination or fluorescent antibody titers may be of confirmatory value. The possibility of melioidosis should be kept in mind in any unexplained suppurative disease, especially cavitating pulmonary disease, in a patient living in, or recently returned from, Southeast Asia.

2. **Occurrence** — Clinical disease is uncommon, generally occurring in individuals who have had intimate contact with soil and water. It may appear as a complication of an overt wound or may follow aspiration of water. Cases have been recorded in, but probably not restricted to, Southeast Asia, Iran, Northeast Australia, Ecuador, Panama, New Guinea, Guam, and Aruba. In certain of these areas, 5-20% of agricultural workers have demonstrable antibodies but no history of overt disease.

3. **Infectious agent** — *Pseudomonas pseudomallei (Loefflerella whitmori)*, Whitmore's bacillus.

4. **Reservoir** — Various animals, including sheep, goats, horses, swine, monkeys and rodents (and a variety of animals in zoological gardens) can become infected. There is no evidence that they are important reservoirs except in transfer of the agent to new foci. The organism is saprophytic in certain soils and waters.

5. **Mode of transmission** — By contact with contaminated soil or water through overt or inapparent skin wounds, by aspiration or ingestion of contaminated water, or by inhalation of dust from soil.

6. **Incubation period** — Can be as short as 2 days. However,

several months or years may elapse between the presumed exposure and the appearance of clinical disease.

7. **Period of communicability** — Man-to-man transmission, except by direct inoculation, has not been proved. Laboratory infections are uncommon.

8. **Susceptibility and resistance** — Disease in man is uncommon even among persons in endemic areas who have close contact with soil or water containing the infectious agent. Many patients become infected following severe injuries or burns or have a history of diabetes or other systemic disease.

9. **Methods of control** —

   A. *Preventive measures:* Unknown.

   B. *Control of patient, contacts, and the immediate environment:*
      1) *Report to local health authority:* Optional report, Class 3B (see Preface).
      2) *Isolation:* Wound isolation precautions.
      3) *Concurrent disinfection:* Safe disposal of sputum and wound discharges.
      4) *Quarantine:* None.
      5) *Management of contacts:* None.
      6) *Investigation of contacts and source of infection:* Human carriers are not known.
      7) *Specific treatment:* In vitro tests show susceptibility to sulfonamides, chloramphenicol and tetracyclines. A favorable outcome may be expected in many subacute and chronic cases. The method of treatment for septicemic cases has not been established, although recovery has been recorded following administration of drug combinations such as tetracycline and chloramphenicol in heroic amounts.

   C. *Epidemic measures:* Not applicable to man; a sporadic disease.

   D. *International measures:* None, although livestock should be examined for evidence of disease when being moved to non-endemic areas.

GLANDERS

Glanders is a highly communicable disease of horses, mules, and donkeys; it has disappeared from most areas of the world, although enzootic foci are known to exist in Mexico and Eastern Asia.

Human infection has occurred rarely and sporadically and almost exclusively in those whose occupations involve contact with animals, or work in laboratories. Infection with the etiological organism, *Pseudomonas mallei (Mallemyces mallei)*, the glanders bacillus, cannot be differentiated serologically from *P. pseudomallei;* differentiation from melioidosis can only be accomplished by characterization of the isolated organism. Prevention depends on control of glanders in the equine species and care in handling causative organisms. Cases in man have been infrequent, even among those having close association with infected animals.

∝⋖⋗

MENINGITIS, ASEPTIC

(Viral meningitis, Serous meningitis, Nonbacterial or Abacterial meningitis)

1. **Identification**—A common, usually nonfatal, clinical syndrome with multiple viral etiologies, characterized by sudden onset of febrile illness with signs and symptoms of meningeal involvement, spinal fluid findings of pleocytosis, (usually mononuclear but may be polymorphonuclear in early stages), increased protein, normal sugar, and absence of bacteria. Active illness seldom exceeds 10 days. Transient paresis and encephalitic manifestations may occur. Paralysis is unusual. Residual signs lasting a year or more may include weakness, muscle spasm, insomnia and personality changes. Recovery is usually complete. A morbilliform rash resembling rubella characterizes certain types caused by echoviruses and coxsackieviruses. Vesicular and petechial rashes occur. Gastrointestinal and/or respiratory symptoms may be associated with the enterovirus groups.

Under optimal conditions, specific identification, using serologic and isolation techniques, can be made in more than half of the infections. Viral agents may be isolated in early stages from specimens of blood, throat washings, stool, or spinal fluid by tissue culture techniques or animal inoculation.

Differential diagnosis: Various diseases caused by nonviral agents may mimic aseptic meningitis, such as inadequately treated pyogenic meningitis, tuberculous or cryptococcal meningitis or meningitis caused by other fungi, cerebrovascular syphilis, and lymphogranuloma venereum. Postinfectious and postvaccinal reactions require differentiation, including sequelae to measles, mumps, varicella and variola, and post-rabies and post-smallpox vaccination; these syndromes are usually encephalitic in type. Leptospirosis, listeriosis, lymphocytic choriomeningitis, viral hepatitis, infectious mononucleosis, influenza and other diseases may produce the same clinical syndrome and require differentiation (see Index).

2. **Occurrence** — Worldwide, usually as sporadic cases, occasionally in epidemics as infections with coxsackievirus, echovirus or other viruses. Actual incidence is unknown. Commonly observed when other forms of meningitis are not present in the community; seasonal increase in late summer and early autumn.

3. **Infectious agents** — Caused by a wide variety of infectious agents, many of which are associated with other specific diseases. Many viruses are capable of producing the syndrome. A third or more of the cases have no demonstrable agent. Mumps may be responsible for about 25% or more of cases in epidemic periods. In U.S.A., enteroviruses (picornaviruses) cause most cases; coxsackievirus group B, types 2, 3, 4, and 5 cause about one-third and echovirus types 2, 5, 6, 7, 9 (most), 10, 11, 14, 18 and 30, about 50%. Poliovirus, coxsackievirus group A, types 2, 3, 7, and 9, arboviruses, measles, herpes simplex and varicella viruses, lymphocytic choriomeningitis virus, adenovirus and others are responsible for sporadic cases. The incidence of specific types varies with geographic locality and time. (Leptospira may be responsible for up to 20% of cases of aseptic meningitis in various areas of the world, including the U.S.A.)

4. **Reservoir, 5. Mode of transmission, 6. Incubation period, 7. Period of communicability, 8. Susceptibility and resistance** — Vary with the specific infectious agent. (Refer to specific diseases.)

9. **Methods of control** —

   A. *Preventive measures:* Depend upon etiology. (See specific disease.)

   B. *Control of patient, contacts, and the immediate environment:*
   1) *Report to local health authority:* In selected endemic areas (U.S.A.); in many countries not a reportable disease, Class 3B (see Preface). If confirmed by laboratory means, specify the infectious agent; otherwise report as cause undetermined.
   2) *Isolation:* Specific diagnosis depends upon laboratory data not usually available until recovery. Therefore, isolate all patients during febrile period.

     3) *Concurrent disinfection:* Includes eating and drinking utensils and articles soiled by secretions and excretions of patients.

     4) *Quarantine:* None.

     5) *Immunization of contacts:* See specific diseases.

     6) *Investigation of contacts:* Not usually indicated.

     7) *Specific treatment:* None for the usual causative viral agents.

C. Epidemic measures: See specific diseases.

D. International measures: WHO Collaborating Centres (see Preface).

MENINGITIS, MENINGOCOCCAL

(Cerebrospinal fever, Meningococcal infection, Meningococcemia)

1. Identification—An acute bacterial disease characterized by sudden onset, with fever, intense headache, nausea and often vomiting, stiff neck, and frequently a petechial rash with pink macules or, very rarely, vesicles. Delirium and coma often appear; occasional fulminating cases exhibit sudden prostration, ecchymoses, collapse, and shock at onset. Meningococcemia may occur without extension to the meninges and should be suspected in cases of otherwise unexplained acute febrile illness associated with petechial rash and leucocytosis. Septic monarthritis occurs. Formerly fatality rates exceeded 50% but with early diagnosis, modern therapy and supportive measures, fatality should be less than 10%. In fulminating meningococcemia the death rate remains high despite antibacterial treatment; promptness in instituting therapy is essential. There is variation in morbidity and mortality during endemic and epidemic cycles. Meningococcal infection may be (1) restricted to the nasopharynx, with only local symptoms or asymptomatic, (2) invasive with acutely ill septicemic patients, two-thirds of whom show a petechial rash, sometimes with joint involvement or (3) meningeal, in which the organisms have penetrated into the meninges.

Diagnosis is confirmed by recovery of meningococci from the blood and/or spinal fluid. Microscopic examination of stained smears from petechiae may reveal organisms. Group specific meningococcal polysaccharides also may be identified in spinal fluid by counter-immunoelectrophoresis.

Other purulent meningitides often are secondary to parameningeal or systemic involvement originating from the nose, accessory nasal sinuses, middle ear, or mastoid. The lungs, endocardium, joints, skin or other sites may be involved. Clinical signs and symptoms may be indistinguishable from those caused by meningococci except for the latter's characteristic rash. Differentiation is based on smears and bacteriologic studies. The commoner infectious agents, which vary in frequency with age, are pneumococci, *Haemophilus influenzae*, hemolytic and other streptococci, *Staphylococcus aureus*, *Escherichia coli*; less commonly, but of increasing frequency in recent years, members of the Klebsiella-enterobacter-proteus group, *Listeria monocytogenes*, *Salmonella*, *Pseudomonas aeruginosa*, and others. *H. influenzae* meningitis occurs in infants and young children as a primary suppurative meningitis, usually without evidence of local or general disease other than of the meninges. Several mycoses cause subacute and chronic meningitides. Epidemiologic behavior and control are described under several individual diseases, e.g., the pneumonias, streptococcal diseases, staphylococcal diseases, and mycoses (see index). Aseptic meningitis as well as meningismus due to other conditions must be considered.

2. **Occurrence** — Endemic and epidemic; worldwide. Common in both temperate and tropical climates, with sporadic cases throughout the year in both urban and rural areas; greatest prevalence during winter and spring. At irregular intervals epidemic waves occur, usually lasting 3 to 5 years. Meningococcal infection occurs more commonly in children and young adults, in males more than in females, and more commonly in adults under crowded living conditions, such as in barracks and institutions. Large epidemics have occurred in hot dry regions. A broad area of high incidence has existed for many years in the sub-Sahara region of mid-Africa.

3. **Infectious agent** — *Neisseria meningitidis (N. intracellularis)*, the meningococcus. Group A organisms have caused the major epidemics in the U.S.A. and elsewhere. Presently, Groups C and B are responsible for most cases in the U.S.A. Both groups A and C have been associated with epidemic meningococcal disease in Brazil since 1974. Group A has been associated with the epidemics in Africa. Additional serogroups have been recognized in recent years,

e.g., Groups X, Y and Z. Organisms belonging to these serogroups generally are less virulent, but fatal infections have occurred.

4. **Reservoir** — Man.

5. **Mode of transmission** — By direct contact, including droplets and discharges from nose and throat of infected persons, more often from carriers than cases; usually causes an acute nasopharyngitis or a subclinical mucosal infection; invasion sufficient to cause systemic disease is comparatively rare. Carrier prevalence of 25% or more may exist without clinical cases. During epidemics more than half of a military unit may be healthy carriers of pathogenic meningococci. Indirect contact is of questionable significance because the meningococcus is relatively susceptible to temperature changes and desiccation.

6. **Incubation period** — Varies from 2 to 10 days, commonly 3 to 4 days.

7. **Period of communicability** — Until meningococci are no longer present in discharges from nose and mouth. Susceptible meningococci usually disappear from the nasopharynx within 24 hours after institution of appropriate specific treatment.

8. **Susceptibility and resistance** — Susceptibility to the clinical disease is low and a high ratio of carriers to cases prevails. Type-specific immunity of unknown duration follows even subclinical infections.

9. **Method of control** —

A. *Preventive measures:*

1) Education as to personal hygiene and the necessity of avoiding direct contact or droplet infection.

2) Prevention of overcrowding in living quarters, public transportation, working places and especially in barracks, camps, ships and schools.

3) Group C polysaccharide vaccine has been highly effective in military recruits. Group A polysaccharide vaccine is being tested in children and young adults in tropical areas, with promising preliminary results. However, vaccine for neither Group A nor Group C is indicated as a general measure.

B. *Control of patient, contacts, and the immediate environment:*

1) *Report to local health authority:* Obligatory case report in most states and countries, Class 2A (see Preface).

2) *Isolation:* Until 24 hours after start of chemotherapy.

3) *Concurrent disinfection:* Of discharges from the nose and throat and articles soiled therewith. Terminal cleaning.

4) Quarantine: None
5) Protection of contacts: Close surveillance for early signs of illness to initiate appropriate therapy without delay. Immunization of case contacts is not indicated. Consideration may be given to prophylactic administration of sulfadiazine if the organism is sensitive, or of rifampin to immediate family members of cases.
6) Investigation of contacts: Impractical.
7) Specific treatment: Penicillin given parenterally in adequate doses is the drug of choice. Parenteral ampicillin is effective; chloramphenicol also is effective, but should be reserved for penicillin-sensitive patients. Treatment should begin when presumptive clinical diagnosis is made even though meningococci have not been identified; until specific etiologic agent is identified, ampicillin is the drug of choice because of its effectiveness against *H. influenzae* infections. If the outbreak is shown to be caused by sulfonamide-sensitive strains sulfadiazine may be given intravenously; however, sulfonamide-resistant Groups B and C, and recently Group A strains are commonplace in many parts of the world.

C. *Epidemic measures:*
1) When an outbreak occurs major emphasis must be placed on careful surveillance, early diagnosis, and immediate treatment of suspected cases. A high index of suspicion is invaluable.
2) Assure the separation of individuals and the ventilation of living and sleeping quarters of all persons who are especially exposed to infection because of their occupation or congested living conditions.
3) When the epidemic strain is sulfonamide-sensitive, mass chemoprophylaxis of a closed community with sulfadiazine (0.5 g for children, 1.0 g for adults, every 12 hours, for 4 doses) reduces carrier rate and limits spread of the disease. Because of the current widespread prevalence of sulfonamide-resistant meningococcal strains throughout the world, sulfonamide prophylaxis should not be instituted unless fewer than 5% of the strains obtained from a statistically valid sample of the carrier population show sulfonamide resistance (resistant strains are those resistant to more than 0.1 mg. % of sulfadiazine). Rifampin (600 mg. orally once daily for 5 days) reduces the carrier rate and limits

spread of disease when the entire community is treated, but its use has been associated with appearance of resistant strains. When mass prophylaxis of a community is not feasible, it may be advisable to administer prophylaxis to all intimate contacts, such as persons sharing the same lodging or giving mouth to mouth resuscitation to patients before definitive treatment of the patient was established. Penicillin is not effective against nasopharyngeal carriers.

D. International measures: WHO Reference Centres (see Preface).

MOLLUSCUM CONTAGIOSUM

1. Identification—A viral disease of the skin which results in pearly pink to white papules with a prominent central pore. The papules vary in size from less than 1 mm to 10 mm. There are usually multiple lesions, most frequently in the genital area in adults; may occur anywhere on children. The eruption usually clears spontaneously in 6-9 months.

2. Occurrence—Worldwide. Nearly 90% of adults have antibodies demonstrable with immunofluorescence or immunodiffusion techniques.

3. Infectious agent—A member of the poxvirus group.

4. Reservoir—Man.

5. Mode of transmission—Usually by direct contact, but transmission by fomites is possible. A rising incidence in venereal disease clinics suggests sexual transmission.

6. Incubation period—Two to seven weeks.

7. Period of communicability—Unknown, but probably as long as lesions persist.

8. Susceptibility and resistance—Any age may be affected, but usually occurs in small children. In prepubertal children males are four times as susceptible as females.

9. Methods of control—

A. Preventive measures: Avoidance of contact with affected patients.

B. Control of patient, contacts, and the immediate environment:
None.

1) *Report to local health authorities:* Official report not ordinarily justifiable, Class 5 (see Preface).

2) *Isolation:* Generally not indicated. Infected children may be excluded from close contact sports such as wrestling.

3) *Concurrent disinfection:* None.

4) *Quarantine:* None.

5) *Immunization of contacts:* None.

6) *Investigation of contacts and source of infection:* Examination of sexual partners where applicable.

7) *Specific treatment:* Rarely indicated. Curettage with local anesthesia. Freezing with liquid nitrogen has some advocates.

MONONUCLEOSIS, INFECTIOUS

(Glandular fever, Monocytic angina)

1. Identification — An acute syndrome due to Epstein-Barr (EB) virus, characterized by fever, sore throat (often with exudative pharyngo-tonsillitis), lymphadenopathy (especially posterior cervical), lymphocytosis exceeding 50% (including 10 percent or more abnormal forms), abnormalities in liver function tests (mainly serum glutamic-oxalo-acetic transaminase [SGOT]), and an elevated heterophile antibody titer. In children, the disease is generally mild and difficult to recognize. Jaundice occurs in about 4% of infected young adults and splenomegaly in 50 percent. Duration is from 1 to several weeks; rarely fatal. A heterophile antibody-negative syndrome resembling infectious mononucleosis may be due to cytomegalovirus, another herpes virus, or toxoplasmosis.

Laboratory diagnosis includes examination of blood smears for abnormal lymphocytes, tests for elevated sheep or horse cell heterophile antibodies after absorption of serum with guinea pig kidney or the beef cell hemolysin test, and liver function tests. An indirect immunofluorescence test against the EB virus may be helpful in heterophile antibody-negative cases. EB virus has been associated with, but not yet proved to be the cause of African Burkitt lymphoma and of nasopharyngeal cancer. High antibody titers have also been found in 30-40 percent of patients with Hodgkin's disease, systemic lupus erythematosus and sarcoidosis.

2. **Occurrence**—Infection is worldwide, but classical infectious mononucleosis occurs primarily in developed countries where the age of infection is delayed until age 15-25; most commonly recognized in college students and hospital personnel. Common and widespread in early childhood in developing countries.

3. **Infectious agent**—Epstein-Barr (EB) virus, closely related to that of other herpes viruses morphologically, but distinct serologically.

4. **Reservoir**—Man and perhaps other primates.

5. **Mode of transmission**—Probably person-to-person, spread by an oral-pharyngeal route. Kissing may facilitate spread among young adults; pharyngeal excretion may persist up to a year after infection. May also occur via blood transfusion in susceptible recipients.

6. **Incubation period**—From 2 to 6 weeks.

7. **Period of communicability**—Unknown but presumably may be long in view of protracted pharyngeal excretion of virus.

8. **Susceptibility and resistance**—Susceptibility to EB virus is general, but incidence of clinical disease is greatest among older children and young adults. Infection appears to confer a high degree of resistance; resistance from unrecognized childhood infection may account for low communicability among adults.

9. **Methods of control**—

A. *Preventive measures:* None.

B. *Control of patient, contacts, and the immediate environment:*
  1) *Report to local health authority:* No individual case report, Class 4 (see Preface).
  2) *Isolation:* None.
  3) *Concurrent disinfection:* Of articles soiled with nose and throat discharges.
  4) *Quarantine:* None.
  5) *Immunization of contacts:* None.
  6) *Investigation of contacts:* For the individual case, of little value.
  7) *Specific treatment:* None.

C. *Epidemic measures:* Field investigation of epidemics should be undertaken with the hope of adding to knowledge of the disease.

D. *International measures:* None.

MUCORMYCOSIS
(Phycomycosis, Zygomycosis)

1. **Identification** — A group of mycoses caused by fungi of the family *Mucoraceae* of the class *Zygomycetes*. These fungi have an affinity for blood vessels, causing thrombosis and infarction. The craniofacial form of the disease usually presents as nasal or paranasal sinus infection, most often during ketoacidotic episodes of diabetes mellitus. Gangrene of the turbinates, perforation of the hard palate, gangrene of the cheek, or orbital cellulitis, proptosis, and ophthalmoplegia may occur. Infection may penetrate to the frontal lobe of the brain, causing infarction. In the pulmonary form of disease, the fungus causes thrombosis of pulmonary blood vessels and infarcts of the lung. In the gastrointestinal form, mucosal ulcers or thrombosis and gangrene of stomach or bowel may occur.

Diagnosis is confirmed by microscopic demonstration of distinctive broad, nonseptate hyphae in biopsies and by culture of biopsy tissue. Wet preparations and smears may be examined. Cultures alone are not diagnostic because these *Zygomycetes* are frequent in the environment as bread or fruit molds.

2. **Occurrence** — Infection is worldwide. Incidence is increasing because of longer survival of patients with diabetes mellitus and certain blood dyscrasias, especially leukemia.

3. **Infectious agent** — Species of *Rhizopus*, especially *Rhizopus oryzae* and *Rhizopus arrhizus*, have caused most of the craniofacial cases of mucormycosis from which the fungus has been cultured. Probably *Mucor* and *Rhizopus* species are the chief causes of the pulmonary and gastrointestinal mucormycosis. *Mortierella*, *Cunninghamella*, and *Absidia*, species have been reported from a few human cases of mucormycosis.

4. **Reservoir** — Members of the Family *Mucoraceae* are common saprophytes in the environment.

5. **Mode of transmission** — By inhalation or ingestion of fungus by susceptible individuals. Direct inoculation by minor trauma; intravenous catheters or cutaneous burns are occasionally implicated.

6. **Incubation period** — One or 2 days. Fungus spreads rapidly in susceptible tissues.

7. **Period of communicability** — Not directly transmitted from man or animal to man.

8. **Susceptibility and resistance** — The rarity of infection in

healthy individuals despite the abundance of *Mucoraceae* in the environment indicates natural resistance. Corticosteroid and immunosuppressive therapy predispose. Malnutrition predisposes to the gastrointestinal form.

9. **Methods of Control —**

   A. *Preventive measures:* Optimal control of diabetes mellitus.

   B. *Control of patient, contacts, and the immediate environment:*

      1) *Report to local health authority:* Official report ordinarily not justifiable, Class 5 (see Preface).
      2) *Isolation:* None.
      3) *Concurrent disinfection:* Ordinary cleanliness. Terminal cleaning.
      4) *Quarantine:* None.
      5) *Immunization of contacts:* None.
      6) *Investigation of contacts:* Ordinarily not profitable.
      7) *Specific treatment:* In cranial form, control of diabetic acidosis; amphotericin B (Fungizone) and resection of necrotic tissue have been helpful.

   C. *Epidemic measures:* Not applicable, a sporadic disease.

   D. *International measuress:* None.

PHYCOMYCOSIS designates all infections caused by *Phycomycetes*. This includes mucormycosis, subcutaneous phycomycosis and rhinoentomophthoromycosis. The latter two have been recognized principally in tropical and subtropical Asia and Africa, are not characterized by thromboses or infarction, do not usually occur in association with serious preexisting disease, do not usually cause disseminated disease, and seldom cause death.

SUBCUTANEOUS PHYCOMYCOSIS is a granulomatous inflammation caused by *Basidiobolus meristosporus (B. haptosporus)*, a ubiquitous fungus occurring in decaying vegetation, soil and the gastrointestinal tract of reptiles. Disease presents as a firm subcutaneous mass, fixed to the skin, principally in children and adolescents, more commonly in males. Infection may heal spontaneously. Recommended therapy is oral potassium iodide.

RHINOENTOMOPHTHOROMYCOSIS usually originates in the nasal mucosa and presents as nasal obstruction or swelling of the nose or adjacent structures. Lesions of the mucosa of the palate and pharynx also occur. Disease is uncommon, occurs principally in adult males. Recommended therapy is oral potassium iodide or intravenous amphotericin B (Fungizone). The infectious agent, *Entomophthora coronata*, occurring in soil and decaying vegetation, also causes disease in insects. For both subcutaneous phycomycosis and rhinoentomophthoromycosis, incubation period and mode of transmission are unknown. Man-to-man transmission does not occur.

MUMPS
(Infectious parotitis)

1. **Identification** — An acute viral disease characterized by fever, and by swelling and tenderness of one or more salivary glands, usually the parotid, and sometimes the sublingual or submaxillary glands. Orchitis occurs in 15-25% of males and oophoritis in about 5% of females past puberty; pancreatitis, neuritis, arthritis, mastitis, and pericarditis may occur. The central nervous system is frequently involved, either early or late in the disease. Transient hearing loss is common; rarely, permanent deafness may occur. Orchitis and meningoencephalitis due to mumps virus may occur without involvement of a salivary gland. Death is exceedingly rare.

Serological tests are of value in confirming diagnosis. Virus may be isolated in chick embryo or cell cultures from saliva, blood, urine and cerebrospinal fluid during the acute phase of the disease.

2. **Occurrence** — Mumps is of less regular occurrence than other common communicable diseases of childhood, such as measles and chickenpox. About one-third of exposed susceptible persons have inapparent infection. Winter and spring are seasons of greatest prevalence.

3. **Infectious agent** — The virus of mumps, a myxovirus antigenically related to the parainfluenza group.

4. **Reservoir** — Man.

5. **Mode of transmission** — By droplet spread and by direct contact with saliva of an infected person.

6. **Incubation period** — 12 to 26 days, commonly 18 days.

7. **Period of communicability** — The virus has been isolated from saliva from 6 days before salivary gland involvement to as long as 9 days thereafter, but the height of infectiousness occurs about 48

hours before swelling commences. Urine may be positive for as long as 14 days after onset of illness. Inapparent infection is not uncommon and can be communicable.

8. **Susceptibility and resistance**—Susceptibility is general. Immunity is generally lifelong and develops after inapparent as well as clinical attacks. The currently available skin test is not a reliable index of immunity.

9. **Methods of control**—

    A. *Preventive measures:* Live attenuated vaccine prepared in chick embryo cell culture is available either as a single vaccine or in combination with rubella and measles live virus vaccines. It causes no reactions and solid immunity develops in more than 95% of recipients with no evidence of loss of protection in the several years that this vaccine has been in use. Vaccine may be administered any time after 1 year of age. Special effort should be made to immunize all persons with no definite history of mumps as they approach maturity. Vaccine is contraindicated in immunosuppressed individuals.

    B. *Control of patient, contacts, and the immediate environment:*
        1) *Report to local health authority:* Selectively reportable, Class 3C (see Preface).
        2) *Isolation:* For 9 days from onset of swelling; less if swelling has subsided.
        3) *Concurrent disinfection:* Of articles soiled with secretions of nose and throat.
        4) *Quarantine:* None.
        5) *Immunization of contacts:* It is not known whether immunization after exposure to natural mumps protects; however, immunization is not contraindicated under such conditions. Mumps hyperimmune globulin is of questionable effectiveness when administered following exposure, but should be considered for patients with immuno-deficiencies for whom the vaccine is contraindicated.
        6) *Investigation of contacts:* Not profitable.
        7) *Specific treatment:* None.

    C. *Epidemic measures:* Immunization of susceptibles, especially those at risk of exposure.

    D. *International measures:* None.

NOCARDIOSIS

1. **Identification**—A chronic bacterial disease often originating in the lungs, with hematogenous spread to produce abscesses of brain, subcutaneous tissue and other organs; high fatality rate. The frequent occurrence of *Nocardia asteroides* in chronic pulmonary disease of other origin may represent a mild form of nocardiosis. Several species of *Nocardia*, including *N. asteroids*, cause mycetoma (see p. 188).

Microscopic examination of stained smears of sputum, pus or spinal fluid reveals gram positive, partially acid-fast, branching hyphae; confirmation is by culture.

2. **Occurrence**—An occasional sporadic disease in man and animals in all parts of the world. No evidence of age, sex, or racial differences.

3. **Infectious agent**—*Nocardia asteroides*, an aerobic actinomycete.

4. **Reservoir**—Soil.

5. **Mode of transmission**—Direct contact with contaminated soil, sometimes through minor wounds and abrasions; pulmonary infections presumably occur through inhalation of organisms suspended in dust.

6. **Incubation period**—Unknown; probably weeks.

7. **Period of communicability**—Not directly transmitted from man or animals to man.

8. **Susceptibility and resistance**—Unknown. Endogenous or iatrogenic adrenal hypercorticism probably predisposes. *N. asteroids* occurs as an opportunistic pulmonary pathogen in the immunologically compromised host (leukemia, lymphoma, transplant recipient).

9. **Methods of Control**—

   A. *Preventive measures:* None.

   B. *Control of patient, contacts, and the immediate environment:*
      1) *Report to local health authority:* Official report not ordinarily justifiable, Class 5 (see Preface).
      2) *Isolation:* None.
      3) *Concurrent disinfection:* Of discharges and contaminated dressings.
      4) *Quarantine:* None.
      5) *Immunization of contacts:* None.
      6) *Investigation of contacts:* Not profitable.

7) *Specific treatment:* Sulfonamides in high doses are effective in systemic infections if given early and for prolonged periods. Some isolates of *N. asteroides* are sensitive to ampicillin, minocycline, erythromycin, cycloserine or other antibiotics; one of these drugs is sometimes given in addition to sulfonamides.

C. *Epidemic measures:* Not applicable, a sporadic disease.

D. *International measures:* None.

ONCHOCERCIASIS
(River Blindness)

1. **Identification**—A chronic, nonfatal filarial disease with fibrous nodules in skin and subcutaneous tissues, particularly of the head and shoulders (America) or pelvic girdle and lower extremities (Africa). The female worm discharges microfilariae which migrate through the skin, causing intense pruritic rash, altered pigmentation, edema and atrophy of the skin. Loss of skin elasticity is responsible for hanging groin and sometimes hernia. Microfilariae frequently reach the eye, causing visual disturbances and blindness; they may be found in organs and tissues other than skin and eye, but their clinical significance is not yet clear; also may be found in the urine in heavy infections.

Laboratory diagnosis is by superficial biopsy of skin with demonstration of microfilariae in fresh preparations by microscopic examination; by excision of nodules and finding adult worms; in ocular manifestations, by observation with ophthalmic microscope of microfilariae in cornea, anterior chamber of vitreous body, or by finding microfilariae in the urine. The Mazzotti test (administration of 25 mg. of diethylcarbamazine) produces characteristic pruritis; it may be positive in low density infections when microfilariae are difficult to demonstrate.

Differentiation from other filarial disease, including filariasis (see p. 113), and other diseases is required in endemic areas.

2. **Occurrence**—Geographical distribution in the Western Hemisphere is limited to Guatemala (principally above the western slope of the continental divide), southern Mexico (states of Chiapas and Oaxaca), northern Venezuela, very small areas in Columbia,

and recently from the state of Amazonas in Brazil; in Africa south of the Sahara, in an area extending from Senegal to Ethiopia down to Angola in the west and Tanzania in the east; also occurs in Yemen. In some localities, almost all of the population is infected and is much afflicted with associated blindness.

3. **Infectious agent**—*Onchocerca volvulus*, a nematode worm.

4. **Reservoir**—Infected persons. Can be transmitted to chimpanzees and has been found in nature in gorillas.

5. **Mode of transmission**—By the bite of infected female black-flies of the genus *Simulium;* in the Americas mainly *S. ochraceum, S. metallicum,* and possibly other species; in Africa, *S. damnosum, S. neavei* and *S. woodi.* Microfilariae picked up by a vector feeding on an infected person penetrate thoracic muscles of the vector, develop into infective larvae, migrate to the proboscis, and are liberated in the skin of another person during a subsequent bloodmeal.

6. **Incubation period**—Microfilariae can be found in the skin about 1 year or more after infection.

7. **Period of communicability**—Man infects flies as long as living microfilariae occur in the skin i.e., for 10-15 years if untreated. In Africa, vectors are infective after 6 days; in Guatemala measurably longer, up to 14 days because of lower temperatures. Not directly transmitted from man to man.

8. **Susceptibility and resistance**—Susceptibility is universal; reinfection may occur; severity of disease depends on cumulative effects of the infections.

9. **Methods of control**—

   A. *Preventive measures:*
      1) Avoid bites of *Simulium* flies by wearing protective clothing and headgear as much as possible, or by use of an insect repellent, such as diethyltoluamide.
      2) Control of vector larvae in rapidly running streams and in artificial waterways by biodegradable insecticides such as methoxychlor or Abate. Aerial spraying may be required to ensure coverage of breeding places in large scale control operations.
      3) Provision of facilities for diagnosis and treatment.

   B. *Control of patient, contacts, and the immediate environment:*
      1) *Report to local health authority:* Official report not ordinarily justifiable, Class 5 (see Preface).
      2) *Isolation:* None.

3) Concurrent disinfection: None.

4) Quarantine: None.

5) Immunization of contacts: None.

6) Investigation of contacts: A community problem. (See 9A).

7) Specific treatment: Diethylcarbamazine (Hetrazan) is useful but may cause severe reactions due to destruction of microfilariae; does not kill adult worms. Suramin, (Naphuride, Antrypol), which is available in the U.S.A. from the Center for Disease Control, Atlanta, GA. (see Preface), kills the adult worms and leads to gradual disappearance of microfilariae; undesirable reaction may occur and require close medical supervision. Neither drug is suited to mass treatment. Excision of nodules to eliminate adult worms may reduce symptoms.

C. Epidemic measures: In areas of high prevalence make concerted effort to reduce incidence, taking measures listed under 9A.

D. International measures: Coordinated programs entered into by neighboring countries where the disease is endemic, based mainly on anti-blackfly measures applied systematically over large enough ecological zones to limit reinvasion of flies from untreated areas. WHO Collaborating Centres (see Preface).

PARAGONIMIASIS

(Pulmonary distomiasis, Endemic hemoptysis, Lung fluke disease)

1. Identification—Clinical manifestations of this trematode disease depend on the path of migration and the organs parasitized. Lungs are most frequently involved; symptoms are cough and hemoptysis. Worms become surrounded by an inflammatory reaction which eventually organizes into a fibrous, cystic lesion. Roentgenographic findings often closely simulate pulmonary tuberculosis. Localization in other organs is not infrequent, with worms maturing in sites such as the brain, subcutaneous tissues, intestinal wall, lymph nodes, or genitourinary tract. Infection usually lasts for many years, and the infected person may appear surprisingly well.

The sputum generally contains flecks of orange-brown pigment, sometimes diffusely distributed, in which masses of worm eggs are seen microscopically, establishing the diagnosis. Eggs are swallowed and thus are also found in feces. Serological tests are helpful aids, but cross reactions occur, especially with *Clonorchis sinensis*.

2. **Occurrence**—Extensive in the Far East, particularly Korea, Japan, and Taiwan; scattered foci in Philippines, parts of mainland China, Southeast Asia, Africa and South America.

3. **Infectious agent**—*Paragonimus westermani*, a trematode, in the Orient; *P. africanus* in Africa, *P. szechuanensis* in China; other species in the Americas.

4. **Reservoir**—Man, dog, cat, pig, and wild carnivores are definitive hosts and act as reservoirs.

5. **Mode of transmission**—Infection occurs when the raw or partially cooked flesh of fresh water crabs such as *Eriocheir* and *Potamon* and of crayfish such as *Cambaroides* containing infective larvae (metacercariae) is ingested. The larvae emerge in the duodenum, then penetrate the intestinal wall, migrate through the tissues, become encapsulated, usually in the lungs, and develop into egg-producing adults. Eggs leave the definitive host via sputum and feces, gain access to fresh water, and embryonate in 2 to 4 weeks. A larva (miracidium) hatches and penetrates a suitable fresh water snail *(Semisulcospira, Thiara* or other species) and undergoes a cycle of development of approximately 3 months. Larvae (cercariae) emerge from the snail and penetrate and encyst in fresh water crabs and crayfish. Pickling of these crutaceans in wine, brine or vinegar, as is common practice in the Orient, does not kill the cysts.

6. **Incubation period**—Flukes mature and begin to lay eggs approximately 6 weeks after man ingests infective larvae. The interval until symptoms appear is long, variable, poorly defined and depends on the organ involved.

7. **Period of communicability**—Eggs may be discharged by the human host for 20 years or more; duration of infection in mollusk and crustacean hosts is unknown. Not directly transmitted from man to man.

8. **Susceptibility and resistance**—Susceptibility is general. Increased resistance possibly develops as a result of infection.

9. **Methods of Control—**

A. *Preventive measures:*
   1) Education of people in endemic areas concerning the life cycle of the parasite.
   2) Stress thorough cooking of crustacea.
   3) Sanitary disposal of sputum and feces.
   4) Control of snails by molluscacides is feasible in some areas, as well as destruction of crabs. Dinitro-o-cyclohexylphenol is effective against both amphibian and aquatic snails.

B. *Control of patient, contacts, and the immediate environment:*
   1) *Report to local health authority:* Official report not ordinarily justifiable, Class 5 (see Preface).
   2) *Isolation:* None.
   3) *Concurrent disinfection:* Of sputum and feces.
   4) *Quarantine:* None.
   5) *Immunization of contacts:* None.
   6) *Investigation of contacts:* None.
   7) *Specific treatment:* Bithionol, available in U.S.A. from the Center for Disease Control, Atlanta, GA, (see Preface), gives good results and is the drug of choice. Both emetine hydrochloride and chloroquine (Aralen) produce clinical improvement and occasional cure.

C. *Epidemic measures:* In an endemic area, occurrence of small clusters of cases or even sporadic infections is an important signal for examination of local waters for infected snails, crabs and crayfish and determination of reservoir mammalian hosts.

D. *International measures:* None.

PARATYPHOID FEVER

1. **Identification—** A generalized bacterial enteric infection, often with abrupt onset, continued fever, enlargement of spleen, sometimes rose spots on trunk, usually diarrhea, and involvement of lymphoid tissues of the mesentery and intestines. While clinically similar, the fatality rate is much lower than for typhoid fever. Many

mild attacks exhibit no more than fever or a transient diarrhea, while some are asymptomatic. (See Salmonella gastroenteritis, p. 276).

Laboratory confirmation and individual type identification are by bacteriologic examination of blood, feces and urine.

2. Occurrence—Sporadically or in limited outbreaks. Probably more frequent than reports suggest. In U.S.A., paratyphoid fever is infrequently identified; of the 3 varieties, paratyphoid B is commonest, A less frequent and C extremely rare. In Western Europe, the incidence of paratyphoid A and B is somewhat greater, while in Eastern Europe and Asia C is common.

3. Infectious agents—*Salmonella paratyphi A (S. enteritidis* bioserotype Paratyphoid A), *S. schottmuelleri (S. paratyphi B, S. enteritidis* serotype Paratyphoid B), (*S. paratyphi C, S hirschfeldii, S. enteritidis* serotype Paratyphoid C), all of human origin; a number of phage types can be distinguished. A bacteremic infection with similar clinical reaction may be induced by any salmonella pathogenic for man and animals.

4. Reservoir—Man. An outbreak occurred in England in which dairy cows were infected and excreted *S. schottmuelleri* organisms in milk and feces.

5. Mode of transmission—Direct or indirect contact with feces or urine of patient or carrier. Spread is by food, especially milk, milk products and shellfish, usually contaminated by hands of a carrier or missed case. Under some conditions, flies may be vectors. A few outbreaks are related to water supplies, including swimming waters.

6. Incubation period—1-3 weeks for enteric fever, and 1-10 days for gastroenteritis; somewhat longer for paratyphoid A than for B and C.

7. Period of communicability—As long as the infectious agent persists in excreta; usually from appearance of prodromal symptoms, throughout illness, and for varying periods after recovery. Commonly 1-2 weeks; some of those infected may become permanent carriers.

8. Susceptibility and resistance—Susceptibility is general. Partial species-specific immunity usually follows recovery.

9. Methods of control—

   A. *Preventive measures:* Same as those listed under Typhoid Fever, 9A, 1-9 (see pp. 351-352). Vaccines against paratyphoid fever have not proved to be effective.

B. Control of patient, contacts, and the immediate environment:

1) *Report to local health authority:* Case report in most states and countries, both suspect and confirmed infections, Class 2A (see Preface).

2) *Isolation:* Exclusion of infected persons from food handling, from patient care, and from occupations involving nursing care of young children and the elderly until cultures of feces are free from *Salmonellae* for at least 3 successive days. Whenever possible stool specimens, rather than rectal swabs, should be obtained for culture.

3) *Concurrent disinfection:* Of feces and urine and of articles soiled therewith. In communities with modern and adequate sewage disposal systems, feces can be discharged directly into sewers without preliminary disinfection. Terminal cleaning.

4) *Quarantine:* Family contacts should not be employed as food handlers during periods of contact with patient or carrier or until at least two cultures of fecal specimens are found to be free of *Salmonellae.*

5) *Immunization of contacts:* None.

6) *Investigation of contacts:* Bacteriological investigation, especially of family contacts, for unrecognized mild cases and carriers. (See (2) above).

7) *Specific treatment:* For overt enteric fever or septicemia, chloramphenicol is the drug of choice; ampicillin is the preferred alternative. If it is necessary to use other antibiotics, sensitivity tests should be performed.

C. *Epidemic measures:* Those for Typhoid Fever, 9C (p. 353).

D. *International measures:* WHO Collaborating Centres (see Preface).

PEDICULOSIS
(Lousiness)

1. Identification—Infestation of the head hair, the hairy parts of the body, or clothing, especially along the seams of inner surfaces, with adult lice, larvae, or nits (eggs). Crab lice usually infest the pubic area; they may infest eyelashes.

2. Occurrence—Worldwide. The head louse is common in outbreaks among school children.

3. Infesting agents—*Pediculus humanus capitis,* the head louse, *P. humanus corporis,* the body louse, and *Phthirus pubis,* the crab louse. Lice of lower animals do not infest man.

4. Reservoir—Infested persons.

5. Mode of transmission—Direct contact with an infested person and indirectly by contact with their personal belongings, especially clothing and headgear. Crab lice are usually transmitted by intimate contact.

6. Incubation period—Under optimum conditions the eggs of lice hatch in a week, and sexual maturity is reached in approximately 2 weeks.

7. Period of communicability—While lice remain alive on the infested person or in his clothing, and until eggs in hair and clothing have been destroyed.

8. Susceptibility and resistance—Any person may become lousy under suitable conditions of exposure. Repeated infestations often result in dermal hypersensitivity.

9. Methods of control—

    A. Preventive measures:
1) Avoid physical contact with infested individuals and their belongings and clothing.
2) Health education of the public in the value of using hot water and soap to maintain cleanliness, and laundering of clothing in hot water (60°C 20 min.) or dry cleaning to destroy nits and lice.
3) Direct inspection of head hair and, when necessary, of body and clothing particularly of children in schools, institutions and summer camps to detect cases early.

    B. Control of infested persons, contacts, and the immediate environment:
1) *Report to local health authority:* Official report not ordinarily justifiable; school authorities should be informed, Class 5 (see Preface).
2) *Isolation:* Not necessary after application of effective insecticide.
3) *Concurrent disinfection:* Of members of family or group, to include clothing, bedding and other appropriate vehicles of transmission (e.g. cosmetic articles).

   4) Quarantine: None.
   5) Immunization of contacts: Does not apply.
   6) Investigation of contacts: Examination of household and other close personal contacts, with concurrent treatment as indicated.
   7) Specific treatment: 1% malathion dusting powder is effective for body and head lice: gamma benzene hexachloride (Lindane), 1% dusting powder or 1% shampoo (Kwell), is the agent of choice in U.S.A. The insecticide Abate, which is nontoxic to man, is also effective and is recommended by WHO for use in areas where strains of pediculi are resistant to malathion, as a 2% dusting powder.

 C. Epidemic measures: Mass treatment as recommended in 9B7.

 D. International measures: None.

PINTA
(Carate, Tian, Lota, Azul)

 1. Identification — An acute and chronic nonvenereal treponematosis. Within 7 to 60 days after skin infection a scaling papule appears, usually on the hands, legs or dorsum of the feet, with satellite lymphadenopathy (bubo). In 5 to 12 months a maculopapular, erythematous secondary rash appears and may evolve into tertiary lesions, the dyschromic stage, with achromic or pigmented (blue, pink, yellow, violet) spots of variable size, mainly on distal portions of extremities but often including trunk and face. In rare instances the untreated disease may be fatal.

 Organisms demonstrable in lesions by dark-field examination. Serologic tests for syphilis usually become reactive during secondary rash and thereafter behave as in venereal syphilis.

 2. Occurrence — Frequent among dark-skinned people of tropics and sub-tropics; in the Western Hemisphere especially prevalent in Mexico, Colombia, Venezuela, and Ecuador. Predominantly a disease of childhood.

 3. Infectious agent — *Treponema carateum*, a spirochete.

 4. Reservoir — Man.

5. Mode of transmission — Unknown; evidence suggests transmission by direct and indirect contact with initial skin lesions and those of early dyschromic stage; location of primary lesions suggests trauma. Various biting and sucking arthropods have been implicated; venereal and congenital transmission rarely reported.

6. Incubation period — Three to 60 days.

7. Period of communicability — Unknown; potentially communicable while skin lesions are active, sometimes for many years.

8. Susceptibility and resistance — Undefined; presumably as in other treponematoses. Rare in white persons, suggesting some natural resistance, but not distinguished clearly from factors of personal hygiene and social and economic status.

9. Methods of control —

A. *Preventive measures:* Those applicable to other nonvenereal treponematoses apply to pinta, see Yaws 9A (pp.   ).

B. *Control of patient, contacts, and the immediate environment:*
   1) *Report to local health authority:* In selected endemic areas; in most countries not a reportable disease, Class 3B (see Preface).
   2) *Items 2 to 7:* Same as for Yaws. See 9B (p. 371).

C. *Epidemic measures:* See Yaws 9C (p. 371).

D. *International measures:* See Yaws 9D (pp. 371-372).

⚭

PLAGUE
(Pest, Black Death)

1. Identification — An infectious disease characterized classically by lymphadenitis, septicemia and petechial hemorrhages, often with toxemia, high fever, shock, restlessness, staggering gait, mental confusion, prostration, delirium and coma. Plague occurs mainly in three clinical forms: (a) *Bubonic plague,* the most common, with acutely inflamed and painful swellings of lymph nodes draining the site of the original infection. Secondary invasion of the blood may lead to localized infection in diverse parts of the body, including the meninges. A secondary, often terminal pneumonia has special significance as the source of primary pneumonic plague in contacts. (b) *Primary septicemic plague*, proved by blood smear or blood culture, is rare; this may be a form of bubonic plague in which the bubo is obscure and may include pharyngeal and tonsillar infections. (c) *Primary pneumonic plague* is the most serious and highly infectious form; it may occur in localized and sometimes devastating epidemics. Untreated bubonic plague has a case fatality rate commonly reported to be about 50%; occasionally it is no more than a localized infection of short duration (pestis minor), and fully virulent plague organisms have been recovered from throat cultures of asymptomatic contacts of plague patients. Untreated primary septicemic plague and pneumonic plague are usually fatal. Modern therapy materially reduces fatality from bubonic plague; pneumonic and septicemic plague also respond if recognized and treated early.

Diagnosis is confirmed by demonstrating the causal agent in fluid from buboes, in blood, in spinal fluid or in sputum.

2. **Occurrence** — Sylvatic (wild rodent) plague is known to exist in the western third of U.S.A., in large areas of South America, in North Central and Southern Africa, in the Near East, in Iranian Kurdistan and along the frontier between Yemen and Saudi Arabia, in Central and Southeast Asia and in Indonesia. Plague in man in the U.S.A. is limited and sporadic, following exposure to wild rodents or their fleas. Urban plague has been controlled in most of the world. Rural bubonic plague of rat origin, until recently a serious health problem in India and Burma, is now relatively rare. Since 1962 South Vietnam has experienced a marked increase in plague, with several thousand cases of bubonic plague, both urban and rural, and scattered outbreaks of pneumonic plague. In many areas of the world, plague continues to be potentially dangerous because of vast areas of persisting wild rodent infection and contact of wild rodents with domestic rats.

3. **Infectious agent** — *Yersinia pestis (Pasteurella pestis)*, the plague bacillus.

4. **Reservoir** — Wild rodents are the natural reservoirs of plague; numerous species of rodents in many parts of the world are subject to periodic epizootics. Lagomorphs (rabbits) and, rarely, carnivores may also be a source of infection to humans.

5. **Mode of transmission** — Bubonic plague is transmitted by the bite of an infective flea (especially *Xenopsylla cheopis*, the oriental rat flea), or by handling infected tissues, or from contact with the pus from an infected animal. Pneumonic plague and pharyngeal plague are spread by the airborne route by inhalation of exhaled droplets from patients with primary pneumonic plague or from

patients with bubonic plague who develop terminal plague pneumonia. Accidental infections may occur among laboratory workers.

6. Incubation period—From 2 to 6 days in bubonic plague; 2 to 4 days in pneumonic plague; may be shorter, rarely longer.

7. Period of communicability—Bubonic plague is not directly transmitted from person to person except through terminal plague pneumonia. Fleas may remain infected for days or weeks or months under suitable conditions of temperature and humidity, or may clear themselves of infection. Fleas are highly infective when the esophagus is blocked by a bacterial mass so that the ingested blood is regurgitated; "blocked" fleas usually are short-lived, 3 to 4 days. Pneumonic plague is usually highly communicable under climatic or social conditions which lead to overcrowding, especially in unsanitary dwellings.

8. Susceptibility and resistance—Susceptibility is general. Immunity after recovery is relative.

9. Methods of control—

   A. Preventive measures:

      1) Education of the public in endemic areas on mode of transmission and the importance of denying food and shelter to rats by control of food, garbage and refuse.

      2) Periodic surveys of rat populations should be done to determine the effectiveness of sanitary programs or to evaluate the potential for epizootic plague. Rat suppression by poisoning or trapping (see 9B6 below) may be necessary as a short term emergency measure. Surveillance of natural foci should be done by bacteriologic testing of wild rodents and their fleas and by serologic studies of rodent and carnivore populations in order to define areas of plague activity and its public health importance.

      3) Active immunization with a vaccine of killed bacteria confers protection in most recipients for several months when administered in a primary series of 2 or 3 doses; booster injections are necessary for continued protection. Vaccination of persons traveling or living in areas of high incidence and of laboratory workers handling plague bacilli is justifiable but should not be relied upon as the sole preventive measure.

      4) Rat control on ships and docks and in warehouses by rat proofing or periodic fumigation, combined when neces-

sary with destruction of rats and their fleas in vessels and in cargoes before shipment, especially containerized cargoes, and upon arrival from plague locations.

B. Control of patient, contacts, and the immediate environment:

1) *Report to local health authority:* Case report of suspect and confirmed cases universally required by International Health Regulations, Class 1 (see Preface).

2) *Isolation:* Rid patient, and especially his clothing and baggage, of fleas with an insecticide of tested effectiveness against local fleas, and hospitalize if practical; ordinary hospital isolation precautions suffice for patients with bubonic plague; *strict isolation with precautions against airborne spread is required for patients with primary pneumonic plague or patients developing plague pneumonia* until the second day after antibiotic therapy has been established, if the patient responds clinically. (See 9B7 below.)

3) *Concurrent disinfection:* Of sputum and purulent discharges, and articles soiled therewith and with urine and feces of patients. Terminal cleaning. Bodies of persons dying of plague should be handled with strict aseptic precautions.

4) *Quarantine:* For contacts of bubonic plague, disinfestation with insecticide powder such as 2% diazinon or 1% Malathion, and surveillance for 6 days. For close contacts of pneumonic plague, dust with insecticide powder if indicated, institute chemoprophylaxis (see 9B5) and maintain surveillance for 6 days, observing closely for developing illness; hospitalize and start additional therapy (see 9B7) as soon as fever or other clinical symptoms appear. (Contacts who have been taking antimalarial prophylaxis should continue this.)

5) *Protection of contacts:* The management of contacts should concentrate on surveillance and close observation, with prompt institution of specific treatment at first appearance of fever or other signs of disease. When pneumonic plague is diagnosed, or suspected, close contacts (including nurses and other hospital attendants) should be given chemoprophylaxis and observed closely, including recorded temperatures at least 4 times daily. Other contacts should be observed closely and chemoprophylaxis considered at the termination of exposure. Chemoprophylaxis for adults may be effected with

broad-spectrum antibiotics such as tetracycline (1.0 g per day) or sulfadiazine (2.0 to 3.0 g per day) for 6 days. Post-exposure immunization is not useful.

6) *Investigation of contacts and source of infection:* Search for infected rodents and fleas or persons exposed to pneumonic plague. Flea control should precede or be done concurrently with anti-rat measures, using an insecticide with residual effect on local fleas. Dust rat runs and harborages in and about known or suspected plague premises or areas. Disinfest by dusting, or spray the houses, outhouses and household furnishings in the same areas with an effective insecticide. Dust the persons and clothing of immediate contacts and all other residents in the immediate vicinity. Suppress rat populations by energetic campaigns of poisoning or trapping and with vigorous concurrent measures to reduce rat harborages and food sources.

7) *Specific treatment:* Streptomycin, tetracyclines, and chloramphenicol used early are highly effective. Results are good, even in pneumonic plague, if therapy is begun within 8 to 24 hours after onset, but poor thereafter. Streptomycin-resistant organisms have been described. After a satisfactory response to drug therapy some patients will show a self-limited brief febrile episode on the 5th or 6th day, unaccompanied by any other evidence of illness. However, reappearance of fever at any time, in association with other clinical or laboratory evidence of disease, may indicate that the infectious agent is resistant, or that a complication has developed, such as secondary pneumonia due to other bacteria; sputum should be examined by stained smear and cultured immediately. Penicillin or other appropriate antibiotics may then be indicated. (The penicillins are not effective against plague. When other antibiotics are not available, use sulfonamides.)

C. *Epidemic measures:*
1) Investigate all deaths, with autopsy and laboratory examinations when indicated. Develop and carry out case-finding intensively. Establish the best possible provision for diagnosis and treatment. Alert all existing medical facilities to report cases immediately and utilize diagnostic and therapeutic services fully. Provide adequate laboratory services, kits containing appropriate

bacteriologic transport media, and adequate supplies of effective antibiotics.

2) Avoid public hysteria by appropriate informational and educational releases through the news media.

3) Institute intensive flea control in expanding circles from known foci.

4) Supplement rodent destruction within all affected areas.

5) Administer broad-spectrum antibiotics or sulfadiazine prophylactically to all medical, nursing and public health personnel exposed to definite and repeated risk of infection, if they cannot be kept under close and frequent observation.

6) Restrict hospital personnel and family contacts to the premises when patients with pneumonic plague are under treatment.

7) Protect field workers against fleas by weekly dusting of clothing with insecticide powder to which fleas are sensitive. Daily application of insect repellents is a valuable adjunct.

8) A single dose of avirulent living plague bacillus vaccine (not available in the U.S.A.) has proved of variable benefit among residents of endemic areas; there are no generally accepted standards for safety and potency testing of such a vaccine, and available strains vary from too reactogenic to inadequately protective. Killed vaccine (see 9A3) affords temporary protection, and booster doses are required.

D. *International measures:*

1) Telegraphic notification by governments to WHO and to adjacent countries of the first imported, first transferred or first nonimported case of plague in any area previously free of the disease. Report newly discovered or reactivated foci of plague among rodents.

2) Measures applicable to ships, aircraft, and land transport arriving from plague areas are specified in International Health Regulations, 1969, WHO*, Geneva.

3) All ships should be free of rodents, or periodically deratted.

4) Ratproofing of buildings of seaports and airports; application of appropriate insecticide with residual effect every 6 months; deratting with effective rodenticide.

---

*Second Annotated Edition, 1974.

5) International travelers: Plague-infected persons or suspects are not permitted to depart from a country. International regulations require that prior to their departure on an international voyage from an area where there is an epidemic of pulmonary plague, those exposed to infection shall be placed in isolation for 6 days after last exposure. On arrival, travelers may be disinsected and kept under surveillance for a period of not more than 6 days reckoned from the date of arrival. No country currently requires immunization against plague for entry. Because protection by vaccines is brief, immunization should be completed just preceding anticipated exposure. (See 9A3 above.)

6) WHO Collaborating Centres (see Preface).

PLEURODYNIA, EPIDEMIC

(Bornholm disease, Epidemic myalgia, Devil's grip)

1. **Identification**—An acute viral disease characterized by sudden onset with severe paroxysmal pain localized in the chest or abdomen, usually accompanied by fever and frequently by headache. The chest pain may be intensified by movement. The location of the characteristic pain tends to be more abdominal than thoracic in infants and young children, while the reverse applies in older children and adults. Most patients recover within one week of onset; relapses may occur frequently; no fatalities have been reported. Localized epidemics are characteristic. It is important to differentiate from more serious medical or surgical conditions. Complications occur relatively infrequently and include orchitis, pericarditis, and aseptic meningitis. During outbreaks of epidemic pleurodynia, cases of group B coxsackievirus myocarditis of the newborn have been reported occasionally. While myocarditis in adults is a rare complication the possibility should always be considered.

Diagnosis is aided by culture of virus from throat washings and feces, and by rise in titer of type-specific neutralizing antibodies in paired sera obtained early and late in illness.

2. **Occurrence**—An uncommon disease occurring in summer and

early autumn; usually seen in children and young adults, but may occur at all ages. Multiple cases in a household are frequent, but single cases do occur. Outbreaks have been reported in Europe, Australia, New Zealand and North America.

3. Infectious agents—Group B coxsackievirus, types 1, 2, 3, 4, and 5, have been associated with the illness.

4. Reservoir—Man.

5. Mode of transmission—Probably contact with an infected person or with articles freshly soiled with the feces or throat discharges of an infected person, who may or may not have symptoms. Group B coxsackieviruses have been found in sewage and on flies and mosquitoes, though the relationship to transmission of human disease is not clear.

6. Incubation period—Usually 3 to 5 days.

7. Period of communicability—Apparently during the acute stage of disease.

8. Susceptibility and resistance—Susceptibility is probably general, and presumably a type-specific immunity results from infection.

9. Methods of control—

    A. Preventive measures: None.

    B. Control of patient, contacts, and the immediate environment:
        1) Report to local health authority: Obligatory report of individual cases, Class 3B.
        2) Isolation: Ordinarily limited to respiratory secretion and fecal excretion precautions. Because of the remote possibility of myocarditis in the newborn, if a patient in a maternity unit or nursery develops an illness which suggests group B coxsackievirus infection, these precautions should be instituted at once. Similarly, individuals, including medical personnel, with suspected group B coxsackievirus infections should be excluded from visiting maternity and nursery units, women near term and infants.
        3) Concurrent disinfection: Prompt and safe disposal of respiratory discharges and of feces. Articles soiled therewith should be disinfected.
        4) Quarantine: None.
        5) Immunization of contacts: None.
        6) Investigation of contacts: Of no practical value.
        7) Specific treatment: None.

C. *Epidemic measures:* General notice to physicians of the presence of an epidemic and the necessity for differential diagnosis from more serious medical or surgical emergencies.

D. *International measures:* WHO Collaborating Centres (see Preface).

THE PNEUMONIAS

A. PNEUMOCOCCAL PNEUMONIA

1. Identification—An acute bacterial disease characterized by the sudden onset of a single shaking chill with fever, pain in the chest, usually dyspnea and leucocytosis and a cough productive of "rusty" sputum. X-rays may provide the first evidence of consolidation. Pneumonia can be bronchial rather than lobar, especially in children; vomiting and convulsions have been observed as the first manifestations. Pneumococcal pneumonia is an important cause of death, especially in infants and the aged. Fatality, formerly 20 to 40% for hospitalized patients, has been greatly reduced by antibiotics.

Early etiologic diagnosis is important for therapy. Presumptive diagnosis can be made by demonstrating many gram-positive diplococci in smears of lower respiratory tract secretions. Confirmation is by isolation of pneumococci from blood or lower respiratory tract specimens.

2. Occurrence—Previously a very common disease, particularly in infancy and old age; most frequent in industrial cities and lower economic groups. Occurs in all climates and seasons; incidence is highest in winter and spring in temperate zones. Usually sporadic in U.S.A., but epidemics may occur in institutions. Consistently recurring epidemics have been described in South African mines; common in some native races, e.g., in New Guinea. A rising incidence commonly accompanies epidemics of viral respiratory disease, especially influenza.

3. Infectious agent—*Streptococcus pneumoniae* (pneumococci). Pneumococci of Types I to XXXII account for about 95% of cases.

4. Reservoir—Man. Pneumococci are commonly found in the upper respiratory tract of healthy persons throughout the world.

5. Mode of transmission—By droplet spread; by direct oral contact; or indirectly, through articles freshly soiled with respiratory discharges. Person-to-person transmission is common, but illness among casual contacts and attendants is infrequent.

6. Incubation period—Not well determined; believed to be 1 to 3 days.

7. Period of communicability—Unknown; presumably until discharges of mouth and nose no longer contain pneumococci in appreciable numbers or in virulent form. Penicillin will eliminate the pneumococcus from most patients within 3 days.

8. Susceptibility and resistance—Resistance is generally high, but may be lowered by exposure to a cold, wet environment, by physical fatigue, by alcoholism, by chronic lung disease, or by a preceding viral respiratory infection. Immunity, specific for the infecting serotype, usually follows an attack and may last for months or years.

9. Methods of control—

    A. Preventive measures: Avoid crowding in living quarters whenever practical, particularly in institutions or barracks or on shipboard.

    B. Control of patient, contacts, and the immediate environment:
        1) Report to local health authority: Obligatory report of epidemics; no individual case report, Class 4 (see Preface).
        2) Isolation: Of limited value; institute secretion precautions for duration of illness.
        3) Concurrent disinfection: Of discharges from nose and throat. Terminal cleaning.
        4) Quarantine: None.
        5) Immunization of contacts: None. (See C below)
        6) Investigation of contacts: Of no practical value.
        7) Specific treatment: Penicillin intramuscularly; oral penicillin V is effective in mild cases. Erythromycin is nearly as effective as penicillin and may be substituted in the event of penicillin sensitivity. Many pneumococci are now resistant to tetracyclines.

    C. Epidemic measures: In outbreaks in institutions or in other closed population groups, general hygienic measures may be supplemented by prophylaxis with antibiotics. Immunization with bacterial polysaccharides of prevailing types may be effective in high-risk populations such as mine workers; effectiveness is under evaluation.

D. International measures: None.

B. BACTERIAL PNEUMONIA, OTHER THAN PNEUMOCOCCAL

1. Identification—An acute febrile disease with pulmonary involvement evidenced by varying respiratory symptoms, and physical signs and positive X-ray findings. Occasionally occurs in association with viral infections of the respiratory tract, particularly influenza. Most often occurs as a superinfection following broad-spectrum antibiotic therapy or as a complication of chronic lung disease, aspiration of gastric contents or tracheostomy. Fatality is generally high, but varies with infectious agent and age of patient.

2. Occurrence—Worldwide in distribution; a frequent disease in infancy and old age especially in the debilitated and those with host defenses altered by antibiotic therapy or surgical manipulation of the respiratory tract. Usually sporadic, but epidemics occur in association with influenza, measles and acute undifferentiated viral respiratory diseases.

3. Infectious agents—Various pathogenic bacteria commonly found in the mouth, nose and throat, such as *Staphylococcus aureus Klebsiella pneumoniae* (Friedlander bacillus), *Haemophilus influenzae,* and *Streptococcus pyogenes* (group A hemolytic streptococci). In recent years pneumonios caused by coliform bacteria and *Pseudomonas* species have become increasingly common, especially by *Pseudomonas aeruginosa,* and *Escherichia coli.*

4. Reservoir—Man.

5. Mode of transmission—Direct by droplet spread or oral contact; indirectly, through articles freshly soiled with discharges of infected persons.

6. Incubation period—Variable, usually short, 1 to 3 days.

7. Period of communicability—Unknown; probably while the infectious agent is present in discharges of noses and throats of patients. For many agents, antibiotic therapy greatly decreases the period of communicability.

8. Susceptibility and resistance—Resistance is generally high, except in debilitated persons; infection is often secondary to viral infections or other factors compromising host defenses. Specific immunity varies with the infectious agent. Immunization is not feasible.

9. Methods of control—

A. *Preventive measures:*
1) Good personal hygiene; avoid crowding in institutions and hospitals; prevent unnecessary or inappropriate use of antibiotics, and carry out scrupulous disinfection of equipment used for respiratory care.
2) Immunization against influenza (p. 161) and chemo-prophylaxis for streptococcal infections (p. 310) may be useful in closed or limited general populations.

B. *Control of patient, contacts, and the immediate environment:*
1) *Report to local health authority:* Obligatory report of epidemics but not individual case report, Class 4 (see Preface). Identification of an accompanying or pre-ceding epidemic of acute respiratory disease is of public health significance.
2) *Isolation:* Strict isolation for staphylococcal and streptococcal pneumonias, secretion precautions for others.
3) *Concurrent disinfection:* Of discharges from mouth and nose and of articles soiled therewith, especially equipment used for respiratory care. Terminal cleaning.
4) *Quarantine:* None.
5) *Immunization of contacts:* None.
6) *Investigation of contacts:* Generally of no practical value, however, contacts of streptococcal pneumonia should be searched for and treated.
7) *Specific treatment:* For streptococcal pneumonia, the same as for pneumococcal; for staphylococcal pneumonia penicillinase-resistant penicillins or cepha-losporins, unless the organism can be shown to be sus-ceptible to penicillin G. Sensitivity tests with the isolated organism are important in selecting the most suitable antibiotic. Effective antibiotics: for *H. influenzae,* ampicillin; for *K. pneumoniae,* kanamycin alone or combined with a cephalosporin or gentamicin; for coliform organisms, ampicillin or kanamycin; for *Pseudomonas* species, gentamicin with carbenicillin.

C. *Epidemic measures:* Applicable only in outbreaks in institutions or in other limited or closed population groups when associated with influenza, measles, or other respiratory infections. Immunization of adults against influenza, and of infants and children against measles, may be useful. Individual chemoprophylaxis is not of proved value.

D. International measures: None.

C. MYCOPLASMAL (PPLO) PNEUMONIA
(Primary atypical pneumonia, Eaton agent pneumonia)

1. Identification—A febrile upper respiratory infection which sometimes progresses to bronchitis or pneumonia. Onset is gradual, with headache, malaise, cough, and usually substernal, but not pleuritic, pain. Sputum, scant at first, may increase later. Early patchy infiltration of the lungs, revealed by X-ray examination, is often more extensive than clinical findings suggest. In severe cases pneumonia may progress from one lobe to another. Leucocytosis may occur after the first week in approximately one-third of cases. Duration of illness varies from a few days to several weeks. Secondary bacterial infection and other complications are infrequent and fatalities are rare.

Diagnosis is based on rise in complement-fixing antibody titers between acute phase and 3 week sera. Development of cold hemagglutinins during early convalescence or of agglutinins for *Streptococcus MG,* or both, supports diagnosis and may occur in one-half to two-thirds of cases. The infectious agent may be cultured on special agar.

Differentiation is required from pneumonitis due to adenoviruses, respiratory syncytial virus, the viruses of influenza, varicella, parainfluenza, and measles and the agents of psittacosis, Q fever, certain mycoses and tuberculosis.

2. Occurrence—Worldwide; sporadic, endemic and occasionally epidemic, especially in institutions and military populations. Attack rates are 5 to over 50 per 1000 per annum in military and 1 to 3 per 1000 per annum in civilian populations. Incidence is greatest during fall and winter months in temperate climates, with much variation from year to year and in different geographic areas. No selectivity for race or sex. Occurs at all ages, but recognized disease is most frequent among school children and young adults.

3. Infectious agent—*Mycoplasma pneumoniae,* (Eaton agent), a member of the pleuropneumonia-like group of organisms (PPLO).

4. Reservoir—Man.

5. Mode of transmission—Probably by droplet inhalation or by oral contact with an infected person or with articles freshly soiled with discharges of nose and throat. Secondary cases of pneumonia among contacts and attendants are infrequent, although a mild respiratory disease may occur.

6. **Incubation period** — 14 to 21 days.

7. **Period of communicability** — Probably less than 10 days; occasionally longer with persisting febrile illness.

8. **Susceptibility and resistance** — Clinical pneumonia occurs in about 3 to 30% of infections with *M. pneumoniae*, depending on age. Attack varies from mild afebrile upper respiratory disease to febrile illness involving the upper or lower respiratory tract. Duration of immunity is indefinite, but resistance has been correlated with humoral antibodies, which remain for 1 or more years.

9. **Methods of control** —

   A. *Preventive measures:* Avoid crowding in living and sleeping quarters whenever possible, especially in institutions, in barracks and on shipboard.

   B. *Control of patient, contacts, and the immediate environment:*
      1) *Report to local health authority:* Obligatory report of epidemics; no individual case report, Class 4 (see Preface).
      2) *Isolation:* None.
      3) *Concurrent disinfection:* Of discharges from nose and throat. Terminal cleansing.
      4) *Quarantine:* None.
      5) *Immunization of contacts:* None.
      6) *Investigation of contacts:* Of no practical value.
      7) *Specific treatment:* Tetracycline antibiotics and erythromycin give good results, especially in severe mycoplasmal pneumonia; erythromycin is preferred for children to avoid tetracycline staining of immature teeth. The infectious agent is highly resistant to penicillin, and variably and in lesser degree, to streptomycin.

   C. *Epidemic measures:* No reliably effective measures for control are available.

   D. *International measures:* WHO Collaborating Centres (see Preface).

D. PNEUMOCYSTIS PNEUMONIA
   (Interstitial plasma-cell pneumonia)

1. **Identification** — A subacute, pulmonary disease occurring

early in life, especially in ill or premature infants; often fatal. Also occurs in older children and adults as an opportunistic infection associated with debilitating conditions, disease of immune mechanisms and the use of immunosuppressants. Clinically, there is progressive dyspnea, tachypnea, cyanosis, and pallor with or without fever or auscultatory signs. Chest X-ray reveals diffuse increased density and areas of emphysema. Postmortem examination reveals heavy airless lungs, thickened alveolar septa, and foamy material containing clumps of parasites in the alveolar spaces.

Diagnosis is established by demonstration of the causative agent in material from lung biopsy, in smears of tracheobronchial mucus, or in histological sections or impression smears from affected lungs stained with Gomori's methenamine silver nitrate method. There are no satisfactory cultural or serological methods.

2. Occurrence—The disease has been recognized in England, Europe, North America and Australia; may be endemic and epidemic in infants in some hospitals and institutions. The organism was first seen in animals in South America.

3. Infectious agent—*Pneumocystis carinii,* an organism of uncertain classification, but generally regarded as a protozoan.

4. Reservoir—Suspected but unknown organisms have been demonstrated in lungs of many animals, including man, but the epidemiological significance of these potential sources is not proved.

5. Mode of transmission—Unknown.

6. Incubation period—Analysis of institutional outbreaks among infants indicates 1 to 2 months.

7. Period of communicability—Unknown.

8. Susceptibility and resistance—Susceptibility is enhanced by prematurity, by chronic debilitating illness, or by disease or therapy in which immune mechanisms are impaired.

9. Methods of control—

    A. Preventive measures: None known.

    B. Control of patient, contacts, and the immediate environment:
        1) Report to local health authority: Official report ordinarily not justifiable, Class 5 (see Preface).
        2) Isolation: Isolation wards have been used in European institutional outbreaks in infants. Prudence would suggest removal of high risk patients from the environment of suspected cases.
        3) Concurrent disinfection: Insufficient knowledge.

  4) Quarantine: None.

  5) Immunization of contacts: None.

  6) Investigation of contacts: None.

  7) Specific treatment: Pentamidine isethionate (Lomidine) is useful. It is available in the U.S.A. from the Center for Disease Control, Atlanta, GA., (see Preface), on an investigational basis. Sulfadiazine plus pyrimethamine also is effective.

 C. Epidemic measures: Knowledge of source of organism and mode of transmission is so incomplete that there are no generally accepted measures.

 D. International measures: None.

E. OTHER PNEUMONIAS

Among the known viruses, the adenoviruses, respiratory syncytial virus, the parainfluenza viruses, and probably others as yet unidentified, have the capacity to induce a pneumonitis. Because these infectious agents cause upper respiratory disease more often than pneumonia, they are presented under Respiratory Disease; Acute Viral, (p. 262). See also viral pneumonia of measles, chickenpox, and influenza (pp. 196, 69, and 159). Pneumonia is also caused by infection with chlamydia (psittacosis) and rickettsiae (Q fever). It can also be associated with the invasive phase of nematode infections such as ascariasis and with aspergillosis.

POLIOMYELITIS
(Infantile paralysis)

 1. **Identification**—An acute viral illness with severity ranging from inapparent infection to nonparalytic and paralytic disease. Symptoms include fever, headache, gastrointestinal disturbance, malaise and stiffness of neck and back, with or without paralysis. The virus invades the alimentary tract; viremia may then follow with invasion of central nervous system and selective involvement of motor cells resulting in flaccid paralysis, most commonly of the lower extremities. Paralysis of muscles of respiration and swallowing may threaten life. Site of paralysis depends upon location of nerve cell destruction in spinal cord or brain stem, but is charac-

teristically asymmetrical. Nonparalytic poliomyelitis is one of the causes of aseptic meningitis (see p. 202). Incidence of inapparent infection usually exceeds clinical cases by more than a hundred fold. Fatality rate for paralytic cases varies from 2 to 10% in epidemics and increases markedly with age.

Poliovirus can be isolated by tissue culture from feces or throat secretions early in the course of infection; a rising titer of complement-fixing or neutralizing antibodies denotes recent infection. Genetic marker tests to differentiate wild from vaccine strains should be performed where warranted.

The differential diagnosis of nonparalytic poliomyelitis includes other forms of acute non-bacterial meningitis, purulent meningitis, tuberculous meningitis, brain abscess, leptospirosis, lymphocytic choriomeningitis, infectious mononucleosis, the encephalitides, and toxic encephalopathies.

Paralytic poliomyelitis can usually be recognized on clinical grounds, but can be confused with post infectious polyneuritis and other paralytic conditions. Other enteroviruses (ECHO and coxsackie, especially type A7) can cause an illness simulating paralytic poliomyelitis, though usually less severe and with negligible residual paralysis. Tick-bite paralysis occurs uncommonly, but worldwide, affecting man and animals, to give a flaccid ascending motor paralysis. In northwestern U.S.A., *Dermacentor andersoni* is most frequently involved; also other ticks in the east and south, mainly in spring and early summer. Patient usually recovers promptly when tick is removed.

2. Occurrence — Worldwide. Before large-scale immunization programs were carried out, the highest incidence of clinically recognizable disease was in temperate zones and the more developed countries. Occurs as sporadic cases and in epidemics; more common during summer and early autumn in temperate climates, but with wide variations from year to year and from region to region. Fairly large areas may experience low incidence for several years, with ultimate reappearance in large numbers. Characteristically a disease of children and adolescents; all ages are affected where artificial or natural immunity has not been acquired, with paralytic illness proportionately more frequent among older persons. Improved living standards may be associated with emergence of paralytic poliomyelitis, as illustrated by increasing incidence in regions with decreasing infant mortality rates. Severe epidemics, formerly uncommon, now occur in lesser developed areas with increasing frequency, mainly involving young children. In such areas, antibodies to all 3 types of poliovirus are generally present by school age. In countries where artificial immunization has been

widely practiced, paralytic cases are chiefly among the least vaccinated groups, mainly preschool children of lower social classes. The use of vaccines has resulted in a marked decrease in overall incidence of paralytic disease; in the U.S.A. in 1974, there were only 14 cases (of whom 3 were vaccine associated) and in England in 1972, only 3 paralytic cases were notified.

3. **Infectious agent** — Poliovirus types 1, 2 and 3; all types cause paralysis but type 1 has been most commonly involved.

4. **Reservoir** — Man, most frequently persons with inapparent infections, especially children.

5. **Mode of transmission** — Direct contact with pharyngeal secretions or feces of infected persons through close association. In rare instances milk has been a vehicle. No reliable evidence of spread by other foods, insects or virus-contaminated sewage; water is rarely if ever involved. Whether feces or pharyngeal secretions have the greater importance in transmission has not been determined and may vary according to environmental circumstances. Virus is more easily detectable, and for a longer period, in feces than throat secretions, but epidemiologic evidence suggests that oral-oral spread may be more important than fecal-oral spread where sanitation is good.

6. **Incubation period** — Commonly 7 to 12 days, with a range from 3 to 21 days.

7. **Period of communicability** — Poliovirus is demonstrable in throat secretions as early as 36 hours and in the feces 72 hours after infection in both clinical and inapparent cases. Virus persists in the throat for approximately one week and in the feces for 3 to 6 weeks or longer. Cases are most infectious from 7 to 10 days before and after the onset of symptoms.

8. **Susceptibility and resistance** — Susceptibility to infection is general but few infected persons develop paralysis. Type-specific resistance of long duration follows both clinically recognizable and inapparent infection. Second attacks are rare and result from infection with poliovirus of a different type. Infants born of immune mothers have transient passive immunity. Tonsillectomy increases the risk of bulbar involvement. Trauma and injection of precipitated antigens or certain other insoluble substances may provoke paralysis in an already infected but symptomless person, the paralysis tending to be localized in the affected limb or appearing there first. Excessive muscular fatigue in the prodromal period may likewise predispose to paralytic involvement. An increased

susceptibility to paralytic poliomyelitis is associated with pregnancy.

9. Methods of control—

A. *Preventive measures:*

1) Active immunization of all susceptible persons against the 3 types of poliovirus. Give priority to ages with highest incidence and to selected groups at unusual risk. Follow by maintenance program to cover all infants. Two methods are available; immunization by either method may begin as early as 6 weeks of age although the suppressive effect of maternal antibody on immune response is avoided if started at age 6 to 8 months.

a) Oral poliovirus vaccines provide a high level of immunity by causing an alimentary infection with attenuated polioviruses. They are administered by mouth, usually in the form of trivalent combinations of the 3 types. The generally accepted pattern in the U.S.A. is to start as early as age 6 to 12 weeks, with 2 doses of trivalent vaccine fed at an interval of 6 to 8 weeks and a third dose 6 to 12 months later. Variations of this schedule are based on national preferences, e.g. in Canada, 3 initial doses at 4 to 8 week intervals and a fourth 6 to 12 months later; in the United Kingdom, 3 doses of trivalent vaccine are recommended at intervals of 6 to 8 weeks between the 1st and 2nd doses and 4 to 6 months between the 2nd and 3rd doses; in Australia, the 3 doses are given with minimal interval of 8 weeks. Some countries start with type 1 vaccine, followed in 6 to 8 weeks with the 2nd and 3rd doses of trivalent vaccine.

b) Formalin-inactivated poliovirus vaccine also provides protection but is less effective in preventing subsequent alimentary infection. Where used, a basic series of 4 injections, preferably initiated in early infancy, is recommended, the first 3 about 6 weeks apart, the fourth 6 months or more after the third. In Sweden, 2 doses are given 2-4 weeks apart for primary vaccination and booster doses are given 1 and 4-5 years later. To maintain optimal antibody levels, regular booster doses every few years appear to be needed.

c) Additional booster doses of vaccine are indicated with the threat of an epidemic, or travel to a high risk area and at the time of entering school. If a child was not previously immunized at school age, a full series is given.

2) Education of the public on the advantages of immunization in early childhood, and on modes of spread.

B. *Control of patient, contacts, and the immediate environment:*

1) *Report to local health authority:* Obligatory case report as a *Disease under Surveillance by WHO,* Class 1. Each case is to be designated as paralytic or nonparalytic. Supplemental reports giving vaccine history, virus type, severity and persistence of residual paralysis 60 days or longer after onset are necessary measures for effective control.

2) *Isolation:* Hospital isolation precautions for not more than 7 days. Of little value under home conditions because spread of infection is greatest in the prodromal period.

3) *Concurrent disinfection:* Of throat discharges and feces and of articles soiled therewith. In communities with modern and adequate sewage disposal systems, feces and urine can be discharged directly into sewers without preliminary disinfection. Terminal cleaning.

4) *Quarantine:* Of no community value because of large numbers of unrecognized infections in the population.

5) *Protection of contacts:* Vaccination of familial and other close contacts contributes little to immediate control; ordinarily the virus is widely spread among them by the time the first case is recognized. In countries with a low prevalence, occurrence of a single non-vaccine associated paralytic case in a community should be regarded as sufficient cause for initiating an oral immunization program for children in the community.

6) *Investigation of contacts:* Thorough search for sick persons, especially children, to assure treatment of unrecognized and unreported cases. Footdrop, scoliosis and other deformities resulting in functional impairment may be late manifestations of initially mild or inapparent illness.

7) *Specific treatment:* None; attention during the acute illness to the complications of paralysis; may require expert knowledge, especially for patients in need of respiratory assistance.

C. *Epidemic measures:*

1) Institute mass vaccination with oral vaccine at the

earliest indication of an outbreak. Use monovalent vaccine of the same virus type causing the outbreak, if available. If typing facilities are not available, use trivalent vaccine.

2) Organize mass vaccination campaigns to achieve the most rapid and complete immunization of epidemiologically relevant groups, especially younger children. Locate vaccination centers in relation to population densities, taking advantage of normal social patterns; schools often meet these criteria.

3) With the use of mass immunization, it is no longer necessary to disrupt community activities by closing schools and other places of population aggregation.

4) Postpone elective nose and throat operations and other elective immunizations until after the epidemic has ended.

5) Provide facilities in strategically located centers for specialized medical care of acutely ill patients and rehabilitation of those with significant paralysis.

D. International measures:

1) Poliomyelitis is a *Disease Under Surveillance by WHO*. National health administrations are expected to inform WHO of outbreaks promptly by telegram or telex, and to supplement these reports as soon as possible with details of the source, nature and extent of the epidemic and of the identity of the type of epidemic virus involved.

2) Susceptible international travelers visiting areas of hyperendemic prevalence should be adequately immunized.

3) WHO Collaborating Centres (see Preface).

PSITTACOSIS
(Ornithosis, Parrot fever)

1. Identification—An acute generalized infectious disease with fever, headache and early pneumonic involvement; cough is initially absent or non-productive; when present sputum is mucopurulent, not copious; anorexia is extreme; constipation common; pulse usually slow in relation to temperature; lethargy; occasional relapses. Human infections may be severe but are usually mild in character. Death is rare.

Laboratory diagnosis is by demonstrating significant increase in complement-fixing antibodies during convalescence; or, under suitably safe laboratory conditions only, by isolation of the infectious agent from sputum, blood or postmortem tissues in mice, eggs, or tissue culture. Recovery of the agent may be difficult, especially if the patient has received broad spectrum antibiotics. Early antibiotic therapy may also delay or prevent the development of complement-fixing antibodies; however, with an appropriate history, a titer of at least 1:16 is considered diagnostic.

2. Occurrence — Worldwide, as sporadic cases or as household outbreaks among persons exposed to sick or seemingly healthy birds. In U.S.A. a disease of persons associated with pet shops, aviaries, pigeon lofts, poultry farms, and poultry processing and rendering plants; largely occupational.

3. Infectious agent — *Chlamydia (Bedsonia) psittaci.*

4. Reservoir — Parakeets, parrots, pigeons, turkeys, domestic fowl, and other birds; occasionally man. Apparently healthy birds can be carriers and occasionally shed the infectious agent.

5. Mode of transmission — Infection is usually acquired by inhaling the agent from desiccated droppings of infected birds in an enclosed space, e.g., in homes, in pigeon lofts, or in poultry processing and rendering plants. Direct contact with infected birds on squab, turkey and duck farms is a possible source; household birds a frequent source; laboratory infections occur. Transmission from man to man is rare but personnel attending psittacosis patients may be infected.

6. Incubation period — From 4 to 15 days, commonly 10 days.

7. Period of communicability — Primarily during the acute illness, especially with paroxysmal coughing. Diseased as well as seemingly healthy birds may shed the agent intermittently and sometimes continuously for weeks or months.

8. Susceptibility and resistance — Susceptibility is general; older adults have a more severe illness; one attack does not confer complete immunity.

9. Methods of control —

    A. Preventive measures:

        1) Regulation of importation and traffic of birds of the parrot family to prevent or eliminate infections by appro-

priate antibiotic treatment. Prevent exposure of previously noninfected birds to potentially infected birds or
birds of unknown history.

2) Surveillance of pet shops and aviaries where psittacosis
has occurred or where birds epidemiologically linked to
cases were obtained. Infected birds should be treated or
destroyed and the premises thoroughly cleaned.

3) Psittacine birds offered in commerce should be raised
under psittacosis-free conditions and handled in such
manner as to prevent infection. Tetracycline-impreg-
nated birdseed or mash can be effective in controlling
disease in parakeets, parrots and pigeons if properly administered to ensure adequate intake.

4) Education of the public in the danger of household or
occupational exposure to infected birds of the parrot
family.

B. *Control of patient, contacts, and the immediate environment:*

1) *Report to local health authority:* Obligatory case report
in most states and countries, Class 2A (see Preface).

2) *Isolation:* Important during acute febrile stage.
Personnel caring for patients with a cough should wear
suitable masks.

3) *Concurrent disinfection:* Of all discharges. Terminal
cleaning.

4) *Quarantine:* None.

5) *Immunization of contacts:* None.

6) *Investigation of contacts and source of infection:* Trace
origin of suspected birds. Kill suspect birds and immerse
bodies in 2% phenolic or equivalent disinfectant. Place in
a plastic bag, close securely, and ship frozen (on dry ice)
to nearest competent laboratory. Buildings housing
infected birds should not be used by man until
thoroughly cleaned and aired.

7) *Specific treatment:* Antibiotics of the tetracycline
group, continued for 10 to 14 days after temperature returns to normal.

C. *Epidemic measures:* Ordinarily not applicable to man because cases are usually sporadic or confined to family outbreaks. The epidemic problem concerns birds. Report outbreaks of ornithosis in flocks of turkeys to state agriculture
and health authorities. Large doses of tetracyclines will
suppress but may not eliminate infection in poultry flocks.
Identify susceptible employees on farms and in processing

plants by serologic tests; workers preferably should be restricted to those with demonstrated antibodies.

D. International measures: Reciprocal compliance with national regulations to control importation of psittacine birds.

Q FEVER

1. **Identification**—An acute febrile rickettsial disease; onset may be sudden, with chilly sensations, retrobulbar headache, weakness, malaise, and severe sweats; much variation in severity and duration. A pneumonitis occurs in most cases, with cough, scanty expectoration, chest pain, and minimal physical findings. Chronic endocarditis, hepatitis, and generalized infections have been reported; inapparent infections occur. Fatality of untreated patients is less than 1% and with treatment is negligible except in aged persons and individuals who develop endocarditis.

Laboratory diagnosis is by complement-fixation or agglutination tests, with demonstration of rise in antibody between acute and convalescent stages; recovery of the infectious agent from blood of patients is diagnostic but is hazardous to laboratory workers.

2. **Occurrence**—Reported from all continents; endemic in many areas. In the U.S.A. endemic in several states, affecting especially veterinarians, dairy workers, and farmers; rare in many areas where infection exists enzootically in animals; explosive epidemics have occurred among workers in diagnostic laboratories, stockyards, meat packing and rendering plants.

3. **Infectious agent**—*Coxiella burneti (Rickettsia burneti)*, an organism with unusual viability in the free state.

4. **Reservoir**—Ticks, wild animals (bandicoots), cattle, sheep, and goats are natural reservoirs, with infection inapparent.

5. **Mode of transmission**—Commonly by airborne dissemination of rickettsiae in dust in or near premises contaminated by placental tissues, birth fluids and excreta of infected animals, in establishments processing infected animals or their by-products, and in necropsy rooms. Also contracted by direct contact with infected animals or other contaminated materials such as wool, straw, fertilizer, and the laundry of exposed persons. Raw milk from infected cows may be responsible for some cases.

6. **Incubation period**—Dependent on size of infecting dose; usually 2 to 3 weeks.

7. **Period of communicability**—Direct transmission from man to man is rare.

8. **Susceptibility and resistance**—Susceptibility is general. Immunity following recovery from clinical illness is probably permanent.

9. **Methods of Control**—

   A. Preventive measures:

      1) Health education on sources of infection and the necessity for hygienic practices such as pasteurization of milk; adequate disinfection and disposal of animal products of conception and strict hygienic measures in cow sheds and barns (dust, urine, feces, rodents) during epizootics.

      2) Pasteurization of milk from cows, goats and sheep at 62.9°C (145°F) for 30 minutes, or at 71.6°C (161°F) for 15 seconds by the high-temperature short-time method, or boiling of milk, inactivate rickettsiae.

      3) Immunization with inactivated vaccine prepared from *C. burneti* infected yolk sac is useful in protecting laboratory workers and might be considered for others in hazardous occupations. Immunization should be preceded by a sensitivity test with a small dose of vaccine to avoid severe local reactions.

   B. Control of patient, contacts, and the immediate environment:

      1) *Report to local health authority:* In U.S.A. in areas where disease is endemic; in many countries not a reportable disease, Class 3B (see Preface).

      2) *Isolation:* None.

      3) *Concurrent disinfection:* Of sputum and blood, and articles freshly soiled therewith. Precautions at postmortem examination.

      4) *Quarantine:* None.

      5) *Immunization of contacts:* Unnecessary.

      6) *Investigation of contacts and source of infection:* Search for history of contact with cattle, sheep and goats, consumption of raw milk, or direct or indirect association with a laboratory handling *C. burneti.*

      7) *Specific treatment:* Tetracyclines administered orally and continued for several days after patient is afebrile; reinstitute if relapse occurs.

C. *Epidemic measures:* Outbreaks are generally of short duration; control measures are essentially limited to elimination of sources of infection, observation of exposed persons and antibiotic therapy for those becoming ill.

D. *International measures:* Control of importation of goats, sheep, and cattle. WHO Collaborating Centres (see Preface).

RABIES
(Hydrophobia)

1. **Identification**—An almost invariably fatal acute encephalomyelitis; onset is with a sense of apprehension, headache, fever, malaise, and indefinite sensory changes, often referred to site of a preceding local wound resulting from a bite of a rabid animal. The disease progresses to paresis or paralysis; spasm of muscles of deglutition on attempts to swallow leads to fear of water (hydrophobia); delirium and convulsions follow. Usual duration is 2 to 6 days, sometimes longer; death is apparently due to respiratory paralysis.

Diagnosis is confirmed by specific fluorescent antibody staining of corneal impressions, mucosal scrapings, frozen skin sections or brain biopsy for presence of intracytoplasmic virus, and viral isolation by intracerebral mouse inoculation.

Related viruses exist in Africa, two of which (Mokola and Duvenhage) are associated with fatal rabies-like human illness. At least some of these illnesses would be diagnosed by the standard fluorescent antibody test as rabies. Post-exposure treatment recommended for rabies probably would be ineffective. Other diseases resulting from bites of animals include pasteurellosis *(Pasteurella multicida* and *P. haemolytica)* from cat and dog bites; B-virus from monkey bites; encephalitis, especially due to other rhabdoviruses such as Mokola virus, tularemia, rat-bite fever, cat-scratch fever and possibly tetanus.

2. **Occurrence**—Uncommon in man; primarily a disease of animals. Occurs throughout the world. Rabies-free areas at present include Australia, New Zealand, Japan, Hawaii, Taiwan and other Pacific Islands, some of the West Indies, England and Ireland, and Norway and Sweden. Urban rabies is a problem of dogs and occa-

sionally other pets; sylvatic or rural rabies is a disease of wild carnivores and bats, with sporadic disease among dogs and livestock. In the U.S.A., wildlife rabies is increasing, especially in skunks, foxes, bats and raccoons.

3. **Infectious agent**—Rabies virus, a rhabdovirus.

4. **Reservoir**—Many wild and domestic *Canidae,* including dogs, foxes, coyotes, wolves and jackals; also cats, skunks, raccoons, mongooses, and other biting mammals. Vampire and fruit-eating bats are infected in South and Central America and Mexico, while infected insectivorous bats are found in the U.S.A., Canada and Europe. Rabbits, squirrels, chipmunks, rats and mice are rarely infected and their bites rarely, if ever, call for rabies prophylaxis.

5. **Mode of transmission**—Virus-laden saliva of a rabid animal is introduced by a bite (rarely by a scratch or other fresh break in the skin). Transmission from man to man is not confirmed, though saliva of the infected human may contain virus. Airborne spread to man has been demonstrated in caves where bats are roosting, but rarely occurs. Transmission from infected vampire bats to domestic animals is common. In the U.S.A. the role of indigenous bats in the transmission of rabies to other animals in the wild has not been established.

6. **Incubation period**—Usually 2 to 8 weeks, occasionally shorter or much longer; depends on extent of laceration, site of wound in relation to richness of nerve supply and distance from brain, amount of virus introduced, protection provided by clothing, and other factors.

7. **Period of communicability**—In dogs and most other biting animals, for 3 to 5 days before onset of clinical signs, and during the course of the disease. Bats may shed virus for weeks without evidence of illness; some other wildlife species for a longer period before onset of symptoms.

8. **Susceptibility and resistance**—Most warm-blooded animals are susceptible. Natural immunity in man is unknown.

9. **Methods of Control**—

   A. *Preventive measures:*
      1) After animal bites, prevention of rabies is based on physical removal of the virus and specific immunological procedures.
         a. Treatment of local wound; The most effective rabies prevention is immediate and thorough cleansing and flushing with soap and water, or detergent and water, or preferably quarternary ammonium compounds of

all types of wounds caused by a bite or scratch of an animal with rabies or suspected rabies. The wound should not be sutured; if suturing is unavoidable for cosmetic or tissue support reasons, up to one-half of a total dose of hyperimmune serum (See 9A, lb below) should be thoroughly infiltrated around and beneath the bite wound before suturing; sutures should be loose and interfere as little as possible with free bleeding and drainage.

b. Specific prevention of rabies in man is by administration of antirabies serum and vaccine as soon as possible after exposure. *Antiserum:* Human rabies immune globulin, if available, should be used; if serum of animal origin is used, an intradermal or subcutaneous test dose should precede its administration to detect allergic sensitivity. A single dose of 20 I.U. per kg body weight of human rabies immune globulin, or 40 I.U. of serum of animal origin is given. Half should be infiltrated around the wound, if possible, and the rest should be given intramuscularly. *Vaccine:* Vaccines presently commercially available should be given in 21 doses initially, either 1 dose daily for 21 days or 2 doses daily for 7 days followed by 1 dose daily for an additional 7 days. Reinforcing doses are given on the 10th, 20th and 90th days following completion of the initial series. Serum may be omitted after nonbite exposures to escaped dogs or cats, but 14 doses of duck embryo vaccine, the only vaccine available in U.S.A., should be given. The following is a guide to prophylaxis in different circumstances:

1) If the animal is apprehended it may be killed and its brain immediately examined by the fluorescent antibody technique if the animal's owner and health authorities concur; this may avoid unnecessary treatment. Otherwise, the animal should be apprehended, confined, and observed for 10 days; the decision to administer serum and vaccine immediately after exposure or during the observation period should be weighed by the behavior of the animal, the presence of rabies in the area, and the circumstances of the bite.

2) If attack was unprovoked, the animal was not apprehended, and rabies is known to be present in

that species in the area, administer serum and vaccine.

3) Rabies vaccination carries a small risk of post vaccinal encephalitis; serum from a non-human source produces serum sickness in many recipients. These risks must be weighed against the risk of contracting rabies. No treatment is indicated unless the skin is broken or a mucosal surface has been contaminated by the animal's saliva. The schedule of inoculations may be reduced to 5 daily doses plus a reinforcing dose 20 days later, if the patient has had a previous full course of antirabic inoculations or had developed neutralizing antibody after pre-exposure immunization (9A7). If severe sensitivity appears in the course of vaccination, consult the Health Department for alternative vaccines. (See Post-Exposure Antirabies Guide below).

c. Management of an animal bite, adapted from Sixth Report of the WHO Expert Committee on Rabies by the USPHS Advisory Committee on Immunization Practices, is summarized thus:

CHECKLIST OF TREATMENTS
FOR ANIMAL BITES

1. Cleanse and Flush Wound Immediately (First Aid).

2. Thorough Wound Cleansing Under Medical Supervision.

3. Antirabies Serum and/or Vaccine as indicated.

4. Tetanus Prophylaxis and Antibacterial Treatment when Required.

5. No Sutures or Wound Closure Advised Unless Unavoidable.

2) Registration and licensing of all dogs; under some circumstances collection and destruction of ownerless animals and strays may be indicated. Preventive vaccination of all dogs and cats; attenuated live vaccines, administered intramuscularly, confer longer lasting immunity than most inactivated vaccines. Education of pet owners and the public that restrictions for dogs and cats are necessary, i.e., keep on leash in congested areas when not confined on owner's premises; that strangely acting or sick animals of any species, domestic or wild,

POST-EXPOSURE ANTIRABIES GUIDE

The following recommendations are only a guide. They should be used in conjunction with knowledge of the animal species involved, circumstances of the bite or other exposure, vaccination status of the animal and presence of rabies in the region.

Species	Animal and Its Condition Condition at Time of Attack	Treatment Kind of Exposure Bite	Non-Bite*
Wild Skunk Fox Raccoon Bat	Regard as Rabid	S + V[1]	S + V[1]
Domestic Dog and Cat	Healthy	None[2]	None[2]
	Escaped (unknown)	S + V	V[3]
	Rabid	S + V[1]	S + V[1]
Other	Consider individually—See Rationale and discussion in text.		

* Scratches, abrasions or open wounds; no penetration of the skin by teeth.
V Rabies Vaccine (Duck Embryo Vaccine, Killed, is vaccine of choice)
S Antirabies Serum
1 Discontinue vaccine if fluorescent antibody (FA) tests of animal killed at time of attack are negative.
2 Begin S V at first sign of rabies in biting dog or cat during holding period (10 days).
3 14 Doses of DEV

(Adapted from "Recommendations of Public Health Service Advisory Committee on Immunization Practices," June 1972.)

may be dangerous and should not be picked up or handled; that it is necessary to report such animals and animals that have bitten a person or another animal to the police and/or the local health department; that confinement and observation of such animals is a preventive measure against rabies, and that wild animals should not be kept as pets unless they have been vaccinated with inactivated vaccine and subjected to at least 30 days quarantine.

3) Detention and clinical observation of dogs or other animals known to have bitten a person or showing suspicious signs of rabies for 7 to 10 days. Domestic animals need not be killed until existence of rabies is reasonably established by clinical signs but, if possible, wild animals should be sacrificed upon suspicion of rabies and the brain examined for evidence of rabies. Rabid dogs and cats usually show a change in behavior, with excitability or paralysis, followed by death; if the animal was infective at the time of bite, signs of rabies will follow, usually within 5 days.

4) Immediate submission to a laboratory of intact heads, packed in ice, of animals that die of suspected rabies. Confirmation of rabies is by demonstration of viral antigen by fluorescent antibody testing or of Negri bodies.

5) Unvaccinated dogs or cats bitten by known rabid animals should be destroyed immediately; if detention is elected, hold animal in an approved pound or kennel for at least 6 months. If previously vaccinated, revaccinate and detain (leashing and confinement) for at least 90 days.

6) Institution of cooperative programs with wildlife conservation authorities for reducing numbers of fox, skunk, and other wildlife hosts of sylvatic rabies in enzootic areas.

7) For pre-exposure immunization for individuals at high risk, e.g., veterinarians and wild life conservation personnel in enzootic areas, staff of quarantine kennels, laboratory and field personnel working with rabies, give two 1.0 ml doses of non-nervous tissue vaccine one month apart and a third dose after 6-7 months (preferred in the USA), or give three 1.0 ml doses at five day intervals followed by a fourth dose one month after the last (recommended by WHO). Serum should be tested

for antirabies antibodies (available through State Health Department laboratories in USA) four weeks after the basic immunization series; if negative, reinforcing doses are repeated until antibodies are demonstrated. If risk of exposure continues, booster doses are given every 1-3 years. If bitten by an animal suspected of being rabid, it is suggested that a daily dose of vaccine be given for 5 days, followed by a single dose given 20 days later; if no known antibody response has been previously demonstrated the full post-exposure prophylaxis must be given (see par. 9A1 above).

B. *Control of patient, contacts, and the immediate environment:*

1) *Report to local health authority:* Obligatory case report required in most states and countries, Class 2A (see Preface).

2) *Isolation:* Strict isolation for duration of the illness.

3) *Concurrent disinfection:* Of saliva and articles soiled therewith. Immediate attendants should be warned of the hazard of infection from saliva and should wear rubber gloves and protective gowns.

4) *Quarantine:* None.

5) *Immunization of contacts:* Contacts of a patient with rabies need not be vaccinated unless an open wound or mucous membrane has been exposed to the patient's saliva.

6) *Investigation of contacts and source of infection:* Search for rabid animal and for persons and other animals bitten.

7) *Specific treatment:* For clinical rabies, intensive supportive medical care.

C. *Epidemic (epizootic) measures:* Applicable only to animals. A sporadic disease in man.

1) Establishment of area control under authority of state laws, public health regulations and local ordinances, in cooperation with appropriate wildlife conservation and animal health authorities.

2) Widespread vaccination of dogs, preferably with an attenuated live vaccine, through officially sponsored intensified programs providing mass immunization at temporary and emergency stations. For protection of other domestic animals, vaccines at the proper level of attenuation for each animal species, or suitable inactivated vaccines, must be used.

3) Strict enforcement of regulations requiring collection, detention and destruction of ownerless or stray dogs, and of unvaccinated dogs found off owner's premises.
4) Encourage reduction in the dog population by castration, spaying and drugs.

D. International measures:
1) Strict compliance by common carriers and by travelers with national laws and regulations that institute quarantine or require vaccination of dogs.
2) WHO Collaborating Centres (see Preface).

RAT-BITE FEVER

Two diseases are included under the general term of rat-bite fever; one is caused by *Streptobacillus moniliformis*, the other by *Spirillum minor*. Because they are similar in clinical and epidemiological behavior, and because it is seen occasionally in the U.S.A., *Streptobacillus moniliformis* is presented in detail. Variations manifested by *Spirillum minor* infection are noted under that disease.

A. *STREPTOBACILLUS MONILIFORMIS* DISEASE
(Haverhill fever)

1. Identification—Usually there is a history of a rat bite within 10 days which heals normally. An abrupt onset with chills and fever, headache and muscle pain is shortly followed by a maculo-papular rash most marked on the extremities. One or more joints usually then become swollen, red and painful. Bacterial endocarditis and focal abscesses may occur late in untreated cases, with a fatality rate of 7-10%.

Laboratory confirmation is by isolation of the organism by inoculation of material from primary lesion or lymph node, blood, joint fluid, or pus into the appropriate bacteriological medium or into laboratory animals (guinea pigs or mice which are not naturally infected). Serum antibodies may be detected by agglutination tests.

2. Occurrence—Distribution is worldwide, though an uncommon disease in North and South America and most European countries;

it is the usual form of rat-bite fever in U.S.A. Recent cases in the U.S.A. have followed bites by laboratory rats.

3. **Infectious agent**—*Streptobacillus moniliformis (Streptothrix muris rattis, Haverhillia multiformis, Actinomyces muris).*

4. **Reservoir**—An infected rat, rarely other rodents (squirrel, weasel).

5. **Mode of transmission**—Infection is transmitted by secretions of mouth, nose, or conjunctival sac of an infected animal, most frequently introduced by biting. Sporadic cases without reference to bite have been recorded. Blood from an experimental laboratory animal has infected man. Actual contact with rats is not necessary; infection has occurred in persons working or living in rat-infested buildings. Some outbreaks have been traced to contaminated milk or milk products.

6. **Incubation period**—Three to 10 days, rarely longer.

7. **Period of communicability**—Not directly transmitted from man to man.

8. **Susceptibility and resistance**—No information.

9. **Methods of control**—

   A. *Preventive measures:*
      1) Reduction of rat population.
      2) Ratproofing of dwellings.

   B. *Control of patient, contacts, and the immediate environment:*
      1) *Report to local health authority:* Obligatory report of epidemics; no individual case report, Class 4 (Preface).
      2) *Isolation:* None.
      3) *Concurrent disinfection:* None.
      4) *Quarantine:* None.
      5) *Immunization of contacts:* None.
      6) *Investigation of contacts and source of infection:* Not practicable.
      7) *Specific treatment:* Penicillin or tetracyclines. Treatment should continue for 7 to 10 days.

   C. *Epidemic measures:* Grouped cases presenting the typical symptoms require search for epidemiologic evidence of a relation to milk supply.

   D. *International measures:* None.

B. *SPIRILLUM MINOR* DISEASE—SODOKU

A sporadic rat-bite fever, Sodoku, caused by *Spirillum minor (S. minus Spirochaeta morsus muris),* is the common form of rat bite fever in Japan and the Far East. Incidence is no greater there than in western counties. Untreated, the fatality rate is approximately 10%. Clinically, *Spirillum minor* disease differs from *Streptobacillus* disease in the usual absence of arthritic symptoms, and the rash commonly consists of reddish or purplish plaques. The incubation period is generally longer, 1 to 3 weeks, usually more than 7 days, and the previously healed bite wound reactivates when symptoms appear. Laboratory methods are essential for differentiation; animal inoculation is used for isolation of the spirillum.

∽

RELAPSING FEVER

1. **Identification** — A systemic spirochetal disease in which periods of fever lasting 2 to 9 days alternate with afebrile periods of 2 to 4 days; the number of relapses varies from 2 to 10 or more. Each pyrexial period terminates by crisis. The total duration of the louse-borne disease averages 13 to 16 days; the tick-borne disease usually lasts longer. Transitory petechial rashes are common during the initial period of fever. The overall fatality rate in untreated cases is between 2 and 10%; it sometimes exceeds 50% in the epidemic louse-borne disease.

Diagnosis is by demonstration of the infectious agent in darkfield preparations of fresh blood or stained thick blood films, or by inoculation of laboratory rats or mice intraperitoneally with blood taken during the pyrexial period.

2. **Occurrence** — Characteristically epidemic where spread is by lice, and endemic where spread is by ticks. Louse-borne relapsing fever occurs in limited localities in Asia, Eastern Africa (Ethiopia and the Sudan), North and Central Africa, and South America. Epidemics are common in wars, in famine, or in other situations where malnourished, overcrowded populations with poor personal hygiene enhance multiplication and wide dissemination of the louse vector. The endemic tick-borne disease is widespread throughout tropical Africa; foci exist in Spain, Northern Africa, Saudi Arabia, Iran, India, and parts of central Asia, as well as in North and South America. Louse-borne relapsing fever has not been reported in the U.S.A. for many years; human cases and occasional outbreaks of tick-borne disease occur in limited localities of several western

states. An outbreak in 1973 was restricted to the north rim of the Grand Canyon in Arizona.

3. Infectious agent—*Borrelia recurrentis*, a spirochete. Many different strains have been described, related to area of isolation and vector rather than to inherent biologic differences. Cross-protection occurs between louse and tick-borne strains. Strains isolated during a relapse often show antigenic differences from those of an immediately preceding paroxysm.

4. Reservoir—For louse-borne disease, man; immediate source of infection is an infective louse. The natural reservoir of some tick-borne relapsing fevers in the U.S.A. is wild rodents, principally ground squirrels and prairie dogs, and ticks through transovarian transmission.

5. Mode of transmission—Not directly transmitted from man to man. Epidemic relapsing fever is acquired by crushing an infective louse, *Pediculus humanus*, over the bite wound or an abrasion of the skin. Man also is infected by the bite or coxal fluid of an argasid tick, principally *Ornithrodoros turicata* and *O. hermsi* in the U.S.A., *O. rudis* and *O. talaje* in Central and South America, *O. moubata* in tropical Africa, and *O. tholozani* in the Near and Middle East. Ticks feed, usually at night, rapidly engorge, and promptly leave the host.

6. Incubation period—Five to 15 days; usually 8 days.

7. Period of communicability—The louse becomes infective 4 to 5 days after ingestion of blood from an infected person and remains so for life (20 to 40 days). Infected ticks can live without feeding for several years and remain infective during this period.

8. Susceptibility and resistance—Susceptibility is general. Duration of immunity after clinical attack is unknown; probably less than 2 years.

9. Methods of control—

   A. Preventive measures:
     1) Louse control, by measures prescribed for louse-borne typhus fever (see pp. 355-356).
     2) Tick control, especially in living quarters, and rest houses by sealing hiding places in walls and floors and/or by spraying with effective residual agents, such as BHC or Bajon.

   B. Control of patient, contacts, and the immediate environment:
     1) Report to local health authority: Obligatory report of louse-borne relapsing fever under International Health

Regulations (1969)* WHO, Class 1 (see Preface). Tick-borne disease, in selected endemic areas, Class 3B (see Preface).

2) *Isolation:* None, provided the patient, his clothing, all household contacts, and the immediate environment have been deloused or freed from ticks.

3) *Concurrent disinfection:* None, if proper disinfestation has been carried out.

4) *Quarantine:* Exposed louse-infested susceptibles may be released after application of a residual insecticide; otherwise, quarantine for 9 days.

5) *Immunization of contacts:* None.

6) *Investigation of contacts and source of infection:* For the individual tick-borne case search for sources of infection; for louse-borne, unprofitable because this calls for a community-wide effort (see 9C following).

7) *Specific treatment:* Tetracyclines.

C. *Epidemic measures:* When reporting has been good and cases are few, application of insecticides with residual effect to contacts of all reported cases. Where infection is known to be widespread, systematic application of an effective residual insecticide to all persons in the community.

D. *International measures:*
1) Telegraphic notification by governments to WHO and to adjacent countries of the occurrence of an outbreak of louse-borne relapsing fever in an area previously free of the disease, regardless of source.

2) As of January, 1971, louse-borne relapsing fever ceased to be a quarantinable disease under international regulations, but the measures outlined in paragraph (1) above should be continued because it is now a *Disease under Surveillance by WHO,* in accordance with a Resolution of the 22nd World Health Assembly.

---

* Second Annotated Edition, 1974.

RESPIRATORY DISEASE, ACUTE VIRAL
(Excluding influenza)

Numerous acute respiratory illnesses of known and presumed viral etiology are grouped here under the general title of Respiratory Disease, Acute Viral. Clinically they are of two forms: the more severe febrile illnesses, such as pneumonia, bronchiolitis and croup, which are sometimes fatal, and the less severe nonfebrile common colds. These respiratory syndromes are associated with a large number of viruses and each virus is capable of producing a wide spectrum of acute respiratory illnesses. The diseases caused by known viruses have important epidemiological attributes in common, such as reservoir and mode of spread. Their clinical characteristics cannot be distinguished from those of diseases of presumed but unidentified viral origin. Many of the viruses invade any part of the respiratory tract; others show a predilection for certain anatomical sites, which may be influenced by epidemiological factors. Some predispose to bacterial complications, occasionally serious. Morbidity and mortality from acute viral respiratory diseases are especially significant in pediatric practice; in adults the relatively high incidence and resulting disability, with consequent economic loss, make diseases of this group a major public health problem.

Several other nonbacterial infections of the respiratory tract are presented separately because they are sufficiently uniform in their clinical and epidemiological manifestations and occur in such regular association with specific infectious agents as to be recognized as disease entities. Psittacosis, influenza, herpangina, and epidemic pleurodynia are examples (pp. 245, 159, 147 and 231 respectively).

A. ACUTE FEBRILE RESPIRATORY DISEASE

1. **Identification**—Viral diseases of the respiratory tract are characterized by fever and one or more constitutional reactions such as chills or chilliness, headache or general aching, malaise, and anorexia; in infants by occasional gastrointestinal disturbances. Localizing signs also occur at various sites in the respiratory tract, either alone or in combination, such as rhinitis, pharyngitis or tonsillitis, laryngitis, laryngotracheitis, bronchitis, bronchiolitis, pneumonitis, or pneumonia. Symptoms and signs usually subside in 2 to 5 days without complications; infection may, however, extend or be complicated by bacterial sinusitis, otitis media, pneumonitis, or persistent bronchitis, depending on age, virus involved, prior experience with the same or related infectious agents, season of year

and other environmental factors. White blood counts are usually low and respiratory bacterial flora are within normal limits unless modified by secondary infections. Commonly diagnosed clinical syndromes include upper respiratory infection (URI), and acute respiratory disease (ARD).

Specific diagnosis requires isolation of the virus from respiratory secretions in appropriate cell or organ cultures and/or antibody studies of paired sera. Differentiation has minor usefulness in management of sporadic undifferentiated respiratory disease. In outbreaks or in continuing high incidence, it is important to identify the cause in a representative sample of typical cases and by appropriate clinical and laboratory methods to rule out other diseases, e.g., mycoplasmal pneumonia, Q fever, and streptococcal infection, for which specific treatment may be effective.

Practical management of acute respiratory disease depends on the differentiation of viral infections from disease entities for which specific measures are available.

2. Occurrence—Worldwide. Seasonal in temperate zones, with greatest incidence during fall and winter and occasionally spring. In large communities, some viral illnesses are constantly present, usually with little seasonal pattern (e.g., parainfluenza virus type 3 and adenovirus type 1); others tend to occur in sharp outbreaks (e.g., respiratory syncytial virus). Annual incidence is high, particularly in infants and children. During autumn, winter and spring, attack rates for preschool children may average 2% per week as compared to 1% for school children and 0.5% for adults. Incidence depends upon proportion of susceptibles infected and virulence of the agent. Many pathogens may be prevalent in a community, but one or another commonly predominates for a few weeks at a time. Under special host and environmental conditions, certain viral infections may disable 3/4 of a population within a few weeks, e.g., outbreaks of adenovirus types 4 or 7 in military recruits or adenovirus type 3 (pharyngo-conjunctival fever) in children attending summer camps.

3. Infectious agents—Parainfluenza virus, types 1, 2, 3, and 4; respiratory syncytial virus; adenovirus, types 1, 2, 3, 4, 5, 7, 14, and 21; rhinoviruses; certain coronaviruses; certain types of coxsackievirus groups A and B, echoviruses, and *Mycoplasma pneumoniae* are considered etiologic agents of acute febrile respiratory illnesses. Some of these agents have a greater tendency to cause more severe illnesses than others and certain ones have a predilection for certain age groups and populations. Respiratory syncytial virus, the major viral respiratory tract pathogen of early infancy, produces illness with greatest frequency during the first 6

months of life, is the major known etiologic agent of bronchiolitis, and is a frequent cause of pneumonia, croup, bronchitis, and febrile upper respiratory illness. The parainfluenza viruses (especially type 1) are the major known etiologic agents of croup and also cause bronchitis, pneumonia, bronchiolitis and febrile upper respiratory illness in pediatric populations. Adenoviruses are associated with several forms of respiratory disease; types 4 and 7 are common causes of acute respiratory disease in military recruits. See mycoplasmal pneumonia and the common cold for additional information about some of these agents (pp. 237 and 265).

4. Reservoir—Man. Many known viruses produce inapparent infections; adenoviruses may remain latent in tonsils and adenoids and be reactivated from time to time over many years.

5. Mode of transmission—Directly by oral contact or by droplet spread; indirectly by handkerchiefs, eating utensils or other articles freshly soiled by respiratory discharges of an infected person. Viruses discharged in the feces, including enteroviruses and adenoviruses, may be involved.

6. Incubation period—From a few days to a week or more.

7. Period of communicability—For the duration of active disease; little is known about subclinical or latent infections.

8. Susceptibility and resistance—Susceptibility is universal. Illness is more frequent and more severe in infants and children. Infection induces specific antibodies. Reinfection with respiratory syncytial and parainfluenza viruses is common, but illness from reinfection is generally milder or absent.

9. Methods of control—

   A. *Preventive measures:*

   1) Oral live attenuated adenovirus vaccines have proved effective against type-specific infections in military recruits, but are not now recommended for use in civilian populations.

   2) When possible, avoid crowding in living and sleeping quarters, especially in institutions, in barracks and on shipboard.

   3) Education of the public in personal hygiene, as in covering the mouth when coughing and sneezing and in sanitary disposal of discharges from mouth and nose.

   B. *Control of patient, contacts and the immediate environment:*

   1) *Report to local health authority:* Obligatory report of epidemics; no individual case report, Class 4 (see Preface).

2) *Isolation:* No established value. Infected persons should avoid direct and indirect exposure of others, particularly young children, feeble or aged persons, or patients with other illnesses. Isolation, insofar as can be accomplished by rest in bed during the acute stage, is advised.
3) *Concurrent disinfection:* Of eating and drinking utensils; sanitary disposal of nose and mouth discharges.
4) *Quarantine:* None.
5) *Immunization of contacts:* None.
6) *Investigation of contacts:* Unprofitable.
7) *Specific treatment:* None. Indiscriminate use of antibiotics is to be discouraged. These valuable therapeutic agents should be reserved for identified bacterial complications such as pneumonia, tracheobronchitis, otitis, and sinusitis.

C. *Epidemic measures:* No effective measures known. Isolation may be helpful in institutions; procedures such as ultraviolet irradiation, aerosols and dust control have not proved useful. Avoid crowding. (See 9A2 above).

D. *International measures:* WHO Collaborating Centres (see Preface).

B. THE COMMON COLD

1. Identification — Acute catarrhal infections of the upper respiratory tract characterized by coryza, lacrimation, irritated nasopharynx, chilliness and malaise lasting 2 to 7 days. Fever is uncommon in children and rare in adults. No fatalities reported, but disability is important because it affects work performance, industrial and school absenteeism, and predisposes to more serious bacterial complications such as sinusitis, otitis media, laryngitis, tracheitis and bronchitis. White blood counts usually are low and bacterial flora of the respiratory tract are within normal limits in the absence of secondary infections.

Cell or organ culture studies of nasal secretions may demonstrate a known virus in 20-35% of cases. Specific clinical, epidemiologic and other manifestations aid differentiation from similar diseases due to toxic, allergic, physical or psychologic stimuli.

2. Occurrence — Worldwide, both endemic and epidemic. In temperate zones, incidence rises in fall, winter and spring. Many persons, except in small isolated communities, have 1 to 6 colds yearly. Incidence highest in children under 5 years; gradual decline with increasing age.

3. Infectious agents—Rhinoviruses, of which there are as many as 89 recognized serotypes plus one subtype, are the major known etiologic agents of the common cold in adults. Coronaviruses such as 229E and OC43 also appear to be important etiologic agents of common colds in adults; they appear to be especially important in the winter and early spring when the prevalence of rhinoviruses is low. Other known respiratory viruses account for a small proportion of common colds in adults. In infants and children parainfluenza viruses, respiratory syncytial virus, adenoviruses, certain enteroviruses, and probably coronaviruses, cause common cold-like illnesses.

4. Reservoir—Man.

5. Mode of transmission—Presumably by direct oral contact or by droplet spread; indirectly by articles freshly soiled by discharges of nose and mouth of an infected person.

6. Incubation period—Between 12 and 72 hours, usually 24 hours.

7. Period of communicability—Nasal washings taken 24 hours before onset and for 5 days after onset have produced symptoms in experimentally infected volunteers.

8. Susceptibility and resistance—Susceptibility is universal. Inapparent and abortive infections occur; frequency of healthy carriers is undetermined, but known to be rare with some viral agents, notably rhinoviruses. The frequently repeated attacks may be due to transient homologous immunity, to the multiplicity of agents or to other causes. Artificial immunization is not available.

9. Methods of control—

   1) Report to local health authority: Official report not ordinarily justifiable, Class 5 (see Preface).
   2) Other control measures as for Section A. Acute Febrile Respiratory Disease 9A, B and C.

RICKETTSIAL FEVERS, TICK-BORNE
(Spotted Fever Group)

The rickettsial diseases of the spotted fever group are clinically similar and are caused by closely related rickettsiae. They are transmitted by species of *Ixodid* ticks, which are widely distributed throughout the world; species vary markedly by geographical area. Similar control measures are applicable for all of the rickettsial fevers and the broad-spectrum antibiotics are effective therapeutically.

Complement-fixation tests, using group-specific spotted fever antigens, become positive in the 2nd week; the Weil-Felix reactions with Proteus OX-19 and Proteus OX-2 become positive with less regularity. Definitive identification of a particular rickettsia is essentially a research procedure; the need rarely arises because the diseases do not overlap in geographic distribution.

A. ROCKY MOUNTAIN SPOTTED FEVER
(New World spotted fever, Tick-borne typhus fever)

1. **Identification** — This prototype disease of the spotted fever group is characterized by sudden onset, with moderate to high fever which ordinarily persists for 2 to 3 weeks, headache, chills, and conjunctival injection. A maculopapular rash, appearing on the extremities about the 3rd day, soon includes the palms and soles and spreads rapidly to most of the body; petechiae and hemorrhages are common. The fatality rate is about 20% in the absence of specific therapy; with prompt treatment death is uncommon.

2. **Occurrence** — Throughout the United States, during spring and summer. Most cases are reported in southeastern states, prevalence is less in Rocky Mountain region. Commonest in wooded suburban areas of the Piedmont Plateau. In western United States adult males are infected most frequently, while in the east incidence is higher in children. The difference relates to conditions of exposure to infected ticks. Fatality increases with age. Infection also occurs in western Canada, western and central Mexico, Panama, Colombia, and Brazil.

3. **Infectious agent** — *Rickettsia rickettsi.*

4. **Reservoir** — Infection in nature is maintained by transovarian and transstadial passage in ticks. The organisms can be transmitted to various rodents and other animals, which assists in maintaining the disease cycle.

5. **Mode of transmission**—Ordinarily by bite of an infected tick. Several hours (4 to 6) of attachment of the tick are required before the rickettsia become reactivated and infection in man can occur. Contamination of skin with crushed tissues or feces of the tick also may cause infection. In eastern and southern United States the common vector is the dog tick, *Dermacentor variabilis;* in northwestern United States, the wood tick, *D. andersoni;* in southwestern United States, occasionally the Lone Star tick, *Amblyomma americanum.* The rabbit tick, *Haemaphysalis leporispalustris* is infected in nature but usually does not feed on man.

6. **Incubation period**—From 3 to about 10 days.

7. **Period of communicability**—Not directly transmitted from man to man. The tick remains infective for life, commonly as long as 18 months.

8. **Susceptibility and resistance**—Susceptibility is general. One attack probably confers lasting immunity.

9. **Methods of control**—

   A. *Preventive measures:*
      1) Avoid tick-infested areas when feasible; search total body area every 3 to 4 hours for attached ticks, if working or playing in infested area; remove ticks from the person promptly and carefully without crushing by gentle steady traction to avoid leaving mouth parts in the skin; protect hands when removing ticks from man or animals. Tick repellents such as diethyltoluamide and dimethylphthalate may be of value.
      2) Measures designed to reduce tick populations are generally impractical. In selected land areas, direct application of chlordane, dieldrin, lindane, diazinon or benzene hexachloride gives excellent control of some vectors.
      3) Vaccines containing killed *R. rickettsi* may result in lessened severity but antigenicity is weak. Vaccination is generally limited to those persons at high risk, such as persons frequenting highly endemic areas and laboratory workers. Booster doses at yearly intervals are necessary.
      4) Education of the public in mode of transmission by ticks and the means for personal protection.

   B. *Control of patient, contacts, and the immediate environment:*
      1) *Report to local health authority:* In selected areas (U.S.A.); in many countries not a reportable disease, Class 3B (see Preface).

2) Isolation: None.

3) Concurrent disinfection: Carefully remove all ticks from patients.

4) Quarantine: None.

5) Immunization of contacts: Unnecessary.

6) Investigation of contacts and source of infection: Not profitable except as a community measure; see 9C below.

7) Specific treatment: The tetracycline antibiotics or chloramphenicol in daily oral doses until patient is afebrile (usually 3 days) and for 1 or 2 additional days.

C. Epidemic measures: In hyper-endemic areas particular attention should be paid to identification of the tick species involved and of infested areas, and to recommendations in 9A1, 2, 4 above.

D. International measures: WHO Collaborating Centers (see Preface).

B. BOUTONNEUSE FEVER

(Marseilles fever, South African tick typhus, Kenya tick typhus, India tick typhus)

1. Identification—A mild to moderately severe febrile illness of a few days to 2 weeks, characterized by a primary lesion at the site of a tick bite. The lesion (tache noire), usually presents at onset of fever, and is a small ulcer 2-5 mm. in diameter with a black center and red areola; regional lymph nodes are enlarged. A generalized maculopapular erythematous rash appears about the 4th or 5th day, usually involving palms and soles, and persists 6 to 7 days; with antibiotic treatment, fever lasts no more than 2 days. The fatality rate is less than 3%, even without specific therapy.

2. Occurrence—Widely distributed throughout the African continent, in India and in those parts of Europe and the Middle East adjacent to the Mediterranean, Black and Caspian Seas. In more temperate areas, highest incidence is during warmer months when ticks are numerous; in tropical areas throughout the year. Outbreaks may occur when groups of susceptibles are brought into an endemic area.

3. Infectious agent—*Rickettsia conori.*

4. Reservoir—As in Rocky Mountain Spotted Fever.

5. Mode of transmission—In the Mediterranean area, by bite of infected *Rhipicephalus sanguineus,* a dog tick. In South Africa, ticks infected in nature and presumed to be vectors include *Haemaphysalis leachi, Amblyomma hebraeum, R. appendiculatus, Boophilus decloratus,* and *Hyalomma aegyptium.*

6. **Incubation period**— Usually 5 to 7 days.

7. **Period of communicability; 8. Susceptibility and resistance; 9. Methods of control** — As in Rocky Mountain Spotted Fever, except that a vaccine is not employed.

C. QUEENSLAND TICK TYPHUS

1. **Identification**— Clinically similar to Boutonneuse fever.

2. **Occurrence**— Queensland, Australia.

3. **Infectious agent** —*Rickettsia australis.*

4. **Reservoir**— As in Rocky Mountain Spotted Fever.

5. **Mode of transmission**— As in Rocky Mountain Spotted Fever. *Ixodes holocyclus,* infesting small marsupials and wild rodents, is probably the major vector.

6. **Incubation period**— About 7 to 10 days.

7. **Period of communicability; 8. Susceptibility and resistance; 9. Methods of control** — As in Rocky Mountain Spotted Fever, except that a vaccine is not employed.

D. NORTH ASIAN TICK-BORNE RICKETTSIOSIS

(Siberian tick typhus)

1. **Identification**— Clinically similar to Boutonneuse fever.

2. **Occurrence**— Asiatic USSR and the Mongolian People's Republic.

3. **Infectious agent** —*Rickettsia siberica.*

4. **Reservoir**— As in Rocky Mountain Spotted Fever.

5. **Mode of transmission**— By the bite of ticks in the genera *Dermacentor* and *Haemophysalis,* which infest certain wild rodents.

6. **Incubation period**— Two to 7 days.

7. **Period of communicability; 8. Susceptibility and resistance; 9. Methods of control**— As in Rocky Mountain Spotted Fever, except that a vaccine is not employed.

∞

RICKETTSIALPOX
(Vesicular rickettsiosis)

1. **Identification** — Rickettsialpox is characterized by an initial skin lesion, chills, fever, a varicelliform rash, and a mild to severe course. Even without specific therapy, the fatality rate is less than 1%. The initial lesion is a firm red papule appearing about a week in advance of fever, most commonly on covered parts of the body. It becomes vesicular, then covered by a scab, and after about 3 weeks leaves a small pigmented scar. Fever, often preceded by chills, is remittent, with peaks of 39.4°C to 40.6°C (103°F to 105°F) usually lasting less than 1 week. Headache, muscular pain and general malaise are frequent. The secondary rash, manifest 3 to 4 days after onset of fever, is without characteristic distribution, is seldom seen on palms or soles, progresses through papular and papulovesicular stages, lasts less than a week, and leaves no scars. Local lymphadenitis follows the initial lesion.

Specific diagnosis is by complement-fixation test which becomes positive between 2nd and 3rd week of the disease.

2. **Occurrence** — In the U.S.A. cases occurred most years in New York City, principally among residents of apartment houses where mouse, mite and rickettsia maintain a natural cycle of infection; a few cases have been recognized in other cities east of the Mississippi River in the U.S.A. No cases have been reported in USA since 1969. The vector occurs in foci from the Atlantic Coast to Arizona and Utah. The disease also occurs in the USSR in the same pattern as in the U.S.A., but commensal rats also may be involved in the natural cycle. In Equatorial and South Africa, cases clinically and serologically consistent with rickettsialpox are contracted in the bushveld, suggesting involvement of a wild rodent and various mites. *Rickettsia akari* has been recovered from a field mouse in Korea, although the disease in man is unrecognized there.

3. **Infectious agent** — *Rickettsia akari*, a member of the spotted fever group of rickettsiae (see p. 267).

4. **Reservoir** — The infected house mouse (*Mus musculus*), and possibly the vector mite, *Allodermanyssus sanguineus*, in which transovarian passage of rickettsiae occurs; possibly commensal rats in USSR.

5. **Mode of transmission** — From mouse to mouse and from mouse to man by bite of an infective rodent mite, *A sanguineus*. Not directly transmitted from man to man.

6. **Incubation period** — Probably 10 to 24 days.

7. Period of communicability—Duration of infectivity of mouse for mite, and of mite for mouse or man, is unknown.

8. Susceptibility and resistance—Susceptibility appears general; duration of immunity after attack is unknown.

9. Methods of control—

A. Preventive measures: Rodent and mite control by elimination of mice and mouse harborages, including proper care and firing of incinerators in dwellings and application of residual miticides (dieldrin and others) to infested areas. Commercial vaccine is neither available nor currently needed.

B. Control of patient, contacts, and the immediate environment:
  1) Report to local health authority: In selected endemic areas U.S.A.; in most states and countries not reportable, Class 3B (see Preface).
  2) Isolation: None.
  3) Concurrent disinfection: None.
  4) Quarantine: None.
  5) Immunization of contacts: None.
  6) Investigation of contacts and source of infection: Search for mice in dwelling and, if feasible, undertake isolation of rickettsiae from rodents and mites.
  7) Specific treatment: The tetracycline antibiotics. Chloramphenicol is equally effective, but should be used only if necessary.

C. Epidemic measures: When groups of cases occur in the same or adjacent dwellings, apply preventive measures listed under 9A above. Observe all residents and treat promptly if disease develops.

D. International measures: WHO Collaborating Centres (see Preface).

RUBELLA
(German Measles)

1. Identification—A mild febrile infectious disease with a characteristic diffuse punctate and macular rash sometimes resembling that of measles, scarlet fever or both. There may be few or no constitutional symptoms in children but adults may experience a 1-5 day prodrome characterized by low-grade fever, headache, malaise, mild coryza, and conjunctivitis. Post-auricular, suboccipital or post-cervical lymphadenopathy is common but not pathognomonic; occasionally adenopathy is generalized. As many as 20-50% of infections may occur without evident rash. Leukopenia is common and thrombocytopenia occurs but only rarely results in hemorrhagic manifestations. Arthralgia or arthritis complicates a significant percentage of infections, particularly among adult females. Encephalitis is a rare complication.

Congenital Rubella Syndrome occurs among 20-25% or more of infants born to women who have acquired rubella during the first trimester of pregnancy, with decreasing frequency thereafter. This syndrome includes cataracts, microphthalmia, microcephaly, mental retardation, deafness, patent ductus arteriosus with other cardiac defects, thrombocytopenic purpura, hepatosplenomegaly with jaundice, and radiographically distinctive bone defects. Moderate and severe cases of congenital rubella syndrome are immediately recognizable at birth; mild cases having only slight cardiac involvement or partial deafness may not be detected for months or years after birth. These congenital malformations and even fetal death may occur following both clinically manifest and inapparent rubella infection in the pregnant woman in the first trimester.

Differentiation of rubella from measles (rubeola, p. 196), scarlet fever (p. 307) and a number of mild infections of similar nature is often necessary (see erythema infectiosum and exanthem subitum below). In addition, macular and maculopapular rashes occur irregularly in 10-15% of patients with infectious mononucleosis; also observed in infections with certain enteroviruses.

Diagnosis of rubella, especially in pregnant women, should be confirmed by demonstration of an antibody titer rise in sera collected as soon as possible (within 10 days) after onset of a suspect illness or an exposure and 7 to 14 days later. Antenatal infection of the fetus can be confirmed in the newborn by demonstration of specific IgM serum antibodies. From a week before until 2 weeks after onset of rash, virus may be isolated from the pharynx. Blood, urine or stool specimens also may yield virus during a less certain and shorter time period.

2. Occurrence — Worldwide; universally endemic except in remote and isolated communities; most prevalent in winter and spring. Extensive epidemics occur occasionally, e.g. U.S.A. in 1935 and 1964 and Australia in 1940. Primarily a disease of childhood but occurring at somewhat greater frequency among adolescents and

adults than measles or chickenpox. Epidemics and outbreaks are common in institutional, college and military populations.

3. **Infectious agent** — The rubella virus.

4. **Reservoir** — Man.

5. **Mode of transmission** — Nasopharyngeal secretions of infected persons; virus is also recoverable from blood, urine, and feces of infected persons. Infection is by droplet spread or direct contact with patients, or presumably by indirect contact with articles freshly soiled with discharges from nose and throat, and possibly blood, urine, or feces. Airborne transmission may occur. Infants with congenital rubella syndrome, with or without obvious damage from their prenatal infection, excrete the virus and serve as sources of infection to their contacts.

6. **Incubation period** — From 14 to 21 days; usually 18 days.

7. **Period of communicability** — For about 1 week before and at least 4 days after onset of rash. Highly communicable. Infants with congenital rubella syndrome may shed virus for months after birth; the period for shedding is extremely variable.

8. **Susceptibility and resistance** — Susceptibility is general after the early months of life when the infant may be transiently protected by transplacentally acquired maternal immune globulin. Thereafter immunity is acquired by natural infection (one attack is sufficient) or by active immunization. Substantial numbers of young adults remain susceptible for lack of exposure to either of these immunizing experiences.

9. **Methods of control** — Efforts to control rubella are prompted primarily by the hazard of significant congenital defects in the offspring of women who acquire the disease during pregnancy. Therefore, except for routine active immunization no attempt should be made to protect female children in good health against exposure to this disease before puberty with precautions to prevent contact with susceptible pregnant women. The immune status of an individual can be determined by serological test; the vaccine is innocuous when given to an immune person.

A. Preventive measures:
   1) A single dose of live attenuated rubella virus vaccine elicits a significant antibody response in approximately 95% of susceptibles against infection from natural exposure. Vaccine virus may be recovered from the nasopharynx for two or more weeks, beginning a few

days post-inoculation but is not communicable. Vaccine virus may infect the fetus when given inadvertently to a susceptible woman early in pregnancy; its teratogenic potential while less than that of wild strains is unknown, and therefore immunization of women known to be pregnant is strictly contraindicated. In the U.S.A., immunization of all children over 1 year of age is recommended; vaccine is given to women in the childbearing age if serologic tests indicate susceptibility and if there is reasonable likelihood of no pregnancy for the next two months. In some areas, e.g., United Kingdom and Australia, routine immunization is given to girls between 11 and 13 years of age without testing for susceptibility and offered to susceptible women in the immediate postpartum period.

2) Immune serum globulin (human) given after exposure early in pregnancy can not be relied upon to protect the fetus but is sometimes given when abortion is refused. Rubella immune globulin (human), containing very high titers of specific antibody is under clinical trial.

3) In case of natural infection early in pregnancy, or of vaccine given to a susceptible pregnant woman, abortion should be considered because of risk of damage to the fetus.

B. *Control of patient, contacts and the immediate environment:*
   1) *Report to local health authority:* All cases of acquired rubella or of the congenital rubella syndrome should be reported. In U.S.A. report is obligatory; Class 3B (see Preface).
   2) *Isolation:* Only to protect nonimmune (susceptible) women during pregnancy (see 5 below).
   3) *Concurrent disinfection:* None.
   4) *Quarantine:* None.
   5) *Immunization of Contacts:* Active immunization after exposure, while not contraindicated (except in pregnant women), will not prevent infection or illness resulting from that exposure. Passive immunization with immune serum globulin is not indicated (except as in 9A2).
   6) *Investigation of contacts:* Of no practical value except to clarify diagnosis or to identify pregnant female contacts, especially in the first trimester of pregnancy. Such pregnant contacts may be serologically tested for susceptibility and advised according to the results (See 9A2).

    7) Specific treatment: None.

  C. Epidemic measures: The appearance of rubella in a school or comparable population may justify immunization.

  D. International measures: None.

ERYTHEMA INFECTIOSUM (Fifth disease): A mild, non-febrile erythematous eruption occuring in epidemics among children. Characterized clinically by a striking erythema of the cheeks (slapped-faced appearance) and reddening of the skin which occurs, fades and recurs; exaggerated by exposure to sunlight, and unaccompanied by constitutional symptoms. Outbreaks are now recognized more frequently; nonfatal; probably of viral etiology.

EXANTHEM SUBITUM (Roseola infantum): An acute illness, probably of viral etiology, with sudden onset, usually in children under 4 years of age, commonly at about 1 year. A sudden fever, sometimes 40.5°C (105°F) or 41°C (106°F), lasts 3 to 5 days. A maculopapular rash on the trunk and later on the rest of the body ordinarily follows lysis of the fever. The rash fades rapidly. Incidence is greatest in the spring. The incubation period is about 10 days, with unrecognized infections seemingly occur among older children.

SALMONELLOSIS

  1. Identification—Commonly manifested clinically by an acute gastroenteritis, salmonellosis is an acute infectious disease with sudden onset of abdominal pain, diarrhea, nausea and vomiting. Dehydration, especially among infants, may be severe. Fever is nearly always present. Anorexia and looseness of the bowels often persist for several days. Occasionally the clinical course is that of an enteric fever or of septicemia with or without focal infection. Although every *Salmonella* strain is potentially capable of producing any of these clinical symptoms or syndromes, severe illnesses are more likely to be associated with some specific bacterial serotypes. A *Salmonella* infection may begin as acute gastroenteritis and develop into enteric fever or focal infection. The infectious agent rarely may localize in any tissue of the body, producing abscesses and causing arthritis, cholecystitis, endocarditis, meningitis, pericarditis, pneumonia, pyoderma or pyelonephritis. Ordinarily deaths are uncommon except in the very young or very old, or in debilitated persons.

In cases of enteric fever and septicemia, *Salmonella* may be recovered on usual enteric media from feces and from the blood during the acute stages of illness. Fecal excretion of Salmonellae usually persists for several days or weeks beyond the acute phase of illness. Administration of broad spectrum antibiotics may increase the duration of excretion of the organism.

2. **Occurrence** — A common worldwide disease, more extensively reported in North American and European countries; often classified with food poisoning (p. 116) because food is the predominant vehicle of infection. The proportion of cases that are clinically recognizable is small. Diagnosis is largely dependent on diligence and effort in field investigation and in culturing stools. Small outbreaks in the general population usually characterize *Salmonella* gastroenteritis epidemiologically. Large outbreaks in hospitals, institutions for children, restaurants and nursing homes are not infrequent, and usually arise from food contaminated at its source or cross-contaminated during processing, or due to contamination by an undetected carrier.

3. **Infectious agents** — Numerous serotypes of *Salmonella* are pathogenic for both animals and man. Strains of human origin are not considered here (see Typhoid and Paratyphoid Fevers, pp. 220, 349). The types most commonly isolated in the period 1969-1973 in the U.S.A. were *S. typhimurium, S. heidelberg, S. newport, S. infantis, S. enteritidis* and *S. st. paul.* There is much variation in serotypes isolated from country to country; in most countries maintaining Salmonella surveillance, *S. typhimurium* is most commonly reported. Approximately 1500 serotypes are known, but only about 200 different types are detected in any given year.

4. **Reservoir** — Domestic and wild animals, including poultry, rodents and pet animals such as tortoises, turtles, chicks and dogs and cats; also man, i.e., patients and convalescent carriers and especially mild and unrecognized cases. Chronic carriers are rare.

5. **Mode of transmission** — By ingestion of the organism in food contaminated by feces of infected man or animals; also in whole eggs and egg products, frozen and dried whole egg, egg albumin and egg yolk, (especially duck eggs); cracked eggs; in meat and meat

products, in poultry (especially broiler chicken and turkey); and in pharmaceuticals of animal origin. Infection is also disseminated by animal feeds and fertilizers prepared from contaminated meat scraps, tankage, fish meal and bones.

Epidemics of *Salmonella* infection are usually traced to foods such as commercially processed meat products, inadequately cooked poultry or poultry products, raw sausages, lightly cooked foods containing eggs or egg products; unpasteurized milk or dairy products including dried milk; to foods contaminated with rodent feces or by an infected food handler; or to utensils, working surfaces or tables previously used to process or prepare contaminated foods such as meat and poultry products. Sporadic cases also may be related to ingestion of contaminated food and sometimes to direct contact with an infected person. Hospital epidemics tend to be protracted, with organisms persisting in the environment; person-to-person transmission via the hands of personnel is considered the major mode of spread. Infection by inhalation has been considered a possibility. In 1965, a severe epidemic of *S. typhimurium* diarrhea in Riverside, California, which produced more than 15,000 cases, resulted from contamination of the unchlorinated public deep water supply.

6. **Incubation period**—Six to 72 hours, usually about 12 to 36 hours.

7. **Period of communicability**—Throughout course of infection. Extremely variable—usually several days to several weeks; a temporary carrier state occasionally continues for months, especially in infants. Chronic carriers (over 1 year) are rare.

8. **Susceptibility and resistance**—Susceptibility is general and is usually increased by gastrointestinal surgery, or by neoplastic disease or other debilitating conditions. Severity of the disease is related to serotype of the organism, the number of organisms ingested and host factors. Inapparent infections are frequent. There is no active or passive immunization.

9. Methods of control—

   A. *Preventive measures:*

      1) Thorough cooking, preferably controlled by a meat thermometer, of all foodstuffs derived from animal sources, particularly turkeys and other fowl (especially frozen), egg products, and meat dishes. Avoid recontamination within the kitchen after cooking is completed. Avoid raw eggs, as in egg drinks, or homemade ice cream, and the

use of dirty or cracked eggs. Egg products should be pasteurized. Refrigerate prepared foods during storage.

2) Education of food handlers and housewives in the necessity of refrigerating food, washing hands before and after food preparation, maintaining a sanitary kitchen, and protecting prepared food against rodent or insect contamination.

3) Recognition, control and prevention of *Salmonella* infections among domestic animals and pets. Chicks, ducklings and turtles are particularly dangerous.

4) Meat and poultry inspection, with adequate supervision of abattoirs, food processing plants and butcher shops, including feed blending mills.

5) Adequate cooking or heat treatment followed by measures to avoid recontamination of prepared animal feeds (meat meal, bone meal, fish meal, pet food and others), by *Salmonella*.

B. Control of patient, contacts, and the immediate environment:

1) *Report to local health authority:* Obligatory case report, Class 2B (see Preface).

2) *Isolation:* Exclusion of infected persons from food handling, patient care, or occupations involving care of young children and the elderly until stool cultures are salmonella-free on 2 successive specimens collected not less than 24 hours apart and no sooner than 24 hours following discontinuation of antibiotics. Three to 10 gram portions of fecal material should be submitted for culture in preference to rectal swabs.

3) *Concurrent disinfection:* Of feces and of articles soiled therewith. In communities with a modern and adequate sewage disposal system, feces can be discharged directly into sewers without preliminary disinfection. Terminal cleaning.

4) *Quarantine:* None.

5) *Management of contacts:* No immunization available. Family contacts should not be employed as food handlers during period of contact.

6) *Investigation of contacts:* Culture all family contacts, especially those engaged in food handling, patient care, or care of young children or elderly persons. Search for unrecognized mild cases and carriers, including those convalescing.

7) *Specific treatment:* None indicated except rehydration

and electrolyte replacement by vein and/or orally (see cholera p. 74). Antibiotics may prolong the carrier state or lead to resistant strains. However, with continued fever or septicemia, a short course of ampicillin or chloramphenicol therapy should be given, based on the antibiotic sensitivities of the causal organism.

C. Epidemic measures: See Staphylococcal Food Poisoning 9C, p. 118.

D. International measures: WHO Collaborating Centres (see Preface).

. SCABIES

1. **Identification** — An infectious disease of the skin caused by a mite whose penetration is visible as papules or vesicles, or as tiny linear burrows containing the mites and their eggs. Lesions are prominent around finger webs, anterior surfaces of wrists and elbows, anterior axillary folds, belt line, thighs, and external genitalia in men; nipples, abdomen, and lower portion of buttocks in women. Itching is intense, especially at night, but complications are few except as lesions become secondarily infected by scratching.

Diagnosis may be established by locating the female mite in its burrow and identifying it microscopically.

2. **Occurrence** — Widespread and a common disease during time of war, poverty, or social upheaval. Uncommon in communities where frequent bathing is usual. It is endemic in many under-developed countries and in certain social groups in affluent countries.

3. **Infectious agent** — *Sarcoptes scabiei*, a mite.

4. **Reservoir** — Man; *Sarcoptes* of animals can live on man but do not reproduce in the skin.

5. **Mode of transmission** — Transfer of parasites is by direct contact and to a limited extent from undergarments or soiled bedclothes freshly contaminated by infected persons; frequently acquired during sexual contact.

6. **Incubation period** — Several days or even weeks before itching is noticed.

7. **Period of communicability** — Until mites and eggs are

destroyed by treatment, ordinarily after 1 or occasionally 2 courses of treatment a week apart.

8. **Susceptibility and resistance** — No known resistance.

9. **Methods of control** —

   A. *Preventive measures:* Education of the public on the need for maintaining cleanliness of person, garments, and bed-clothes.

   B. *Control of patient, contacts, and the immediate environment:*
      1) *Report to local health authority:* Official report not ordinarily justifiable. Class 5 (see Preface).
      2) *Isolation:* Exclude infected children from school until they and their families have been treated adequately.
      3) *Concurrent disinfection:* Proper laundering of under-wear, sheets, and occasionally of blankets.
      4) *Quarantine:* None.
      5) *Immunization of contacts:* None.
      6) *Investigation of contacts:* Search for unreported or un-recognized cases among companions or household members. Single infections in a family are uncommon.
      7) *Specific treatment:* When multiple areas are involved, a bath followed by application of 1% gamma benzene hexachloride (Kwell), crotamiton (Eurax), tetratethy-lthiruam monosulfide (Tetmosol) in 5% solution twice daily, or an emulsion of benzyl benzoate ointment, to the whole body. The following day a cleansing bath is taken and a change made to fresh clothing and bedclothes. Itching may persist for days and is not to be regarded as a sign of superinfection; this is important, for over-treatment is common. In about 5% of cases a second course of treatment may be necessary after an interval of 7 to 10 days. Close supervision of treatment, including bathing is necessary.

   C. *Epidemic measures:*
      1) Treatment is undertaken on a coordinated mass basis.
      2) Case-finding efforts are extended to screen whole families, military units or institutions.
      3) Soap and facilities for mass bathing and laundering are essential.
      4) Health education of infected persons and others at risk, as well as treatment. Cooperation of civilian or military authorities, often both, is needed.

   D. *International measures:* None.

SCHISTOSOMIASIS
(Bilharziasis)

1. **Identification**— A blood fluke (trematode) infection with adult male and female worms living in veins of the host. Eggs deposited there produce minute granulomata and scars in organs where they lodge. Symptomatology is related to the location of the parasite in the human host; *Schistosoma mansoni* and *Schistosoma japonicum* give rise primarily to intestinal, and *Schistosoma haematobium* to urinary, manifestations. The most important pathologic effects are the complications that arise from chronic infection: liver involvement and portal hypertension occur in the intestinal form, while obstruction and superimposed infection occur in the urinary disease.

Diagnosis depends on the demonstration of eggs in the stool, urine or biopsy specimen; useful immunological tests include the intradermal test (immediate hypersensitivity) and the complement fixation, circumoval precipitin, and indirect fluorescent antibody tests.

This is prevalent among bathers in lakes in many parts of the world, including North America and certain coastal sea water beaches. The larvae of certain other schistosomes of birds and mammals may penetrate the human skin and cause a dermatitis, sometimes known as "swimmer's itch"; these schistosomes do not mature in man.

2. **Occurrence**—*S. mansoni* occurs in Africa, the Arabian peninsula, northeastern and eastern South America and the Caribbean area. *S. haematobium* occurs in Africa, the Middle East, and one or more small foci in India. *S. japonicum* occurs in the Orient (China, Japan, Philippines, Sulawesi, Laos and Thailand). In some endemic areas more than half of the population is affected. None of these species is indigenous to North America. *S. intercalatum* occurs in parts of West Africa, including Camaroon, the Congo and Gabon.

3. **Infectious agents**—*Schistosoma mansoni, S. haematobium, S. japonicum* and *S. intercalatum.*

4. **Reservoir**— Man is the principal reservoir of *S. haematobium, S. intercalatum* and *S. mansoni.* Dogs, cats, pigs, cattle, water buffalo, horses, field mice and wild rats are epidemiologically important animal hosts of *S. japonicum.* Persistence of the disease depends on the presence of an appropriate snail as intermediate host; i.e., members of the genera *Biomphalaria* for *S. mansoni,*

Bulinus for *S. haematobium* and *S. intercalatum,* and *Oncomelania* for *S. japonicum.*

5. **Mode of transmission**—Infection is acquired from water containing larval forms (cercariae) which have developed in snails. The eggs of *S. haematobium* leave the mammalian body mainly with urine, those of *S. mansoni, S. intercalatum* and *S. japonicum* with feces. The egg hatches in water and the liberated larva (miracidium) enters a suitable freshwater snail host. Free-swimming larvae (cercariae) emerge from the snail after several weeks and penetrate human skin, usually while the person is working, swimming, or wading in water; they enter the bloodstream, are carried to blood vessels of the lung, migrate to the liver, develop to maturity, and then migrate to veins of the abdominal cavity. Adult forms of *S. mansoni, S. japonicum* and *intercalatum* usually remain in mesenteric veins; those of *S. haematobium* usually migrate through anastomoses into the pelvic veins. Eggs are deposited in venules and escape into the lumen of bowel or urinary bladder, or lodge in other organs.

6. **Incubation period**—Systemic manifestations usually begin when worms are reaching maturity, 4 to 6 weeks after infection. Eggs usually are found in feces or urine a week or two after onset of symptoms, delay for longer periods is not uncommon.

7. **Period of communicability**—As long as eggs are discharged in urine or feces of infected persons, usually 1 to 2 years, but may be 25 years or longer. Infected snails may give off cercariae for months.

8. **Susceptibility and resistance**—Susceptibility is universal; whether or not resistance develops as a result of infection is controversial.

9. **Methods of control**—

A. *Preventive measures:*

1) Disposal of feces and urine so that eggs will not reach bodies of fresh water containing snail intermediate hosts. Control of animals infected with *S. japonicum* is desirable but usually not practical.

2) Improved irrigation and agricultural practices; reduction of snail habitats by drainage and filling.

3) Treatment of snail breeding places with molluscacides.

4) Provision of cercaria-repellent or protective clothing against cercariae for persons required to enter contaminated water. Brisk toweling of wet skin surfaces.

5) Provision of water for drinking, bathing and washing clothes from sources free from cercariae.

6) Education of people in endemic areas regarding mode of transmission and methods of protection.

7) Mass treatment of infected persons in endemic areas may help to reduce transmission through lessened severity and duration of the disease; in the past this has not materially reduced prevalence.

B. *Control of patient, contacts, and the immediate environment:*

1) *Report to local health authority:* In selected endemic areas; in many countries not a reportable disease, Class 3C (see Preface).

2) *Isolation:* None.

3) *Concurrent disinfection:* Sanitary disposal of feces and urine.

4) *Quarantine:* None.

5) *Immunization of contacts:* None.

6) *Investigation of contacts:* Examine contacts for infection from a common source. Search for source is a community effort, see 9C.

7) *Specific treatment:* For *S. mansoni,* sodium antimony dimercaptosuccinate (Astiban) intramuscularly; for *S. haematobium,* niridazole (Ambilhar) orally; stibophen (Fuadin) intramuscularly is also effective for both species. For *S. japonicum* tartar emetic (sodium antimony tartrate) intravenously must be used. All the above drugs have significant toxic effects. Astiban and Ambilhar are available through the Parasitic Disease Drug Service, Center for Disease Control, Atlanta, Georgia (see Preface).

C. *Epidemic measures:* In areas of high prevalence, determine areas with high snail density and treat with molluscacides. Schistosomes have a high snail host specificity; expert aid is needed to determine which snails to control. Prohibit persons entering contaminated water. Provide clean water, examine population for infection, and treat diseased persons.

D. *International measures:* WHO Collaborating Centres (see Preface).

SHIGELLOSIS
(Bacillary dysentery)

1. **Identification** — An acute bacterial disease primarily involving the large intestine, characterized by diarrhea, accompanied by fever and often vomiting, cramps and tenesmus. In severe cases the stools contain blood, mucus and pus. In the usual outbreak there are mild and asymptomatic infections. The severity of illness and the fatality rate are functions of the age of the patient, of the pre-existing state of nutrition, of the level of sanitation (or the size of the infecting dose), and of the serotype of the organism predominating in the outbreak. For hospitalized patients the fatality rate may exceed 20% in the absence of supportive therapy. *Shigella dysenteriae 1* (Shiga's bacillus) is much more likely to be associated with serious disease, including septicemia, than are other members of the genus.

Bacteriologic diagnosis is by isolation of *Shigella* from feces or rectal swabs. The presence of pus cells in the stool exudate is highly suggestive of this diagnosis.

2. **Occurrence** — Worldwide: two thirds of the cases, and most of the deaths, are in children under 10 years of age. In those populations where malnutrition and poor sanitation coexist, dysentery is a frequent and serious disease that occurs at all ages. Outbreaks are common under conditions of crowding and where sanitation may be poor, such as in many jails, institutions for children, in mental hospitals, and among persons living under field conditions and aboard ships. Shigellosis is an important component of acute epidemic gastroenteritis of tropical populations (see p. 97) but may be endemic in both tropical and temperate climates where living conditions are poor.

3. **Infectious agents** — The genus *Shigella* comprises four species or sub-groups: Group A, *Sh. dysenteriae;* Group B, *Sh. flexneri;* Group C, *Sh. boydii;* Group D, *Sh. sonnei;* Groups A, B and C are further divided into some 30 serotypes, designated by arabic numbers. More than one serotype commonly is present in a community; mixed infections with other intestinal pathogens are not infrequent. In the U.S.A. during 1974 *Sh. sonnei* accounted for over 80% of all isolations reported. There are similar reports from Western Europe and Japan. Antibiotic resistant *Sh. dysenteriae* became epidemic in Central America in 1969 and has continued since 1972 as an endemic problem; introduction elsewhere in the Americas has occurred.

4. **Reservoir** — The only significant reservoir is man. However, significant outbreaks have occurred in primate colonies.

5. **Mode of transmission** — By direct or indirect fecal-oral transmission from a patient or a carrier. Infection may occur after the ingestion of very few organisms. Individuals primarily responsible for transmission are those who fail to cleanse contaminated hands or under their fingernails after defecation. They may then spread infection by direct physical contact with others, or by contaminating food or fomites. Water, milk and fly-borne outbreaks may occur as the result of direct contamination with feces.

6. **Incubation period** — One to 7 days, usually less than 4 days.

7. **Period of communicability** — During acute infection and until the infectious agent is no longer present in feces, usually within 4 weeks of illness. Asymptomatic carriers may transmit disease. The carrier state is usually short but may rarely persist for a year or longer.

8. **Susceptibility and resistance** — Susceptibility is general; the disease is more severe in children than in adults, among whom many inapparent infections may be asymptomatic. The elderly, debilitated individuals, and persons of all ages suffering from malnutrition, are particularly susceptible, and may succumb more often than others. Studies with serotype specific live vaccines have shown evidence of protection against challenge with the homologous strain.

9. **Methods of control** —

   A. *Preventive measures:*
      1) Instruction of patients, convalescents, and carriers in personal hygiene, particularly as to sanitary disposal of feces, hand washing after defecation and before eating, and exclusion of infected persons from handling food.
      2) Education in personal hygiene; encourage breast feeding throughout infancy; scrupulous cleanliness in preparation, handling and refrigeration of all foods, and boiling of milk and water for infant feeding.
      3) Sanitary supervision of processing, preparation and serving of all foods. (See Typhoid Fever 9A6, p. 351).
      4) Sanitary disposal of human feces.
      5) Protection and purification of water supplies. (See Typhoid Fever 9A1, p. 351).
      6) Pasteurization of milk and dairy products or boiling of milk. (See Typhoid Fever 9A4, p. 351).
      7) Control of flies and their breeding areas. (See Typhoid Fever 9A3, p. 351).

8) Travelers to areas with inadequate sanitary facilities should eat only cooked foods served hot, avoid ice, salads and raw vegetables, and only eat fruits which have been washed thoroughly and then peeled by the person who consumes them.

B. Control of patient, contacts, and the immediate environment:
   1) *Report to local health authority:* Case report is obligatory in most states and countries, Class 2B (see Preface). Recognition and report of epidemics has more than usual importance in schools and institutions.
   2) *Isolation:* During acute illness, with rigid personal precautions by attendants; enteric precautions in the handling of feces and fecally stained clothing and bed linen. Patients should not be employed as food handlers until successive fecal samples or rectal swabs, collected 24 hours or more apart, but not sooner than 48 hours following discontinuance of antimicrobials, are found to be free of shigella.
   3) *Concurrent disinfection:* Of feces and contaminated articles. In communities with a modern and adequate sewage disposal system, feces can be discharged directly into sewers without preliminary disinfection. Terminal cleaning.
   4) *Quarantine:* None.
   5) *Management of contacts:* Whenever feasible, contacts should be excluded from food handling and the care of young children during period of contact and until consecutive negative stool cultures are obtained. Thorough hand-washing before handling food or children must be stressed if such contacts are unavoidable.
   6) *Investigation of contacts:* Search for unrecognized mild cases and convalescent carriers among contacts may be unproductive for sporadic cases and seldom contributes to the control of an outbreak. It may generally be confined to food handlers, children in hospitals, and other situations where the spread of infection is particularly likely.
   7) *Specific treatment:* Fluid and electrolyte replacement is the important consideration. Antibiotics which are absorbed from the gastrointestinal tract (ampicillin, tetracyclines, chloramphenicol) have been shown to shorten the duration of illness and positive cultures; however, multi-resistance to antibiotics is common. The

choice of specific agents will vary in different areas as antimicrobial susceptibility patterns differ.

C. *Epidemic measures:*
1) Groups of cases of acute diarrheal disorder should be reported at once to the local health authority, even in the absence of specific identification of the disease agent.
2) Investigation of food, water and milk supplies, general sanitation, and search for unrecognized mild cases and carriers.
3) Prophylactic administration of antibiotics has generally been disappointing, but may be efficacious in association with concurrent control measures.

D. *International measures:* WHO Collaborating Centres (see Preface).

SMALLPOX

1. **Identification**—A systemic viral disease generally with a characteristic exanthem. Onset is sudden, with fever, malaise, headache, severe backache, prostration and occasionally abdominal pain. The 2 to 4 day pre-eruptive illness frequently resembles influenza. The temperature falls and a deep-seated rash appears. This rash passes through successive stages of macules, papules, vesicles, pustules and finally scabs, which fall off at the end of the third to fourth week; fever frequently intensifies after the rash has evolved to the pustular stage. The lesions become evident first on the face and subsequently on the body and extremities, are more abundant on the face and extremities than on the trunk (centrifugal distribution), and are more densely concentrated over irritated areas, prominences and extensor surfaces. Most frequently confused with varicella (chickenpox), smallpox usually can be identified by the clear-cut prodomal illness, by the centrifugal distribution of the rash, by the appearance of all lesions more or less simultaneously, by the similarity of appearance of all lesions in a given area, and by its more deeply seated lesions. In smallpox, vesicles are virtually never seen at the apex of the axilla. In previously vaccinated persons, the rash may be significantly modified to the extent that only a few highly atypical lesions are seen; generally the prodomal illness is not modified.

Two types of smallpox are recognized: *variola minor* (alastrim) and *variola major* (classical smallpox). An intermediate form is present in Africa. In variola major, the fatality rate among the unvaccinated is 20-40% or more; death normally occurs between the 5th and 7th day, occasionally as late as the 2nd week. Approximately 3% of variola major cases experience a fulminating disease characterized by a severe prodrome, prostration and bleeding into the skin and mucous membranes; such hemorrhagic cases are rapidly fatal. The usual rash does not appear and the disease may be confused with severe acute leukemia, meningococcemia or idiopathic thrombocytopenic purpura. In the "flat" variety, observed in 5% of cases, the focal lesions are slow to appear, and the vesicles tend to project only slightly above the surrounding skin and are soft and velvety to the touch. In the few patients with this type who survive, the lesions resolve without pustulation.

Outbreaks of variola minor are normally associated with a fatality rate of 1% or less. Although the rash is similar to that observed in variola major, the patient generally experiences less severe systemic reactions, and "hemorrhagic" and "flat" varieties are rarely observed.

Laboratory confirmation is by isolation of the virus on chorioallantoic membrane or tissue culture from scrapings of lesions, from vesicular or pustular fluid, from crusts, and often from the blood during the febrile pre-eruptive period. A rapid provisional diagnosis is often possible by electron microscopy or the precipitation-in-gel technique.

2. **Occurrence** — Smallpox is a continuing threat to all countries and is introduced to smallpox-free countries by international travelers. Half of the cases occurring in Europe since 1950 have been hospital acquired. The last outbreak in the U.S.A. occurred in 1949 in the Rio Grande Valley in Texas. As of 1975 smallpox has been eradicated from the Americas; the last case was reported from Brazil April 19, 1971. Under a global smallpox eradication program started in 1967 and coordinated by WHO, in 1975 the disease was endemic in only Bangladesh and India in Asia and Ethiopia in Africa, with the expectation that global eradication will be achieved within the year.

3. **Infectious agent** — Variola virus.

4. **Reservoir** — Man.

5. **Mode of transmission** — Transmission normally occurs by close contact with patients through respiratory discharges, lesions of skin and mucous membranes, or material which they have recently contaminated. Airborne spread may occur. Household,

hospital and school contacts are especially at risk. Transmission to laundry workers by bedding and other linens has been frequently observed. Virus may persist for several years in separated scabs but does not appear to be particularly infectious in this form. Inapparent infections are rare and have not been implicated in further disease transmission, but unrecognized cases may lead to extensive secondary spread.

6. **Incubation period**—From 7 to 17 days; commonly 10 to 12 days to onset of illness and 2 to 4 days more to onset of rash.

7. **Period of communicability**—From the development of the earliest lesions to disappearance of all scabs; about 3 weeks. Most communicable during first week.

8. **Susceptibility and resistance**—Susceptibility is universal; permanent immunity usually follows recovery; second attacks are rare.

9. **Methods of control**—

   A. *Preventive measures:*
   1) Effective vaccination, before exposure, prevents the disease. Immunity gradually wanes but virtually complete protection is afforded by revaccination with fully potent vaccine every 3 to 5 years.
   2) Many nations have been kept free of endemic disease for long periods by an alert surveillance and outbreak control program and by vigilance at airports, ports and border crossing points of travelers coming from infected areas. When smallpox has been introduced, intensive case finding and vaccination of direct and indirect contacts can rapidly stop the spread.
   3) In smallpox-free countries, routine primary vaccination usually is recommended after 12 months of age, with revaccination every 5-10 years. In the U.S.A. and other countries where effective surveillance and resources for rapid response to any imported case exists, routine primary vaccination of infants and children is no longer recommended. Where the health systems are not so highly developed, routine vaccination must be continued until global eradication has been achieved. In countries in which smallpox is endemic or in those countries geographically proximate to endemic areas, primary vaccination as soon after birth as possible is advised, with revaccination at 1 year and repeated revaccination every 5 years. Vaccination is required within 3 years for

international travelers under the provisions of the International Health Regulations, (1969).* It is particularly important also for those at special risk, such as clinic and hospital employees (including physicians, nurses, attendants, laboratory, ambulance and laundry workers), and morticians and others handling the dead. Those working in communicable disease wards which might admit smallpox patients should be revaccinated annually.

4) Vaccination is accomplished by inserting potent smallpox vaccine into the superficial layers of the skin. The use of vaccine fully potent at the moment of insertion is the most important (and most neglected) part of the vaccination procedure. Freeze-dried vaccine, which is reconstituted at the time of use, is now generally available; its use assures adequate potency, particularly in tropical areas if reconstituted and handled according to the manufacturer's instructions. Glycerinated vaccine maintains its potency for at least 6 months if kept below freezing at all times before use; if stored below 10ºC (50ºF), it should maintain its potency for at least 14 days. It deteriorates rapidly at ambient temperatures and therefore only freeze-dried vaccine may be used in WHO eradication programs. The preferred site for vaccination is the outer aspect of the upper arm over the insertion of the deltoid muscle. No cleansing of the skin is needed unless the vaccination site is obviously dirty, in which case it should be gently wiped with a cloth or cotton moistened with water, and permitted to dry.

The vaccination techniques of multiple puncture, multiple pressure and jet injection give the highest percentage of successful vaccinations. In the *multiple puncture technique,* a forked (bifurcated) needle is used. The needle is dipped into the vaccine and touched to the surface of the skin. The needle is then held perpendicular to the skin and 15 punctures are made in an up-and-down manner within the smallest possible area—about 3 mm (1/8 inch) in diameter. For primary vaccination when there is no likelihood of current exposure and inspection one week later is feasible, only 2 or 3 strokes are employed. In the *multiple pressure technique,* a small drop of vaccine is placed on the skin and a series of pres-

* Second Annotated Edition, 1974.

sures is made with a sharp needle, held tangentially to the skin, into the smallest possible area, about 3 mm (1/8 inch) in diameter. The strokes are completed in 5 to 6 seconds with an up-and-down motion perpendicular to the skin. In smallpox-free countries, 6-10 strokes are normally used for primary vaccination and 30 for revaccination; in others, 30 strokes are used for both primary and revaccination. A trace of blood should be observed at the vaccination site. In *jet injection* vaccination an intradermal injector deposits about 0.1 ml of a purified, less concentrated vaccine prepared especially for this method.

No dressing should be applied at the time of vaccination by any technique; if the lesion should ooze later, a loose nonocclusive dressing protects the clothing. Vaccination is repeated, as above, 1 week later (6-8 days) unless a "major reaction" is present. A "major reaction" is one which, one week after vaccination, presents a vesicular or pustular lesion, or an area of definite induration or discoloration (often irregular) surrounding any scab or ulcer remaining at the point of vaccine insertion. It is the criterion of successful vaccination, i.e., one in which an immunizing vaccinal infection has occurred. All other responses, including those which are possible but not certainly major reactions, are termed "equivocal reactions" and the individual should be revaccinated, using vaccine of known potency and a more vigorous technique. All primary vaccinations should utimately elicit a Jennerian vesicle, i.e., a major reaction. Revaccinations, except in often vaccinated highly immune groups, should produce major reactions in 80-90% of subjects. Persons with a high level of immunity exhibit a hypersensitivity reaction in the first 2 to 3 days, with erythema and the appearance of papules or frequently vesicles resulting in a scab which may still be present at the end of 1 week. Such a reaction may be induced by both potent or inactivated vaccine and thus immunity cannot be assumed. For this reason, all persons showing equivocal (or doubtful) reactions should be revaccinated again with potent vaccine and proper technique.

Complications and undesirable sequelae of vaccination are unusual. Most are rare and the majority are prevented by observing the contraindications noted below and by using fewer needle insertions in those without immunity. Major complications are (1) encephalitis, very rare in the U.S.A. but somewhat more frequent in some parts of Europe; (2) progressive vaccinia (vaccinia necrosum), exceptionally rare, occurring in individuals with immunological defects which are congenital, a consequence of neoplasms of the reticuloendothelial system, or the result of therapy with immunosuppressive drugs, corticosteroids or radiation; (3) eczema vaccinatum with vaccinial lesions appearing at the site of past or present eczematous lesions. More frequent but minor complications include (1) generalized vaccinia with multiple vaccinial lesions appearing in 5 to 10 days on various parts of the body; (2) autoinoculation of mucous membranes or abraded skin; (3) benign toxic erythema multiforme type eruptions, usually generalized and symmetrical which may frequently occur at the height of the vaccinia, and (4) secondary infections, caused by tetanus and staphylococcal organisms, from contamination of the vaccination site. Vaccinia immune globulin* (VIG), 0.3-0.6 ml/kg body weight, is indicated in the treatment of eczema vaccinatum and progressive vaccinia; it is of questionable value in postvaccinal encephalitis. It may be obtained in the U.S.A. within a few hours by contacting one of the designated consultants listed by the USPHS Center for Disease Control, Atlanta, GA, (see Preface) or commercially. Methisazone (Marboran) also has been reported to be of benefit in treatment of these conditions.

5) Contraindications to vaccination: In endemic areas, the risk of acquiring fatal smallpox far exceeds the danger of vaccination complications. In general, life-threatening acute illness is the only recognized contraindication to vaccination.

In smallpox-free countries, the following are additional contraindications to vaccination: (a) eczema and other forms of chronic dermatitis in the individual to be vaccinated or in a household contact; (b) leukemia; lymphoma or other reticuloendothelial malignancies; (c) dysgammaglobulinemia; (d) patients receiving immunosuppressive drugs such as steroids or antimetabolites or ionizing radiation; (e) pregnancy. In the face of any such

---

* In England, Human Antivaccinia Immunoglobulin.

contraindication, an individual requiring vaccination because of potential exposure in an endemic area should be given vaccinia immune globulin (VIG), 0.3 ml per kg, at the same time as vaccination. If there has been possible exposure to smallpox, vaccination is indicated even if VIG is not available.

B. *Control of patient, contacts, and the immediate environment:*
   1) *Report to local health authority. An epidemiological emergency:* Report definite or suspected cases immediately by telephone or telegraph to local health authorities. Case reports required by International Health Regulations, (1969)*, WHO Class 1 (see Preface).
   2) *Isolation:* Until all scabs have disappeared, preferably under hospital conditions in screened rooms. Strict isolation precautions; infection can be carried outside the hospital by various materials contaminated by the patient, especially on clothing and linen.
   3) *Concurrent disinfection:* Deposit oral and nasal discharges in a paper container and burn. Bedclothes and other fabrics should be sterilized by boiling or autoclaving. Terminal disinfection: The floors, walls and other hard surfaces should be fumigated, or sprayed or mopped with disinfecting agents known to kill poxviruses and allowed to remain for 4 hours before washing with water. Compounds found to be of value include phenolic and quaternary ammonium compounds, formalin and chlorine preparations. When fumigation is practiced, spaces can be disinfected by exposure to moist formalin vapor for 6 hours, or to ethylene oxide. When chemical disinfectants are not available, simpler methods may be used such as copious washing of hard surfaces with soap and water, allowing them to remain undisturbed for 48 hours. Exposure to ultraviolet light or sunlight for several hours is also effective if surfaces are fully exposed.
   4) *Quarantine:* All persons living in the same house with the smallpox patient as well as face-to-face contacts should be promptly vaccinated with known potent vaccine (see 5 below) and placed under daily surveillance for 17 days after last contact with the smallpox patient. Quarantine should be substituted for surveillance of intimate contacts whose cooperation is uncertain. At the

---

* Second Annotated Edition, 1974.

first sign of fever or other illness, the individual should be isolated. Any who refuse vaccination or have not been vaccinated (as determined by absence of vaccination scar) who have been in intimate contact with the patient should be placed under quarantine for the period when disease might appear, i.e., from 10 days after the first, to 17 days after the last contact.

5) *Immunization of contacts:* All contacts, both intimate and casual, should be promptly vaccinated at two sites, employing a known potent vaccine. Previously vaccinated contacts exposed 7 or more days before, as well as all unvaccinated contacts, should receive vaccinia immune globulin (VIG) if available, 0.3 ml/kg body weight (see 9A4 above). Methisazone (Marboran) has been shown to afford protection when given early in the incubation period.

6) *Investigation of contacts and source of infection:* Prompt investigation to determine the source of infection is of the greatest importance. Many outbreaks in smallpox-free areas are diagnosed only after the 3rd or 4th generation of cases. Since inapparent cases of smallpox are rare and do not appear to transmit infection, the source of infection should always be determined. Persons with supposed "chickenpox" or those who have recently experienced pustular or hemorrhagic disease (especially fatal cases) should be considered as the possible sources of infection.

7) *Specific treatment:* None.

C. *Epidemic measures:*

1) Isolation of patients, vaccination of contacts, laboratory confirmation of diagnosis and investigation of source of infection (see 9B above).

2) In smallpox-free areas, vaccination of an entire community should be used *only* when steps taken above do not appear to be successful. In endemic areas and countries geographically proximate, the occurrence of an outbreak may provide excellent motivation for participation in an area-wide mass vaccination program.

3) Immediate publicity, stating frankly and clearly the situation and control measures taken, often can avert panic on the part of the public. At best, however, in normally smallpox-free areas, an increased demand for vaccination can be anticipated and special provision

should be made to supply the needs of physicians and clinics without disrupting the identification, vaccination and surveillance of contacts.

D. *International measures:*

1) Telegraphic notification by governments to WHO and to adjacent countries of the first imported, first transferred, or first nonimported case of smallpox in an area previously free of the disease.

2) Measures applicable to international travelers are specified in International Health Regulations, (1969)* WHO, Geneva. For entry into other countries international travelers may be required to possess an international certificate of vaccination (see Vaccination Certificate Requirements for International Travel, WHO, 1975). The U.S.A. requires this certificate only from travelers who, within the preceding 14 days have been in a country, any part of which is infected. The validity of this certificate extends for 3 years, beginning 8 days after a successful primary vaccination was performed, or for a revaccination, on the date of that revaccination. This must be dated, be signed by a physician, indicate manufacturer and lot number of the vaccine used, and bear a stamp authorized by the national health authority. In the U.S.A., validation of a vaccination certificate can be obtained from most health departments. For individuals for whom vaccination is normally contraindicated, vaccination may be performed while administering VIG at the same time at another site (see 9A4 above). Alternately, a statement signed by a physician may be presented stating that vaccination is contraindicated. Under the International Health Regulation, (1969)* health authorities are requested to take such a statement into consideration when deciding whether or not the traveler should be admitted to the country, placed under surveillance or quarantined; some countries do not waive the requirement and will place the traveler in quarantine.

3) WHO initiated a 10-year global smallpox eradication program in 1967. WHO Collaborating Centers (see Preface).

---

* Second Annotated Edition, 1974.

MONKEYPOX

Isolated cases of vesiculo-pustular disease resembling smallpox have occurred in West Africa and Zaire after smallpox transmission had been interrupted in the area. Man-to-man transmission occurred on two occasions. The virus isolated is identical with monkeypox, a member of the variola-vaccinia group of viruses. Although this virus has been isolated from outbreaks of the disease among captive animals, it has never been isolated in the wild and its natural reservoir is unknown.

SPOROTRICHOSIS

1. Identification—A fungus disease, usually of the skin, which begins as a nodule. As the nodule grows lymphatics draining the area become firm and cord-like and form a series of nodules, which in turn may soften and ulcerate. Arthritis, pneumonitis and other visceral infections are rare. A fatal result is uncommon.

Laboratory confirmation is through cultivation of the pus or exudate, preferably aspirated from an unopened lesion; rarely visualized by direct smear and then only with selective fungus stains. Serologic tests may be helpful.

2. Occurrence—Reported from all parts of the world, in males more frequently than in females, and in adults more than in children; often an occupational disease of farmers, gardeners and horticulturists. No differences in racial susceptibility. The disease is characteristically sporadic, and relatively uncommon. An epidemic among gold miners in South Africa involved some 3,000 persons; fungus was growing on mine timbers. Many animals are susceptible, including horses, mules, dogs, cats, and rats and some other wild animals.

3. Infectious agent—*Sporothrix schenckii (Sporotrichum schenckii)*, a dimorphic fungus.

4. Reservoir—Soil, vegetation, wood.

5. Mode of transmission—Introduction of fungus through skin following pricks by thorns or barbs, the handling of sphagnum moss, or by slivers from wood or lumber. Transmission by inhalation of spores is rare. Outbreaks have occurred among children who had played in baled hay.

6. Incubation period—The lymphatic form may develop one week to 3 months or longer after injury.

7. Period of communicability—Rarely transmitted from man to man. Environment presumably may be contaminated for duration of active lesions.

8. Susceptibility and resistance—Man probably is highly susceptible.

9. Methods of control—

   A. *Preventive measures:* Treatment of lumber with fungicides in industries where disease occurs.

   B. *Control of patient, contacts, and the immediate environment:*
      1) *Report to local health authority:* Official report ordinarily not justifiable, Class 5 (see Preface).
      2) *Isolation:* None.
      3) *Concurrent disinfection:* Of discharges and dressings. Terminal cleaning.
      4) *Quarantine:* None.
      5) *Immunization of contacts:* None.
      6) *Investigation of contacts and source of infection:* Not profitable.
      7) *Specific treatment:* Iodides are effective in lymphocutaneous infection; in other forms, amphotericin B (Fungizone) is more effective.

   C. *Epidemic measures:* In the South African epidemic, mine timbers were sprayed with a mixture of zinc sulfate and triolith. This and other sanitary measures controlled the epidemic.

   D. *International measures:* None.

STAPHYLOCOCCAL DISEASE

Staphylococci produce a variety of syndromes with clinical manifestations that range from a single pustule or impetigo to septicemia and death. A lesion or lesions containing pus is the primary clinical finding, abscess formation the typical pathology. Clinical and epidemiological virulence of strains varies greatly. The most useful index of pathogenicity is an ability to coagulate plasma (coagulase); almost all virulent strains are coagulase-positive.

Staphylococcal disease has distinctly different clinical and epidemiological patterns when seen in the general community, in the hospital nursery or among hospitalized patients. Each will therefore be presented separately. Staphylococcal food poisoning, an intoxication and not an infection, is discussed separately (p. 117); attention here is to staphylococcal infections, local and general.

A. STAPHYLOCOCCAL DISEASE IN THE COMMUNITY

1. Identification — The common skin lesions are impetigo, boils, carbuncles, abscesses and infected lacerations. The basic lesion of impetigo is described in Section B; in addition, a distinctive bullous impetigo (Ritter's disease) is associated with certain strains of phage group II. The other skin lesions are localized and discrete. Constitutional symptoms are unusual; if lesions extend or are widespread, fever, malaise, headache or anorexia may develop. Usually, lesions are uncomplicated but may lead to pneumonitis, lung abscess, osteomyelitis, septicemia, pyarthrosis, meningitis, or brain abscess. In addition to primary lesions of the skin, staphylococcal conjunctivitis and osteomyelitis are relatively frequent. Staphylococcal pneumonia is a well recognized complication of influenza. Patients who develop septicemia or endocarditis frequently (up to 50%) have undergone steroid therapy or have had debilitating illnesses such as leukemia, lymphoma or diabetes. Staphylococcal endocarditis and other complications may result from parenteral infection from use of illicit drugs.

2. Occurrence — Worldwide. Maximal incidence is in areas where personal hygiene (especially the use of soap and water) is neglected and people are crowded. Common among children, especially in warm weather. Occurs sporadically and as small epidemics in families and summer camps, with various members developing recurrent illness due to the same staphylococcal strain.

3. Infectious agent — Various coagulase-positive strains of *Staphylococcus aureus* which may be characterized by phage type antibiotic resistance or serological agglutination; epidemics are caused by relatively few specific strains and these are usually resistant to penicillin G. *S. epidermidis* also may cause septicemia and endocarditis.

4. Reservoir — Man.

5. **Mode of transmission**—The major site of colonization is the anterior nares; 30 to 40% of normal persons carry coagulase-positive staphylococci in their anterior nares. Auto-infection is responsible for at least 1/3 of infections. A person with a draining lesion or any purulent discharge is the most common source of epidemic spread. Transmission is by contact with a person who has either a purulent lesion or who is an asymptomatic (usually nasal) carrier of a pathogenic strain. Some carriers are more effective disseminators of infection than others. The role of contaminated objects has been overstressed. Airborne spread is rare, but has been demonstrated in infants with associated viral respiratory disease.

6. **Incubation period**—Variable and indefinite. Commonly 4 to 10 days.

7. **Period of communicability**—As long as purulent lesions continue to drain or the carrier state persists. Auto-infection may continue for the period of nasal colonization or duration of active lesions.

8. **Susceptibility and resistance**—Immune mechanisms are not well understood. Susceptibility is greatest among the newborn and the chronically ill. Elderly and debilitated persons, as well as those with diabetes mellitus, cystic fibrosis, agammaglobulinemia, agranulocytosis, neoplastic disease and burns are particularly susceptible. Use of steroids and antimetabolites also increases susceptibility.

9. **Methods of control**—

A. *Preventive measures:*
1) Education in personal hygiene, especially hand washing and the importance of avoiding common use of toilet articles.
2) Prompt treatment of initial cases in children and families.

B. *Control of patient, contacts, and the immediate environment:*
1) *Report to local health authority:* Obligatory report of outbreaks in schools, summer camps or other population groups; also any recognized concentration of cases in the community. No individual case report, Class 4 (see Preface).
2) *Isolation:* Not practical in most communities; infected persons should avoid contact with infants and debilitated persons.
3) *Concurrent disinfection:* Place dressings from open

lesions and discharges in paper bag and burn or dispose in other practical and safe manner.

4) *Quarantine:* None.

5) *Immunization of contacts:* None.

6) *Investigation of contacts:* Search for draining lesions; occasionally determination of nasal carrier status of the pathogenic strain among family members is useful.

7) *Specific treatment:* In localized skin infections, systemic antibiotics are not indicated unless infection spreads significantly or complications ensue. For serious staphylococcal infections, employ a penicillinase-resistant penicillin or, when allergy to penicillins is present, use a cephalosporin, or erythromycin, clindamycin, gentamycin, or vancomycin. In serious systemic infections the selection of antibiotics should be governed by results of susceptibility tests carried out on isolates. Prompt parenteral treatment is important. Staphylococci are generally insensitive to sulphonomides unless they are used in combination with trimethoprim in the preparation cotrimoxazole.

C. Epidemic measures:

1) Search for persons with draining lesions and for nasal carriers of the epidemic strain; organisms from nasal carriers should be tested for their bacteriophage reaction and/or antibiotic sensitivity pattern before being identified as the epidemic strain. Those people with organisms similar to the epidemic organisms should if possible be removed from the group and all should be treated with local application of an appropriate antibiotic (i.e., bacitracin). Institute strict personal hygiene. Treat all persons with clinical disease.

2) An unusual or abrupt increase in prevalence of staphylococcal infections in the community suggests the possibility of an unrecognized hospital epidemic.

D. International measures: WHO Collaborating Centres (See Preface).

B. STAPHYLOCOCCAL DISEASE IN HOSPITAL NURSERIES

1. Identification—Impetigo of the newborn (pemphigus neonatorum) and other purulent skin manifestations are the most frequent nursery-acquired staphylococcal diseases; the characteristic skin lesions develop secondary to colonization of nose or umbilicus, conjunctiva, circumcision site or rectum of infants with a pathogenic strain. (Colonization of these sites with usual strains of staphylococci is a normal occurrence in infants and does not imply disease.) Lesions may be distributed anywhere on the body but most commonly in diaper and intertriginous areas; lesions are initially vesicular, rapidly turning seropurulent surrounded by an erythematous base. Rupture of pustules favors peripheral spread. Though less common, a distinctive generalized bullous impetigo (scalded skin syndrome, toxic epidermal necrolysis (Ritter's disease) also occurs. Complications are unusual although furunculosis, breast abscess, staphylococcal pneumonia, septicemia, meningitis, osteomyelitis, brain abscess or other serious disease occasionally has been observed.

2. **Occurrence** — Worldwide. Problems occur mainly in hospitals, are promoted by laxity in aseptic techniques and are exaggerated by development of antibiotic-resistant strains of the infectious agent.

3. **Infectious agent; 4. Reservoir; 6. Incubation period; 7. Period of communicability** — Same as for Staphylococcal Disease in the Community (A above).

5. **Mode of transmission** — Except indirect contact, spread by hands of medical attendants is the primary mode of transmission within hospitals; to a lesser extent, airborne.

8. **Susceptibility and resistance** — Susceptibility among the newborn appears to be general. Infants remain at risk of disease for duration of colonization with pathogenic strains.

9. **Methods of control** —

   A. *Preventive measures:*

      1) Use of aseptic techniques and adequate hand washing before each and every infant contact in nurseries.

      2) A rotational system in the nursery whereby one unit (A) is filled and subsequent babies admitted to a second nursery (B) while the initial unit (A) discharges infants and is cleaned before new admissions. If facilities are present for rooming-in of baby with mother, this reduces risk. Separate facility for isolation of infants with definite or suspect risk.

      3) Surveillance and supervision through an active Hospital Infections Control Committee, including a regular system of reporting, investigating and reviewing all hospital-acquired infections. Illness developing after dis-

charge from hospital also should be investigated and recorded.

4) The value of bacterial interference whereby the newborn is exposed to a nonvirulent strain is under investigation; successful colonization with this strain may prevent colonization by virulent staphylococcal strains. However, there have been several instances where the interfering strain has resulted in disease.

5) Some advocate routine application of antibacterial substances such as Triple Dye (brilliant green, crystal violet, acriflavine) to the unbilical cord stump while the baby is in the hospital.

B. *Control of patient, contacts, and the immediate environment:*

1) Report to local health authority: Obligatory report of epidemics; no individual case report, Class 4 (see Preface).

2) Isolation: Without delay isolate all known or suspect cases in the nursery. Do not permit hospital personnel with minor staphylococcal lesions (pustules, boils, abscesses, paronychia, conjunctivitis, severe acne, otitis externa or infected lacerations) to work in the nursery.

3) Concurrent disinfection; *4) Quarantine;* and *5) Immunization of contacts:* Same as A for Staphylococcal Disease in the Community. (A above)

6) Investigation of contacts and source of infection: See epidemic measures given below.

7) Specific treatment: For localized impetiginous lesions, remove crusts, cleanse skin, treat with bacitracin ointment or wash with an iodophor solution 4 to 6 times daily. Systemic antibiotics are not indicated unless disease is progressing, with fever, malaise or secondary complications. For serious infections, treat as in Section A, preceding paragraph 9B7.

C. *Epidemic measures:*

1) The occurrence of 2 or more concurrent cases of impetigo related to a nursery or a single case of breast abscess in a nursing mother or infant is presumptive evidence of an epidemic and warrants investigation. Culture all lesions and determine antibiotic resistance and phage type of epidemic strain.

2) In a nursery outbreak, institute group isolation and quarantine of cases and contacts until all have been discharged. Before admitting new patients, wash cribs,

beds, isolettes and other furniture with phenolic or iodinated detergents. Autoclave instruments and basins and sterilize mattresses, bedding and diapers.

3) Examine all nurses, aides and attendants, including physicians, for draining lesions anywhere on the body. Culture nasal specimens from all persons in contact with infants. Under circumstances of continuing disease it may become necessary to exclude and treat all carriers of the epidemic strain until cultures are negative. Treatment of asymptomatic carriers is directed at suppression of the nasal carrier state which is usually accomplished by the local application of appropriate antibiotic ointments to the nasal vestibule, rather than through systemic treatment.

4) Investigate adequacy of nursing procedures; emphasize strict aseptic technique. Personnel assigned to isolation and quarantine nurseries must not work with normal newborns.

5) Although prohibited for routine use, preparations containing 3% hexachlorophene may be employed in bathing newborns during an outbreak. Pending further data on potential central nervous system toxicity such bathing should be restricted to normal full-term infants and to no more than three daily baths.

C. STAPHYLOCOCCAL DISEASE IN MEDICAL AND SURGICAL WARDS OF HOSPITALS

1. **Identification** — Lesions vary from a simple furuncle or stitch abscess to an extensively infected bedsore, surgical wound or septic phlebitis, a chronic osteomyelitis or even a fulminating pneumonia, endocarditis or septicemia. Postoperative staphylococcal disease is a constant threat to the convalescence of the hospitalized surgical patient. Wide and sometimes injudicious use of antibiotic therapy has increased the number of antibiotic-resistant staphylococci; its use often promotes false security, with resultant relaxation of aseptic techniques. In over 90% of hospital-acquired staphylococcal disease, the infecting organisms are resistant to penicillin or other commonly used antibiotics. The increasing complexity of surgical operations, with greater organ exposure and more prolonged anesthesia, promotes entry of staphylococci. Staphylococcal enteritis is a serious complication in antibiotic-treated patients.

Verification depends on isolation of *Staphylococcus aureus,* associated with a clinical illness compatible with the bacteriologic findings.

2. **Occurrence** — Worldwide. Staphylococcal infection has become recognized as a major form of acquired sepsis in the general wards of hospitals, though recently it appears to be giving place to infection with gram-negative bacillary organisms. At times, attack rates assume epidemic proportions. Spread to the community may occur when persons infected in the hospital are discharged.

3. **Infectious agent; 4. Reservoir; 5. Mode of transmission; 6. Incubation period; 7. Period of communicability** — Same as for Staphylococcal Disease in the Community. (A above)

8. **Susceptibility and resistance** — Susceptibility is general, but greatest in chronically ill or debilitated patients, those receiving systemic steroid or antimetabolite therapy, and those undergoing major and prolonged surgical operation and convalescence. The widespread use of parenteral injections and continuous intravenous therapy with in-dwelling plastic catheters has opened new portals of entry for infectious agents.

9. **Methods of control** —

A. Preventive measures:
1) Strictly enforced aseptic techniques and programs of monitoring nosocomial infections coordinated through a Hospital Infections Control Committee.
2) Education of hospital medical staff to use common antibiotics for simple infections and reserve certain antibiotics for penicillin-resistant staphylococcal infections (e.g., oxacillin, methicillin).

B. Control of patient, contacts, and the immediate environment:
1) *Report to local health authority:* Obligatory report of epidemics; no individual case report, Class 4 (see Preface).
2) Isolation: Whenever a moderate abundance of staphylococci is known or suspected to be present in sputum or draining pus, the patient should be isolated promptly. Isolation is not required when wound drainage is scanty provided that an occlusive dressing is employed and care is taken in changing dressings to prevent contamination of the environment.
3) *Concurrent disinfection:* Collect and burn dressings; autoclave bedclothing, towels and linens prior to laundering. Terminal cleaning.
4) *Quarantine:* None.
5) *Immunization of contacts:* None.
6) *Investigation of contacts and source of infection:* Not

practical for sporadic cases (see 9C below).

7) *Specific treatment:* Appropriate antibiotics as determined by antibiotic sensitivity tests.

C. *Epidemic measures:*

1) The occurrence of 2 or more cases in epidemiologic association is sufficient to suspect epidemic spread and to initiate investigation.

2) Search for additional cases due to same strain among patients and those recently discharged. Auto-infection is common. Investigate all cases for common factor of exposure. Examine attendants, including physicians, for infected lesions. Culture patients and all related personnel to detect asymptomatic nasal carriers of the epidemic strain; remove infected persons from further contact with patients until free of infection.

3) Review and enforce rigid aseptic techniques. Provide strict isolation for each patient with purulent lesions, where practical; in large outbreaks, group isolation may be unavoidable.

D. *International measures:* WHO Collaborating Centres (see Preface).

STREPTOCOCCAL DISEASES CAUSED BY GROUP A (BETA HEMOLYTIC) STREPTOCOCCI

(Streptococcal sore throat, Scarlet fever, Impetigo, Erysipelas, Puerperal fever.)

1. Identification — Group A (usually beta hemolytic) streptococci cause a variety of diseases. The more frequently encountered conditions are streptococcal sore throat, scarlet fever and streptococcal skin infections (impetigo or pyoderma). Other diseases include puerperal fever, septicemia, erysipelas, cellulitis, mastoiditis, otitis media, pneumonia, and peritonitis. All clinical forms may occur in an endemic situation or in the course of a single outbreak.

Streptococcal sore throat exhibits clinical characteristics which may include fever, sore throat, exudative tonsillitis or pharyngitis, tender cervical adenopathy, and leucocytosis. Injection and edema of the pharynx frequently involve the tonsillar pillars and soft palate, often extending on to the hard palate; petechiae are occasionally seen against the background of diffuse redness. It is important to note that a streptococcal sore throat may occur with a minimum of symptoms, often with only a sore throat, and that lack of tonsillar exudate does not rule in or out the diagnosis of streptococcal sore throat. It may be accompanied by or followed by suppurative sequelae such as otitis media or peritonsillar abscess; also may be followed after intervals of 1 to 5 weeks by nonsuppurative sequelae such as rheumatic fever or acute glomerulonephritis.

Scarlet fever is a form of streptococcal disease which includes a skin rash; it occurs when the infecting strain of streptococcus is a good toxin producer and the patient is not immune to the toxin. Clinical characteristics include all those symptoms occurring with a streptococcal sore throat or, occasionally, a wound or puerperal infection, as well as enanthem, strawberry tongue, and exanthem. The rash is usually a fine erythema, commonly punctate, blanching on pressure, and appearing most often on the neck, chest, in folds of the axilla, elbow and groin, and on inner surfaces of the thighs. Typically, the rash does not involve the face, but there is flushing of the cheeks and circumoral pallor. High fever, nausea, and vomiting often accompany severe infections. During convalescence, a desquamation of the skin is seen at the tips of fingers and toes, less often over wide areas of trunk and limbs, including palms and soles. Severity of the disease has been decreasing in the United States for many years. The fatality rate in some parts of the world, however, is as high as 3%. Scarlet fever may be followed by the same sequelae as may occur with streptococcal sore throat.

Streptococcal skin infection (pyoderma, impetigo) is usually superficial and may proceed through vesicular, pustular, and encrusted stages. Scarlatiniform rash is rare and rheumatic fever does not occur later. Glomerulonephritis, however, may occur later.

Erysipelas is an acute cellulitis characterized by fever, constitutional symptoms, leucocytosis and a red, tender, edematous, spreading lesion of the skin, often with a definite raised border. The central point of origin tends to clear as the periphery extends. Face and legs are common sites. Recurrences are frequent. The disease may be especially severe, with bacteremia, in patients suffering from debilitating disease. Fatality varies greatly with the part of the body affected and whether there is an associated disease. Erysipelas due to group A streptococci is to be distinguished from erysipeloid, caused by *Erysipelothrix rhusiopathiae (insidiosa)*, a localized cutaneous infection seen primarily as an occupational disease of persons handling animals, meat, poultry, and fish.

Streptococcal puerperal fever is an acute disease, usually febrile, accompanied by local and general symptoms and signs of bacterial invasion of the genital tract and sometimes bactereruia in the postpartum or postabortion patient. Fatality from streptococcal puerperal fever is low when adequately treated. Many puerperal infections are caused by organisms other than hemolytic streptococci. They are clinically similar but differentiated bacteriologically and epidemiologically. The infectious agents include: nonhemolytic streptococci, anaerobic streptococci, *Staphylococus aureus*, *Escherichia coli*, *Clostridium perfringens*, *Bacteroides sp.*, and others. Group A streptococci are of primary importance in postpartum infections; the anaerobic organisms, colon bacilli, *Bacteroides sp.*, and staphylococci in postabortion infections. Treatment is by antibacterial agents and appropriate antibiotics. Epidemiologic characteristics and methods of control are those of group A streptococcal infections.

Provisional laboratory diagnosis of group A streptococcal disease is based on morphology of colonies, production of clear or beta hemolysis on blood agar, and inhibition by antibiotic discs containing 0.1 units of bacitracin; definitive diagnosis depends upon specific grouping procedures. However, a few group A strains produce little or no beta hemolysis (these may be nephritogenic). Immunofluorescent techniques are also available for rapid identification. A rise in serum antibody titer (antistreptolysin 0, antihyaluronidase, anti-DNA-ase B) may be demonstrated between acute and convalescent stages of illness.

Streptococci of other groups can produce human disease. Beta hemolytic organisms of group B, an important cause of bovine mastitis, are not infrequently found in the human vagina, and may cause neonatal sepsis and suppurative meningitis. Group D organisms (including enterococci), hemolytic or nonhemolytic, are involved in subacute bacterial endocarditis and urinary tract infections.

2. **Occurrence**—*Scarlet fever* and *streptococcal sore throat* are common in temperate zones, well recognized in semitropical areas and relatively rare in tropical climates. Inapparent infections are as common or more common in the tropics than in temperate zones. In the U.S.A.; they may have endemic, epidemic, or sporadic character. Epidemic occurrence is more frequent in certain geographic

areas, such as New England, the Great Lakes region and the Rocky Mountain area. Group A streptococcal infection due to a limited number of specific M-types, especially type 12, have frequently been associated with the development of acute glomerulonephritis; acute rheumatic fever may occur as a non-suppurative complication following infection with almost any group A serotype. Milk and milk products have been associated most frequently with food-borne out-breaks; recently opened and deviled hard-boiled eggs have become implicated more frequently. Apart from food-borne epidemics, which may occur in any season, the highest incidence is during late winter and spring. The 3 to 12 year age group is most affected; no sex or racial differences in susceptibility have been defined; military and school populations are frequently affected.

Highest incidence of streptococcal *impetigo* occurs in young children in late summer and fall in hot climates.

Geographic and seasonal distributions of *erysipelas* are similar to those for scarlet fever and streptococcal sore throat; most common after 20 years of age, with highest attack rates at 40 to 60 years; also frequent in infants. Occurrence is sporadic, even during epidemics of streptococcal infection.

Reliable morbidity data do not exist for puerperal fever. In the U.S.A. and developed countries generally, morbidity and mortality have declined precipitously since the advent of antibiotics. It is now chiefly a sporadic disease, although epidemics may occur in institutions where aseptic techniques are faulty.

3. **Infectious agent**—*Streptococcus pyogenes*, group A streptococci of approximately 60 serologically distinct types which may vary greatly in geographic and time distributions. In scarlet fever, two immunologically different types of erythrogenic toxin (A and B) have been demonstrated. Frequently, streptococci of groups B, C, D and G are hemolytic.

4. **Reservoir**—Man.

5. **Mode of transmission**—Transmission results from direct or intimate contact with patient or carrier, rarely by indirect contact through transfer by objects or hands. Dried streptococci reaching the air via contaminated floor dust, lint from bed-clothing, handkerchiefs, etc., are viable but probably noninfectious. Nasal carriers are particularly liable to transmit disease. Casual contact rarely leads to infection.

Explosive outbreaks of streptococcal sore throat may follow ingestion of contaminated milk or other food.

6. **Incubation period**—Short, usually 1 to 3 days, rarely longer.

7. Period of communicability — In untreated uncomplicated cases 10-21 days; for untreated conditions with purulent discharges, weeks or months. With adequate penicillin therapy transmission generally is eliminated within 24 hours.

8. Susceptibility and resistance — Susceptibility to streptococcal sore throat and to scarlet fever is general, although many persons develop either antitoxic or type-specific antibacterial immunity, or both through inapparent infection. Antibacterial immunity develops only against the specific M-type of group A streptococcus that induces disease or inapparant infection and lasts for years. Immunity against erythrogenic toxin, and hence to rash, develops within a week of the onset of scarlet fever and is usually permanent. Second attacks of scarlet fever are rare but may occur because of the 2 immunological forms of toxin, or because early antibiotic therapy of the first attack interfered with the formation of antitoxin. Repeated attacks of sore throat or other streptococcal disease due to different types of streptococci are relatively frequent. Both active and passive immunization against erythrogenic toxin are possible but not practical. Passive immunity to streptococcal disease occurs in newborns with transplacental maternal antibodies.

One attack of erysipelas appears to predispose individuals to subsequent attacks; recurrences may be due to streptococcal infection or to hyper-sensitivity.

9. Methods of Control —

  A. *Preventive measures:*
    1) Provision of laboratory facilities for recognition of group A hemolytic streptococci.
    2) Education of the public in modes of transmission, in the relationship of streptococcal infection to rheumatic heart disease and glomerulonephritis, and as to the necessity for completing the course of antibiotic therapy prescribed for the streptococcal infection.
    3) Boiling or pasteurization of milk and exclusion of infected persons from handling milk likely to be contaminated. Milk from any cow with evidence of mastitis should be excluded from sale or use.
    4) Other foods such as deviled eggs should be prepared just prior to serving or be adequately refrigerated at 5°C or lower.
    5) All food handlers should be questioned daily about res-

piratory illness or skin lesions and those with symptoms excluded from work.

6) Strict asepsis in obstetrical procedures, with special attention to possible contamination from mouths and noses of attendants, as well as by hands and instruments. Protection of patient during labor and the postpartum period from attendants, visitors and other patients with respiratory or skin infection.

7) Chemoprophylaxis: Monthly injections of long-acting benzathine penicillin G or daily penicillin orally for persons to whom recurrent streptococcal infection constitutes a special risk, such as individuals who have had rheumatic fever, chorea, or recurrent erysipelas or chronic post-streptococcal glomeruloneplinty who do not tolerate penicillin may be given erythromycin.

B. *Control of patient, contacts, and the immediate environment:*

1) *Report to local health authority:* Obligatory report of epidemics; no individual case report, Class 4 (see Preface).

2) *Isolation:* May be terminated after 24 hours treatment with penicillin or other effective antibiotics; therapy should be continued for 10 days.

3) *Concurrent disinfection:* Of purulent discharges and all articles soiled therewith. Terminal cleaning.

4) *Quarantine:* None.

5) *Immunization of contacts:* None.

6) *Investigation of contacts:* Search for and treat carriers.

7) *Specific treatment:* Penicillin. Several forms are acceptable for treatment i.e., intramuscular benzathine penicillin G (treatment of choice), or procaine penicillin G, or oral penicillin G, or phenoxymethyl penicillin. Therapy should provide for adequate penicillin levels for 10 days. Such treatment ameliorates the acute illness, reduces frequency of suppurative complications, prevents the development of most cases of acute rheumatic fever and many cases of acute glomerulonephritis. Also prevents further spread of the organism. Sulfonamides are not effective in eliminating the streptococcus from the throat and in preventing nonsuppurative complications. Many strains are resistant to the tetracyclines; rheumatic fever may occur after therapy with these drugs. Erythromycin is the preferred treatment for penicillin-sensitive patients.

C. *Epidemic measures:*
   1) Determine the source and manner of spread, as person-to-person, by milk, or food-borne. Outbreaks can often be traced to an individual with a persistent streptococcal infection through identification of the serologic type of the streptococcus.
   2) Under special circumstances, penicillin prophylaxis may be given to limited population groups such as a household or to other intimate contacts, or to those known to have been exposed to contaminated milk or other food, or even to an entire population group (see 9A5).
   3) Prompt investigation of any unusual grouping of cases as to the possibility of contaminated milk or other foods.

D. *International measures:* WHO Collaborating Centres (see Preface).

❦

STRONGYLOIDIASIS

1. **Identification**—A helminthic infection of the duodenum and upper jejunum. Clinical manifestations include dermatitis when larvae of the parasite penetrate the skin; cough and rales, or even pneumonitis when they pass through the lungs; abdominal symptoms when the adult females lodge in the mucosa of the intestine. Symptoms may be mild or severe, depending upon intensity of infection. They include, in order of frequency, pain, usually epigastric and often suggesting peptic ulcer, nausea, weight loss, vomiting, diarrhea, weakness and constipation. Urticaria may occur, especially with reinfection. Rarely, internal autoinfection with increasing worm burden may lead to wasting and death. Eosinophilia is usually moderate in the chronic stage.

Diagnosis is by identifying motile larvae in freshly passed feces, or in fluids obtained by duodenal intubation. Held at room temperature for 24 hours or longer, feces may show developing stages of the parasite, including filariform or infective larvae and free-living nonparasitic male and female adults.

2. **Occurrence**—Geographic distribution closely parallels that of hookworm disease (see p. 10), but indigenous cases occur far beyond the usual distribution of that disease. Prevalence in endemic areas

is not accurately known. May be endemic or epidemic in institutions where personal hygiene is poor.

3. **Infectious agent** — *Strongyloides stercoralis,* a nematode.

4. **Reservoir** — Man and possibly dogs.

5. **Mode of transmission** — Infective (filariform) larvae in moist soil contaminated with feces penetrate the skin, usually of the foot, enter the venous circulation, and are carried to the lungs. They penetrate capillary walls, enter alveoli, ascend the trachea to the epiglottis, and descend the digestive tract to reach the upper part of the small intestine, where development of the adult parasitic female is completed. The female, generally held to be parthenogenetic, lives embedded in the mucosa of the intestine, where eggs are deposited. They hatch and liberate noninfective rhabditiform larvae which migrate into the lumen of the intestine, then leave the host in the feces, and develop either into infective filariform larvae, which may reinfect the host, or into free-living adults. The free-living, fertilized females produce eggs which soon hatch, liberating rhabditiform larvae, which become filariform larvae. The life cycle may occur entirely within the human body, a unique situation in which the worm burden may increase without exposure to an external source. Perianal infection also is possible.

6. **Incubation period** — From penetration of the skin by filariform larvae until rhabditiform larvae appear in feces is about 17 days; incubation period, until symptoms appear, is indefinite and variable.

7. **Period of communicability** — Directly communicable from man to man as long as living worms remain in the intestine; up to 35 years.

8. **Susceptibility and resistance** — Susceptibility to infection is universal. Acquired immunity has been demonstrated in laboratory animals but not man. Patients on immunosuppresive medication may experience massive hyperinfection.

9. **Methods of control** —

   A. *Preventive measures:*
      1) As for Hookworm Disease (see p. 9). Sanitary disposal of human excreta, particularly the use of sanitary privies in rural areas.
      2) Rigid attention to hygienic habits; emphasize the need to wear shoes.

   B. *Control of patient, contacts, and the immediate environment:*
      1) *Report to local health authority:* Official report or-

dinarily not justifiable, Class 5 (see Preface).

    2) Isolation: None.

    3) Concurrent disinfection: Sanitary disposal of excreta.

    4) Quarantine: None.

    5) Immunization of contacts: None.

    6) Investigation of contacts: Members of the same household or institution for evidence of infection.

    7) Specific treatment: Because of the potential for autoinfection, all infections, regardless of worm burden, should be treated. Thiabendazole (Mintezol); pyrvinium pamoate (Povan); pyrvinium embonate.

C. Epidemic measures: Not applicable; a sporadic disease.

D. International measures: None.

SYPHILIS

Two distinctive forms are recognized; one is venereally spread and occurs worldwide; the other, believed by many to be a closely related but different disease, is often referred to as endemic syphilis or bejel. It is usually spread non-venereally and is confined to parts of the world where economic, social and climatic conditions favor its development. Bejel does not occur in U.S.A.

I. VENEREAL SYPHILIS
(Lues)

1. Identification— An acute and chronic treponematosis characterized clinically by a primary lesion, a secondary eruption involving skin and mucous membranes, long periods of latency, and late lesions of skin, bone, viscera, and the central nervous and cardiovascular systems. The primary lesion usually appears about 3 weeks after exposure as a papule at the site of the initial invasion; after erosion, it presents a variety of forms, the most distinctive, although not the most frequent, being an indurated chancre; invasion of blood precedes the initial lesion, and a firm, non-fluctuant, painless satellite bubo commonly follows. Infection without chancre is frequent. After 4 to 6 weeks even without specific treatment, the chancre begins to involute and a generalized secondary eruption may appear, often accompanied by mild constitutional symptoms. Secondary manifestations disappear spontaneously within weeks to as long as 12 months, with subsequent clinical latency of weeks to years. In the early years latency may be interrupted by recurrence of infectious lesions of the skin and mucous membrane or developing lesions of the eye and central nervous system; in later (5 to 20) years, by destructive non-infectious lesions of skin, viscera, bone, and mucosal surfaces. Latency sometimes continues through life and sometimes spontaneous recovery occurs. In other instances, and unpredictably, late disabling manifestations occur in cardiovascular, central nervous or other systems. Actual fatality rates cannot be accurately estimated; prenatal infection is frequently fatal before birth or in infancy. Early acquired syphilis does not result in death or serious disability; late manifestations shorten life, impair health and limit occupational efficiency.

Primary and secondary syphilis are confirmed by dark-field or phase-contrast examination of exudates of lesions or aspirates from lymph nodes (if no antibiotic has been administered), and in all instances by serologic tests of blood and spinal fluid. Tests with nontreponemal antigens should be supplemented by tests employing treponemal antigens, i.e., fluorescent antibody or treponemal immobilization, or treponemal hemagglutination, to aid in exclusion of biologic false-positive reactions. The dark-field examination is indispensable in seronegative primary syphilis.

2. Occurrence—One of the most frequent and widespread communicable diseases, primarily involving young persons between 15 and 30 years of age. Considerable differences in racial incidence are related more to social than to biologic factors; more prevalent in urban than rural areas and in males than in females. Since 1957, early venereal syphilis has increased significantly throughout much of the world.

3. Infectious agent — *Treponema pallidum*, a spirochete.

4. Reservoir — Man.

5. Mode of transmission — By direct contact in heterosexual or homosexual activity with exudates from obvious or concealed moist early lesions of skin and mucous membrane, body fluids and secretions (saliva, semen, blood, vaginal discharges) of infected persons during infectious periods; rarely by kissing or fondling of children. Transmission occurs occasionally through blood transfusion. Infection by indirect contact with contaminated articles is possible, but rarely occurs. Prenatal infection may occur after fourth month of pregnancy through placental transfer.

6. Incubation period — Ten days to 10 weeks, usually 3 weeks.

7. **Period of communicability**—Variable and indefinite. During primary and secondary stages and also in mucocutaneous recurrence; may be intermittently communicable for 2 to 4 years. Extent of communicability through sexual activity during latency period (2 to 4 years) is not established; possible inapparent lesions make this stage potentially infectious. Adequate penicillin treatment usually ends infectivity within 24 hours.

8. **Susceptibility and resistance**—Susceptibility is universal, though only approximately 10% of exposures result in infection. There is no natural immunity. Infection leads to gradually developing resistance against the homologous strain of *Treponema* and to some extent against heterologous strains; immunity may be overcome by a large reinfecting dose or may fail to develop because of treatment in the primary or secondary stage. Superinfection may produce lesions simulating those of the currently existing stage; in late latency, superinfection has special significance by its ability to evolve as benign lesions of the skin and mucous membranes.

9. **Methods of control**—

    A. *Preventive measures:* The following are applicable to all venereally transmitted diseases: syphilis, chancroid, lymphogranuloma venereum, granuloma inguinale, gonorrhea, herpes simplex virus infection type 2, trichomonal vaginitis, candidiasis and diseases caused by *Chlamydia* (Bedsonia) and certain of the mycoplasmas.

        1) General health promotional measures, health and sex education, preparation for marriage, premarital and prenatal examinations, including blood serology as part of general physical examination.

        2) Protection of community by control of prostitution and discouragement of sexual promiscuity, in cooperation with social and law enforcement agencies; by teaching methods of personal prophylaxis applicable before, during and after exposure and by serologic examination of women in both early and late pregnancy.

        3) Provision of facilities for early diagnosis and treatment; encouragement of their use through education of the public about symptoms of the venereal diseases and modes of spread, and through making these services available irrespective of economic status. Intensive case-finding programs, to include interview of patients and tracing of contacts; for syphilis, repeated mass serologic examination of special groups with known high incidence of venereal disease.

4) Emphasis on control of patients with venereal disease in a transmissible stage should not preclude search for persons past that stage to prevent relapse, congenital syphilis, and disability due to late manifestations.

B. *Control of patient, contacts, and the immediate environment:*

1) *Report to local health authority:* Case report of early infectious syphilis is required in all states, and variously in other countries, Class 2A (see Preface); report of positive serology and dark-field examinations by laboratories in some states.

2) *Isolation:* None. To avoid reinfection, patients should refrain from sexual intercourse with previous partners not undergoing treatment.

3) *Concurrent disinfection:* None in adequately treated cases; care to avoid contact with discharges from open lesions and articles soiled therewith.

4) *Quarantine:* None.

5) *Immunization of contacts:* Not applicable.

6) *Investigation of contacts:* Interview of patients and tracing of contacts are fundamental features of a program for control of venereal disease. Trained interviewers obtain best results. The stage of disease determines the criteria for contact-tracing: (a) for primary syphilis, all sexual contacts of preceding 3 months; (b) for secondary syphilis, those of preceding 6 months; (c) for early latent syphilis, those of preceding year, provided time of primary and secondary lesions is not established; (d) for late and late latent syphilis, marital partners and children of infected mothers; (e) for congenital syphilis, all members of immediate family. Contacts of confirmed cases should receive chemotherapy.

7) *Specific treatment:* Long acting penicillin G (PAM, benzathine penicillin or equivalent preparation); in general, large amounts initially on day of diagnosis to assure reasonably effective therapy should the patient fail to return. For example, 2.4 million units of benzathine penicillin is treponemicidal for 3-4 weeks and 7-10 days with PAM and thus usually is effective for both primary and secondary syphilis. Increased dosages for longer periods of therapy are indicated for the late stages of syphilis. Erythromycin or tetracycline antibiotics may be used in penicillin-sensitive persons.

Such patients require extended post-treatment observation and follow-up checks of serological reactions.

C. *Epidemic measures:* Intensification of measures outlined under 9A and 9B, preceding.

D. *International measures:*
1) Appropriate examination of groups of adolescents and young adults moving from areas of high prevalence of treponemal infections.
2) Adherence to agreements among nations (e.g., Brussels Agreement) as to records, provision of diagnostic and treatment facilities, and contact interviewing at seaports for foreign merchant seamen.
3) Provision for rapid international exchange of information on contacts.
4) WHO Collaborating Centers (see Preface).

II. NONVENEREAL SYPHILIS
(Bejel, Dichuchwa, Njovera)

1. Identification — A disease of limited geographical distribution, acute nature, and characterized clinically by an eruption of skin and mucous membrane, usually without an evident initial primary sore. Mucous patches of the mouth are often the first lesions, soon followed by moist papules in folds of skin and by drier lesions of the trunk and extremities. Other early skin lesions are macular or papular, often hypertrophic, and frequently circinate, resembling those of venereal syphilis. Plantar and palmar hyperkeratoses occur frequently, often with painful fissuring; patchy depigmentation and hyperpigmentation of the skin and alopecia are common. Inflammatory or destructive lesions of skin, long bones, and nasopharynx are late manifestations. Unlike venereal syphilis, the nervous and cardiovascular systems are rarely involved. The fatality rate is low.

Organisms are demonstrable in lesions by dark-field examination. Serologic tests for syphilis are reactive in the early stages and remain so for many years of latency, gradually tending toward reversal; response to treatment as in venereal syphilis.

2. Occurrence — A common disease in localized areas where poor economic and social conditions and primitive sanitary and dwelling arrangements prevail. Present in the Balkans and in eastern Mediterranean and Asian countries; numerous foci and Africa, particularly in arid regions.

3. Infectious agent — *Treponema pallidum,* a spirochete.

4. Reservoir — Man.

5. **Mode of transmission** — Direct or indirect contact with infectious early lesions of skin and mucous membranes; latter favored by common use of eating and drinking utensils and generally unsatisfactory hygienic conditions; congenital transmission is rare.

6. **Incubation period** — Two weeks to 3 months.

7. **Period of communicability** — During moist eruptions of skin and until mucous patches disappear; sometimes several weeks or months.

8. **Susceptibility and resistance** — Similar to venereal syphilis.

9. **Methods of control** —

   A. *Preventive measures:* Those of the nonvenereal treponematoses. See Yaws, 9A (pp. 370-371).

   B. *Control of patient, contacts, and the immediate environment:*
      1) *Report to local health authority:* In selected endemic areas; in most countries not a reportable disease; Class 3B (see Preface).
      2) See Yaws 9B (p. 371) for items 2-7, applicable to all nonvenereal treponematoses.

   C. *Epidemic measures:* Intensification of preventive and control activities.

   D. *International measures:* See Venereal Syphilis 9D4 (preceding); and Yaws 9D (p. 371).

TAENIASIS AND CYSTICERCOSIS
(Beef or Pork tapeworm disease)

1. **Identification** — An infection with the adult stage of the beef tapeworm *(Taenia saginata)* or the adult or larval stage of the pork tapeworm (*T. solium*). Clinical manifestations of infection with the adult worm *(taeniasis)* are variable and may include nervousness, insomnia, anorexia, loss of weight, abdominal pain, and digestive disturbances. Many infections are asymptomatic. Taeniasis is a non-fatal disease.

The larval infection with *T. solium*, cysticercosis, is a serious somatic disease that may involve many different organs and tissues. When eggs of the pork tapeworm are swallowed by man they hatch in the small intestine and larval forms (cysticerci) develop in subcutaneous tissues, striated muscles, and other tissues or vital organs of the body. Consequences may be grave when larvae localize in the ear, eye, central nervous system, or heart. In the presence of somatic cysticercosis, psychic symptoms, including epileptiform seizures, strongly suggest cerebral involvement. Cysticerosis is a chronic disease; it may cause serious disability with a relatively high mortality rate.

Infection with an adult tapeworm is diagnosed by identification of proglottids (segments) of the worm or of eggs in feces or on an adhesive cellulose tape swab. Taenia eggs also must be differentiated from vegetative diatoms and eggs of *Hymenolepis nana*, (relatively common, especially in children) and from *H. diminuta* and *Dipylidium caninum* (rare). Specific diagnosis is based on the morphology of gravid proglottids; obtaining the scolex or head confirms the identification and assures elimination of the worm. Eggs of *T. solium* and *T. saginata* cannot be differentiated. Subcutaneous or visceral cysticercosis is recognized by excision of the larval cyst and microscopic examination.

2. **Occurrence**—Cosmopolitan distribution; particularly frequent wherever beef or pork is eaten raw or lightly cooked. Incidence is highest in parts of Africa and Asia, Mexico, Peru and eastern Europe. Where *T. saginata* and *T. solium* coexist, *T. saginata* is by far the commoner. Infection with *T. solium* is rare in the U.S.A. and Canada.

3. **Infectious agents**—*Taenia saginata*, the beef tapeworm of man, intestinal infection with adult worm only; *Taenia solium*, the pork tapeworm of man, intestinal infection with adult worm and somatic infection with the larva (cysticercus) of *T. solium*.

4. **Reservoir**—An infected person whose feces contain eggs, free or within proglottids of the parasite in feces.

5. **Mode of transmission**—For *T. saginata*, by ingestion of raw or inadequately cooked beef containing the infective larva (cysticercus). For *T. solium* (1) by ingestion of raw or inadequately cooked pork containing the infective larva (cysticercus) and subsequent development of the adult worm in the intestine; or (2) by direct transfer of eggs in feces of a person harboring an adult worm to his own or another's mouth, or indirectly through ingestion of food or water contaminated with eggs, resulting in somatic cysticercosis.

6. **Incubation period**—From 8 to 14 weeks.

7. Period of communicability — *T. saginata* is not directly transmitted from man to man but *T. solium* may be; eggs of both species are disseminated in the environment as long as man harbors the worm in the intestine, sometimes 30 to 40 years; eggs may remain viable for months.

8. Susceptibility and resistance — Man is universally susceptible. No apparent resistance follows infection.

9. Methods of control —

A. Preventive measures:

1) Education of the public to prevent soil and water contamination with human feces in rural areas, to avoid use of sewage effluents for pasture irrigation, and to thoroughly cook beef and pork.

2) Adequate inspection of the carcasses of cattle and swine will detect most infected meat; cysticerci in beef may be few. Condemn carcasses of infected animals.

3) Do not allow swine access to latrines or to human feces.

4) Immediate management of persons harboring adult *T. solium* is essential to prevent human cysticercosis. *T. solium* eggs are infective immediately upon exiting the host and are capable of producing a severe and incurable human illness, aggressive measures to protect the patient from himself as well as to protect his contacts are mandatory.

B. Control of patient, contacts, and the immediate environment:

1) *Report to local health authority:* Selectively reportable, Class 3C (see Preface).

2) *Isolation:* Patients with *T. solium* infection should be isolated (enteric precautions) until treated. (See 9A4 above.)

3) *Concurrent disinfection:* Sanitary disposal of feces; for *T. solium* rigid sanitation, with washing of hands after defecating and before eating.

4) *Quarantine:* None.

5) *Immunization of contacts:* None.

6) *Investigation of contacts:* Usually not profitable.

7) *Specific treatment:* For *T. saginata;* niclosamide (Yomesan) (available in the U.S.A. from the Center for Disease Control (CDC), Atlanta, Georgia (see Preface). Quinacrine hydrochloride (atabrine) is also effective and for *T. solium* is the preferred drug because of the theoretical possibility of autoinfection following the use of niclosamide. No specific chemotherapy for cysti-

cercosis; surgical excision is the only satisfactory treatment.

C. Epidemic measures: None.

D. International measures: None.

TETANUS
(Lockjaw)

1. Identification—An acute disease induced by toxin of the tetanus bacillus growing anaerobically at the site of an injury; characterized by painful muscular contractions, primarily of masseter and neck muscles, secondarily of trunk muscles; a common first sign suggestive of tetanus is abdominal rigidity, though rigidity is sometimes confined to the region of injury. History of injury or apparent portal of entry is often lacking. In the absence of effective immunization the fatality rate varies from 35 to 70%, according to age, sex, length of incubation, severity of symptoms geographic area and therapy.

Laboratory confirmation is of little help. The organism is rarely recovered from the site of infection and usually there is no antibody response.

2. Occurrence—Worldwide. Occurs sporadically or in occasional small circumscribed outbreaks; affects all ages. In U.S.A. and most industrial countries, relatively uncommon; more common in agricultural regions and in underdeveloped areas where contact with animal excreta is more likely and immunization is generally insufficient. It is an important cause of death in many countries of Asia, Africa and South America, especially in rural and tropical areas where tetanus neonatorum is prevalent. A hazard in the parenteral use of drugs by addicts.

3. Infectious agent—*Clostridium tetani*, the tetanus bacillus.

4. Reservoir—Soil and intestinal canals of animals, especially horses in which the organism is a harmless normal inhabitant; also man.

5. Mode of transmission—Tetanus spores introduced into the body during injury, usually a puncture wound contaminated with soil, street dust or animal feces, but also through burns and trivial or unnoticed wounds. The presence of necrotic tissue and/or foreign bodies favors growth of the anaerobic pathogen. The majority of cases follow injuries considered too trivial for medical consultation. Tetanus neonatorum usually occurs through infection of the unhealed umbilicus.

6. **Incubation period**—Commonly 4 days to 3 weeks, dependent on character, extent and location of wound; average 10 days. Most cases occur within 14 days, but may be longer.

7. **Period of communicability**—Not directly transmitted from man to man.

8. **Susceptibility and resistance**—Susceptibility is general. Prolonged active immunity is induced by tetanus toxoid; transient passive immunity follows injection of tetanus immune globulin (human) or tetanus antitoxin. Recovery from tetanus does not result in solid immunity; second attacks may occur.

9. **Methods of control**—

   A. *Preventive measures:*
      1) Education as to the value of routine immunization with tetanus toxoid, the kinds of injury liable to be complicated by tetanus, and the need after severe injury for either a booster injection if previously actively immunized, or passive protection by tetanus immune globulin (human) or tetanus antitoxin if not previously immunized.
      2) Active immunization with tetanus toxoid gives the best protection. The initial basic series of three injections is preferably given in infancy or early childhood, together with diphtheria toxoid and pertussis vaccine (see Diphtheria 9A, p. 103).

         Tetanus toxoid is recommended for universal use regardless of age, but is especially important for workers in contact with soil or domestic animals and members of the military forces, policemen and others with greater than usual risk of traumatic injury. Pregnant women should be actively immunized where tetanus neonatorum is prevalent, preferably early, but may be done in the second or even in the third trimester. In the U.S.A. active immunization is by 2 initial doses of alum-precipitated toxoid not less than 4 weeks apart, followed by a third injection about 8 to 12 months later; thereafter, in the absence of injury, booster doses at intervals of 10 years. Tetanus toxoid may be given at any age.
      3) For a person actively immunized against tetanus who has not received a booster in the previous 3 to 5 years, a single booster injection of tetanus toxoid administered

promptly on the day of injury; reactions are infrequent but have been observed, *especially after too frequent boosters.*

4) If there has been no previous active immunization (including recovered cases) and if the patient is seen on the day of injury and there are no compound fractures, gunshot wounds or other wound not readily debrided, passive protection may be induced by injecting 250 units of tetanus immune globulin (human) or 5,000 units of equine or bovine tetanus antitoxin: antibiotics (penicillin) should also be given for 7 days. If delay is greater, or such complications exist, the dose of immune globulin or antitoxin should be at least doubled. The human tetanus immune globulin is preferred because of the rarity of serium reactions. Protection provided by tetanus immune globulin lasts about 21 days; by animal tetanus antitoxin from 3 to 14 days. Active immunization should be started during the protective period of immune globulin or antitoxin by giving the first dose of adsorbed, not fluid, toxoid (9A2) at a different site than used for the immune globulin or antitoxin.

5) Under all circumstances, removal of foreign matter from wounds by thorough cleansing, with debridement of necrotic tissue when present.

6) Licensing of midwives, with provision of professional supervision and education as to methods, equipment and techniques of asepsis in childbirth.

7) Education of mothers, relatives and attendants in the practice of strict asepsis of the umbilical stump of newborn infants; especially important in many lesser developed areas where ashes, cow dung poultices or other contaminated substances are traditionally applied to the cord stump.

B. *Control of patient, contacts, and the immediate environment:*

1) *Report to local health authority:* Case report required in most states and countries, Class 2A (see Preface).

2) *Isolation.* None.

3) *Concurrent disinfection:* None.

4) *Quarantine:* None.

5) *Immunization of contacts:* None.

6) *Investigation of contacts and source of infection:* Case investigation to determine circumstances of injury. In tetanus neonatorum, detailed inquiry into the methods

of umbilical care employed by attendants and/or members of the family at birth. Where applicable search for others involved in the same accident.

7) *Specific treatment:* Tetanus immune globulin (human) intramuscularly, in large doses. Tetanus antitoxin in a single large dose should be given intravenously with appropriate precautions; penicillin in large doses intramuscularly. Maintain an adequate airway; employ sedation as indicated; muscle relaxant drugs together with tracheotomy and mechanically assisted respiration may be necessary to save life. Active immunization should be initiated concurrently with therapy.

C. *Epidemic measures:* In the rare hospital outbreaks make a thorough search for inadequacies in sterilization.

D. *International measures:* Active immunization against tetanus is advised for international travelers.

TOXOPLASMOSIS

1. **Identification**—A systemic protozoan disease. Primary infection seldom gives rise to clinical illness, but may be accompanied by undue fatigue or muscle pains. Rarely acute disease occurs with fever, lymphadenopathy and lymphocytosis persisting for days or weeks; even more rarely it is severe, with generalized muscle involvement, cerebral manifestations and death. Adult chorioretinitis is more frequently associated with chronic infection. A primary infection during the early gestational period of pregnancy may lead to death of the fetus; or later infection to chorioretinitis, brain damage with intra-cerebral calcification, hydrocephaly, microcephaly, fever, jaundice, rash, hepatomegaly and splenomegaly; xanthochromic spinal fluid and convulsions may be evident at birth or shortly thereafter.

Diagnosis is by demonstration of the agent in body tissues or fluids by biopsy or at necropsy or by inoculation of susceptible animals, embryonated eggs or tissue culture. Demonstration of the agent in tissue is more significant when supported by positive clinical and serological findings. The "dye-test", complement fixation, hemagglutination, and indirect fluorescent antibody test are corroborative, and demonstration of specific gamma M (19S) antibodies in infants and titer rises on sequential sera are supplementary. Antibody titers must be critically evaluated since high levels may persist for years without relation to active disease.

2. **Occurrence**—Worldwide in animals and man. Infection in man is common but clinical disease exceptional.

3. **Infectious agent**—*Toxoplasma gondii*, an intracellular coccidian protozoan belonging to the *Sporozoa* and closely related to the genus *Isospora*. The taxonomy and complete life cycle of this parasite are still uncertain. Only felines have been shown to excrete the oocyst form in feces, but evidence indicates that *Felidae* are the definitive hosts of *T. gondii*, and that after infection they excrete oocysts for approximately 10 days; these become infective 1-3 days later.

4. **Reservoir**—Not well understood. Rodents, dogs, cats, swine, cattle, sheep, goats, chickens, and other homeothermic mammals and birds appear to be intermediate hosts of *T. gondii*, without evident species differences in susceptibility; all may carry the invasive stage (trophozoite) of *T. gondii* in tissue.

5. **Mode of transmission**—Unclear for postnatal infections; transplacental infection may occur in women with a primary infection and infection is also possible during delivery. Consumption of raw or undercooked infected meat has been implicated. Laboratory-infected ticks have transmitted infection to experimental animals; experimental and natural transmission of *T. gondii* by cat feces has been demonstrated in small mammals and presumably occurs in man.

6. **Incubation period**—Unknown; 10 to 23 days in one common source outbreak where the vehicle was undercooked meat.

7. **Period of communicability**—Probably not directly transmitted from man to man except in utero. In cats probably during acute stage, possibly longer.

8. **Susceptibility and resistance**—Susceptibility is general. Duration and degree of immunity are unknown but antibody persists for years, probably for life. Patients undergoing immunosuppressive therapy are highly susceptible.

9. **Methods of control**—

    A. Preventive measures: No known specific preventive measures. Suggested measures are thorough cooking of meats and avoidance of cat feces.

    B. Control of patient, contacts, and the immediate environment:
        1) Report to local health authority: Not ordinarily required

but is desirable to facilitate research, Class 3C (see Preface).

2) *Isolation:* None.

3) *Concurrent disinfection:* None.

4) *Quarantine:* None.

5) *Immunization of contacts:* None.

6) *Investigation of contacts:* In congenital cases, determine antibodies in mother and other members of family; in acquired cases, determine contact with infected animals and common exposure of others to suspected infective raw meat or cat feces.

7) *Specific treatment:* In experimental infections of animals, sulfonamides have prophylactic value; when administered early, may have therapeutic effect. Pyrimethamine (Daraprim) combined with triple sulfonamides and folinic acid is the preferred treatment in man. Acute disease responds more favorably to treatment than the chronic forms. Treatment should be accompanied by appropriate hematological control. Duration of treatment should approximate four weeks.

C. *Epidemic measures:* Not applicable—a sporadic disease.

D. *International measures:* None.

TRACHOMA

1. **Identification**—A specific communicable keratoconjunctivitis of insidious or abrupt onset; of long or even lifetime duration if untreated. It is characterized by conjunctival inflammation with lymphoid follicles and papillary hyperplasia, associated with vascular invasion of the cornea (pannus) and in its later stages by conjunctival cicatrization which may lead to gross deformity of the eyelids, progressive visual disability and blindness. Associated bacterial infections, common in many areas, increase communicability and severity, and modify clinical behavior.

Laboratory diagnosis is by demonstration of intra-cytoplasmic inclusion bodies in epithelial cells of conjunctival scrapings by Giemsa or immunofluorescent staining; or by isolation of the agent in cell culture or in chick embryo yolk sac. While in general some microbiologic differences exist, some strains are indistinguishable from those of inclusion conjunctivitis although the two diseases have quite dissimilar epidemiologic patterns.

Other forms of chronic follicular conjunctivitis with scarring and corneal pannus include those found with molluscum nodules of the lid margin, with toxic reaction to chronically administered eye drops, and occasionally to chronic staphylococcal lid margin infection.

2. **Occurrence** — Worldwide, in tropical, subtropical, temperate and cold climates, but with unequal and varying distributions, marked by differences in age of onset, clinical evolution, frequency of spontaneous cure, frequency of disabling sequelae and response to treatment. Trachoma is widespread in the Middle East, in Asia, along the Mediterranean littoral and in parts of Africa and South America; in U.S.A., among Indians and Mexican immigrants of the Southwest. High prevalence is generally associated with poor hygiene, poverty, and crowded living conditions, particularly in dry, dusty regions. Nomadic persons generally have a less severe form than stationary populations.

3. **Infectious agent** — *Chlamydia (Bedsonia) trachomatis* which includes several antigenic types (TRIC agents).

4. **Reservoir** — Man.

5. **Mode of transmission** — By direct contact with ocular discharges and possibly mucoid or purulent discharges of nasal mucous membranes of infected persons, or materials soiled therewith. Flies, especially *Musca sorbens*, may contribute to spread of the disease, but transmission occurs in their absence. Communicability is relatively low.

6. **Incubation period** — Five to 12 days (based on volunteer studies).

7. **Period of communicability** — While active lesions are present in the conjunctivae and adnexal mucous membranes. Concentration of the agent in the tissues is greatly reduced with cicatrization, but increases again with reactivation and when infective discharges recur.

8. **Susceptibility and resistance** — Susceptibility is general; there is no evidence that infection confers immunity. In endemic areas children have active disease more frequently than adults; the severity of disease often is related to environmental conditions. Lack of water and exposure to dry winds, dust and fine sand may contribute to the severity of the disease.

9. **Methods of control—**

   A. *Preventive measures:*
   1) Provision of adequate case-finding and treatment facilities, with emphasis on preschool children.
   2) Education of the public on the need for personal hygiene, especially the risk in common use of toilet articles.
   3) Improved basic sanitation, including availability and use of soap and water; avoid common-use towels.
   4) Conduct epidemiological investigations to determine important factors in occurrence of the disease in each specific situation.
   5) There is no conclusive evidence that vaccines are useful in preventing infection or in reducing the severity of established cases.

   B. *Control of patient, contacts, and the immediate environment:*
   1) *Report to local health authority:* Case report required in some states and countries of low endemicity, Class 2B (see Preface).
   2) *Isolation:* Not practical in most areas where the disease occurs.
   3) *Concurrent disinfection:* Of eye discharges and contaminated articles.
   4) *Quarantine:* None.
   5) *Immunization of contacts:* None.
   6) *Investigation of contacts:* Members of family, playmates and schoolmates.
   7) *Specific treatment:* Oral tetracyclines (treatment of choice) or erythromycin are effective in the active stages of the disease, as are oral sulfonamides. In developing countries where the disease is severe and highly prevalent, mass treatment with topical tetracycline or erythromycin is frequently used.

   C. *Epidemic measures:* In regions of hyperendemic prevalence, mass treatment campaigns have been successful in reducing severity and frequency, when associated with education of the people in personal hygiene and improvement of the sanitary environment.

   D. *International measures:* WHO Collaborating Centres (See Preface).

TRICHINOSIS
(Trichiniasis, Trichinellosis)

1. Identification — A disease caused by migration through the body of larvae of *Trichinella spiralis* and by their encystment in muscles after ingestion of raw or insufficiently cooked, infected meat. Clinical disease in man is highly variable. Usually a mild febrile disease, but can range from inapparent infection to a fulminating, fatal disease. Sudden appearance of edema of upper eyelids is a common early and characteristic sign, usually noted about the 10th or 11th day; is sometimes followed by subconjunctival, subungual and retinal hemorrhages, pain and photophobia. Gastrointestinal symptoms, such as diarrhea, may precede ocular manifestations. Muscle soreness and pain, skin lesions, thirst, profuse sweating, chills, weakness, prostration, and rapidly increasing eosinophilia may shortly follow ocular signs. Fever is usual, remittent, and terminates by lysis after 1 to 3 weeks; sometimes as high as 40°C (104°F). Respiratory and neurological symptoms may appear in the 3rd to 6th week, myocardial failure between the 4th and 8th weeks.

Skin tests, eosinophilia, flocculation and complement-fixation tests may aid in diagnosis. Biopsy of skeletal muscle, not earlier than about 10 days after exposure to infection, frequently provides conclusive evidence by demonstrating the organism.

2. Occurrence — Worldwide but variable in prevalence, depending on practices in eating and preparing pork, and the extent to which the disease is recognized and reported. Necropsy surveys reveal former wide prevalence in U.S.A.; age adjusted rate now only 2.2% or probably lower; cases usually are sporadic and outbreaks localized.

3. Infectious agent — Larva (trichina) of *Trichinella spiralis*, an intestinal roundworm.

4. Reservoir — Swine, dogs and cats, and many wild animals, including fox, wolf, bear, polar bear, marine mammals and rats.

5. Mode of transmission — Eating of raw or insufficiently cooked flesh of animals containing viable encysted trichinae, chiefly pork and pork products, and "beef products" such as hamburger adulterated either intentionally or inadvertently with pork. In the small intestine, larvae develop into mature adults and mate. Gravid female worms then pass larvae, which penetrate the intestinal wall, enter the lymphatics, and are disseminated via the bloodstream throughout the body. The larvae encyst in striated skeletal muscle.

6. **Incubation period** — About 9 days after ingestion by man of infective meat; varies between 2 and 28 days.

7. **Period of communicability** — Not transmitted directly from man to man. Animal hosts remain infective for months, and meat from such animals can cause disease for appreciable periods unless treated to kill the larvae. (See 9A, 4 and 5.)

8. **Susceptibility and resistance** — Susceptibility is universal. Infection is not known to result in acquired immunity.

9. **Methods of Control** —

    A. Preventive measures:
  1) Regulations to assure adequate processing of pork products. In the U.S.A., pork inspection by trichinoscopy is considered to be impractical and costly; it also affords a false sense of security. The digestion technique is useful in slaughter houses.
  2) Pork must be ground in a separate grinder, or the grinder thoroughly cleaned before processing other meats.
  3) Adoption of suitable laws and regulations insuring cooking of garbage and offal before feeding to swine. Incineration or burial of garbage may be cheaper than feeding to swine.
  4) Education as to the need to cook all fresh pork and pork products at a temperature and time sufficient to allow all parts to reach at least 65.6°C (150°F) or until meat changes from pink to grey, which allows a good margin of safety, or unless it is established that these meat products have been processed either by heating, curing or freezing adequate to kill trichinae.
  5) Education of hunters to thoroughly cook bear meat.
  6) Low temperatures maintained throughout infected meat are effective in killing trichinae, i.e., holding at -27°C (-16°F) for 36 hours or at higher temperatures for longer periods of time; at least 20 days storage at -18°C (0°F), the temperature of the home freezer, is required.

    B. Control of patient, contacts, and the immediate environment:
  1) Report to local health authority: Case report desirably required in most states and countries, Class 2B (see Preface).
  2) Isolation: None.
  3) Concurrent disinfection: None.
  4) Quarantine: None.

    5) Immunization of contacts: None.

    6) Investigation of contacts: Check other family members and persons who have eaten suspected meat for evidence of infection.

    7) Specific treatment: Thiabendazole has been used with encouraging results. It is most efficacious in the acute stage of the disease. Corticosteroids are indicated in severe cases.

C. Epidemic measures: Institute epidemiologic study to determine the common food involved. Confiscate remainder of food and correct faulty practices.

D. International measures: None.

∞

TRICHOMONIASIS

    1. Identification — A common, chronic disease of the genitourinary tract in women, characterized by vaginitis, frequently with small petechial or punctate hemorrhagic lesions, and profuse, thin, foamy, yellowish discharge of foul odor. In men, the infectious agent invades and persists in the prostate, urethra, or seminal vesicles, but rarely produces symptoms or demonstrable lesions. Infection also may frequently be asymptomatic in women.

    Diagnosis is through identification of the motile parasite, either by microscopic examination of discharges, or by culture.

    2. Occurrence — Geographically widespread, and a frequent disease of all continents and all peoples, primarily of adults, with highest incidence among females aged 16 to 35 years. In sampled areas of the U.S.A., the prevalence among females has been as high as 50%.

    3. Infectious agent — *Trichomonas vaginalis*, a protozoon.

    4. Reservoir — Man.

    5. Mode of transmission — By contact with vaginal and urethral discharges of infected persons, during sexual intercourse, during passage of infant through the birth canal, and possibly by contact with contaminated articles.

    6. Incubation period — Four to 20 days, average 7 days.

7. **Period of communicability** — For the duration of the infection.

8. **Susceptibility and resistance** — Susceptibility to infection is general, but clinical disease is mainly in females.

9. **Methods of control** —

A. *Preventive measures:* Educate public as to the symptoms and mode of transmission; encourage women with symptoms to seek immediate treatment and to avoid sexual intercourse while infected.

B. *Control of patient, contacts, and the immediate environment:*
  1) *Report to local health authority:* Official report not ordinarily justifiable, Class 5 (see Preface).
  2) *Isolation:* None, avoid sexual relations during period of infection and treatment.
  3) *Concurrent disinfection:* None, the organism cannot withstand drying.
  4) *Quarantine:* None.
  5) *Immunization of contacts:* None.
  6) *Investigation of contacts:* Sexual partner, particularly if infection is recurrent.
  7) *Specific treatment:* Metronidazole (Flagyl) by mouth is effective in both male and female patients. It is contraindicated during the first trimester of pregnancy. Concurrent treatment of sexual partner to prevent reinfection.

C. *Epidemic measures:* None.

D. *International measures:* None.

TRICHURIASIS
(Trichocephaliasis, Whipworm disease)

1. **Identification** — A nematode infection of the large intestine, often asymptomatic and detected only by examination of feces. Heavy infections result in intermittent abdominal pain, bloody stools, diarrhea, and loss of weight. Rectal prolapse may occur in very heavy infections.

Diagnosis is by demonstration of eggs in feces.

2. **Occurrence**—Cosmopolitan, especially in warm, moist regions.

3. **Infectious agent**—*Trichuris trichiura (Trichocephalus trichiurus)*, a nematode; the human whipworm.

4. **Reservoir**—Man.

5. **Mode of transmission**—Indirect; not transmissible from man to man. Eggs passed in feces require a minimum of 3 weeks in soil for embryonation. Ingestion of fully embryonated eggs picked up from contaminated soil is followed by hatching and attachment of the developing worm to the mucosa of the cecum and proximal colon. Egg passage in the feces begins about 90 days after ingestion.

6. **Incubation period**—Indefinite.

7. **Period of communicability**—As long as eggs are in the feces; several years.

8. **Susceptibility and resistance**—Susceptibility is universal.

9. **Methods of control**—

   A. *Preventive measures:*
      1) Provision of adequate facilities for disposal of feces.
      2) Education of all members of the family, particularly children, in the use of toilet facilities.
      3) Encouragement of satisfactory hygienic habits, especially as to washing the hands before handling food and avoidance of ingestion of soil by thorough washing of vegetables and by other means.

   B. *Control of patient, contacts, and the immediate environment:*
      1) *Report to local health authority:* Official report not ordinarily justifiable, Class 5 (see Preface). School health authorities should be advised of unusual frequency in school populations.
      2) *Isolation:* None.
      3) *Concurrent disinfection:* None, sanitary disposal of feces.
      4) *Quarantine:* None.
      5) *Immunization of contacts:* None.
      6) *Investigation of contacts:* Examine feces of all members of family group, especially children and playmates.
      7) *Specific treatment:* Light or moderate infections are self-limited and require no treatment. If treatment is undertaken mebendazole (Vermox) a newly licensed compound, is safe, effective, and the drug of choice. Thiabendazole is less effective, but may be used when

mebendazole is not available; it is contraindicated in pregnancy. Diphetarsone (Bemarsal) also may be used. In severe cases 0.2% hexylresorcinol enemata may be required, but this heroic treatment should only be given in a hospital.

C. *Epidemic measures:* Not applicable.

D. *International measures:* None.

TRYPANOSOMIASIS, AFRICAN
(African sleeping sickness)

1. **Identification** — In the early stages by a chancre at the primary tsetse fly bite site and by fever, intense headache, insomnia, lymph node enlargement (especially posterior cervical), anemia, local edema and rash; later, by body wasting, somnolence, and signs referable to the central nervous system. May run a protracted course of several years or death may follow within a few months; highly fatal.

Diagnosis in early stages is by finding trypanosomes in lymph from punctured nodes and in the blood. In advanced stages trypanosomes may be found in the cerebrospinal fluid. Inoculation of laboratory rats or mice or culture on appropriate media is sometimes useful. An antibody rise may be demonstrated by fluorescent antibody and complement fixation tests; high levels of immunoglobulins, especially IgM, are typical of African trypanosomiasis.

2. **Occurence** — The disease is confined to tropical Africa between 15°N and 20°S latitude, corresponding to the distribution of the tsetse fly; in some endemic regions up to 30% of persons have been infected. The disease is endemic in many African foci; outbreaks can occur when, for any reason, man-fly contact is intensified or when trypanosomes are introduced into a tsetse-infected area by movement of reservoir hosts. Where flies of the *Glossina palpalis* group are the principal vectors, infection occurs mainly along streams as in West and Central Africa; where the vector is *Glossina morsitans*, over wider dry savannas as in East Africa and around Lake Victoria.

3. **Infectious agents** — *Trypanosoma gambiense* and *Trypanosoma rhodesiense*, hemoflagellates. Criteria for species differentia-

tion are not absolute; isolates from cases of virulent, rapidly progressive disease are considered to be *T. rhodesiense*.

4. **Reservoir**—Man is an important reservoir of *T. gambiense*. Wild game, especially bushbuck and antelopes, and domestic cattle are the chief animal reservoirs of *T. rhodesiense*.

5. **Mode of transmission**—By bite of an infective *Glossina*, the tsetse fly. Six species are mainly concerned in nature: *Glossina palpalis*, *G. tachinoides*, *G. morsitans*, *G. pallidipes*, *G. swynnertoni*, and *G. fuscipes*. The tsetse fly, whether male or female, is infected by ingesting blood of a person or animal that contains trypanosomes. The parasite multiplies in the fly for 18 days or longer, according to temperature and other factors, until infective forms develop in the salivary glands. Once infected, a tsetse fly remains infective for life (up to 3 months); infection is not passed from generation to generation in flies; congenital transmission can occur in man. Direct mechanical transmission by blood on the proboscis is possible for *Glossina* and other man-biting flies like horse-flies.

6. **Incubation period**— In *T. rhodesiense* infection usually 2 to 3 weeks; in *T. gambiense* infections usually longer, i.e., may be several months, or even years.

7. **Period of communicability**—To the tsetse fly, as long as the parasite is present in the blood of the infected person or animal; extremely variable in untreated cases, but communicable in late as well as early stages of the disease.

8. **Susceptibility and resistance**—Susceptibility is general. Spontaneous recovery in cases without symptoms of central nervous system involvement is thought to occur but has never been confirmed; occasional inapparent infections occur with both *T. gambiense* and *T. rhodesiense*.

9. **Methods of Control**—

    A. *Preventive measures:*

        1) Selection of appropriate methods of prevention must be based on knowledge of the local ecology of the vectors and infectious agents. Thus, in a given geographic area, priority must be given to one or more of the following:

        a) Destruction of vector tsetse fly habitats by selective brush clearing along certain water courses or around villages. If cleared areas can be reclaimed for agricultural use, a permanent solution to the vector problem may result.

        b) Reduction of fly population by appropriate use of in-

secticides (5% DDT or 3% dieldrin) are effective.
c) Removal of people from fly-infested areas and congregation into larger settlements.
d) Reduction of parasite population by survey of human population for infection and treatment of infected persons.
e) Informing people as to personal measures to protect against biting tsetse flies.
f) Ordinarily, prophylactic medication with pentamidine isethionate* in a single 250-mg dose intramuscularly protects adults for 3 to 6 months against *T. gambiense;* may be used for the indigenous population, but this is not generally recommended for the casual visitor to an endemic area, and not at all for visitors to *T. rhodesiense* infested areas. Pentamidine-resistant strains have developed subsequent to mass prophylaxis using this drug.

B. Control of patient, contacts, and the immediate environment:
1) *Report to local health authority:* In selected endemic areas establish records of prevalence and encourage control measures; not a reportable disease in most countries, Class 3B (see Preface).
2) *Isolation:* Not practicable. Prevent tsetse flies from feeding on patients with trypanosomes in their blood. In some countries legal restrictions are placed on movement of untreated patients.
3) *Concurrent disinfection:* None.
4) *Quarantine:* None.
5) *Immunization of contacts:* None.
6) *Investigation of contacts:* None.
7) *Specific treatment:* Early in the course of infection suramin* or pentamidine* is used; the former is the drug of choice for *T. rhodesiense* infections, while the latter is preferred for *T. gambiense* infections. Melarsoprol* (Mel B) has been used effectively for treatment of advanced cases of either form.

C. Epidemic measures: Mass surveys, treatment of identified

---

*Available in U.S.A. from Center for Disease Control, Atlanta, Georgia, on an investigational basis (see Preface).

cases and tsetse fly control are urgent. If epidemics recur in an area despite control measures, it may be necessary to move whole villages to safer districts. Other measures as in 9A.

D. International measures: Promote cooperative efforts of governments in endemic areas. WHO Collaborating Centres (see Preface).

TRYPANOSOMIASIS, AMERICAN
(Chagas' disease)

1. **Identification**—Acute stages are generally seen in children; chronic manifestations generally appear later in life, although many infected persons have no clinical manifestations. The acute disease is characterized by variable fever, malaise, lymphadenopathy and hepatosplenomegaly. An inflammatory response at the site of infection (chagoma) may last up to 8 weeks. Unilateral bipalpebral edema (Romana's sign) occurs in a significant percentage of acute cases. Life-threatening or fatal manifestations include myocarditis and meningo-encephalitis. Chronic sequelae include myocardial damage with cardiac dilatation and arrhythmias and intestinal tract involvement with megaesophagus and megacolon.

Diagnosis in the acute phase is established by demonstration of the organism in blood (or, rarely, in a lymph node or in skeletal muscle) by direct examination, by culture, by inoculation into rats or mice, or by xenodiagnosis (feeding uninfected triatomid bugs on the patient and finding the parasite in the bug's feces several weeks later). Parasitemia is most intense during febrile episodes early in the course of infection. In the chronic phase xenodiagnosis may be positive but other methods rarely reveal parasites. Serologic tests, such as complement-fixation, fluorescent antibody and direct agglutination are important for individual diagnosis as well as screening purposes. These tests are more sensitive than any of the methods for demonstrating the parasite per se.

2. **Occurrence**—The disease is confined to the Western Hemisphere, with wide geographic distribution in rural Mexico and Central and South America; in some areas highly endemic. In the whole of South America it is estimated that a total of 7 million

people are infected. Two human infections have been reported in U.S.A. (Texas); serologic studies suggest the possible presence of other, but asymptomatic, cases. *Trypanosoma cruzi* has been found in small mammals in Alabama, Arizona, California, Florida, Georgia, Louisiana, Maryland, New Mexico, Texas and Utah.

3. Infectious agents—*Trypanosoma cruzi (Schizotrypanum cruzi),* a protozoan that occurs in man as a hemoflagellate, as well as an intracellular parasite without an apparent flagellum.

4. Reservoir—Reservoirs include infected persons and many domestic and wild animals such as dog, cat, pig, guinea pig, bat, house rat, wood rat, fox, opossum and armadillo.

5. Mode of transmission—By fecal material from infected vectors, i.e., blood-sucking species of *Reduviidae* (cone-nosed bugs), especially from *Triatoma, Rhodnius* and *Panstrongylus*. Infection is through contamination of conjunctiva, mucous membranes, and abrasions or wounds of the skin by fresh infected bug feces. Transmission may occur by blood transfusion and organisms also may pass through the placenta to cause congenital infection. Accidental laboratory infections are not uncommon.

6. Incubation period—About 5 to 14 days after bite of the insect vector; 30-40 days if infected by blood transfusion.

7. Period of communicability—Organisms are present regularly in the blood during the acute period and may persist in very small numbers throughout life in symptomatic and asymptomatic persons. The vector becomes infective 8 to 10 days after biting an infective host and remains so for life (as long as 2 years).

8. Susceptibility and resistance—All ages are susceptible, but in younger persons the disease usually is more severe.

9. Methods of Control—

   A. Preventive measures:
     1) Systematic attack upon vectors through use of effective insecticides with residual action.
     2) Construction or repair of dwellings to eliminate hiding places for the insect vector and shelter for the domestic and wild reservoir animals.
     3) Use of bed nets in houses infested by the vector.
     4) Education of the public as to the mode of spread and methods of prevention.
     5) In endemic areas screen blood donors by complement-fixation or other suitable test to prevent infection by transfusion. Addition of gentian violet (25 ml of 0.5% solution per 500 ml of blood 24 hours before use) will prevent transmission.

B. *Control of patient, contacts, and the immediate environment:*
   1) *Report to local health authority:* In selected endemic areas; not a reportable disease in most countries, Class 3B (see Preface).
   2) *Isolation:* None.
   3) *Concurrent disinfection:* None.
   4) *Quarantine:* None.
   5) *Immunization of contacts:* None.
   6) *Investigation of contacts and source of infection:* Search bedding and rooms for the vector, and examine domestic and wild animals for evidence of infection. All members of the family of a case should be examined.
   7) *Specific treatment:* No drug has proved of value. A nitrofurfurylidine derivative, Bayer 2502, is available from the Center for Disease Control, Atlanta, Georgia, on an investigational basis (see Preface).

C. *Epidemic measures:* In areas of high incidence, field surveys to determine distribution and frequency of vectors and animal hosts.

D. *International measures:* None.

TUBERCULOSIS

1. **Identification** — A chronic mycobacterial disease, which is important as a cause of disability and death in many parts of the world. Primary infection usually goes unnoticed clinically; tuberculin sensitivity appears within a few weeks; lesions commonly become inactive, leaving no residual changes except pulmonary or tracheobronchial lymph node calcifications. May progress, however, to active pulmonary tuberculosis, pleurisy or lympho-hematogenous dissemination of bacilli to produce miliary, meningeal or other extrapulmonary involvement. Serious outcome of primary infection is more frequent in infants and adolescents than in older persons.

Pulmonary tuberculosis generally arises from a latent primary focus and if untreated has a variable and often asymptomatic course, with exacerbations and remissions, but may be cured with chemotherapy. Clinical status is established by presence of tubercle bacilli in sputum, or by progression or retrogression as detected in serial X-rays following a definitive bacteriologic diagnosis. Abnormal X-ray densities indicative of pulmonary infiltration, cavitation, or fibrosis commonly occur before clinical manifestations. Cough, fatigue, fever, weight loss, hoarseness, chest pain and hemoptysis may occur but often are absent until advanced stages.

Presumptive diagnosis is confirmed by demonstration of tubercle bacilli by culture of sputum, tracheobronchial, gastric washings, or other specimens. Smear examination may give a presumptive diagnosis. Repeated examinations often are needed to find bacilli. Persons infected with *M. tuberculosis* and *M. bovis* will react to a low dose tuberculin test (e.g., with the bio-equivalent of 5 International Units). The reaction may be suppressed in critically ill tuberculosis patients and during certain acute infectious diseases, especially measles.

Extrapulmonary tuberculosis is much less common than pulmonary. It includes tuberculous meningitis, acute hematogenous tuberculosis, and involvement of bones and joints, eyes, lymph nodes, kidneys, intestines, larynx, skin or peritoneum. Diagnosis is by recovery of tubercle bacilli from lesions or exudates.

2. Occurrence — Present in all parts of the world; numerous countries have showed downward trends of mortality and morbidity for many years. Mortality rates range from below 5 to 100 deaths per 100,000 population per year. The mortality and morbidity rates increase with age; higher in males than in females; much higher in nonwhites than in whites. In 1974 the reported incidence of new cases in the U.S.A. was 14.2 per 100,000 population. In developed countries prevalence of pulmonary tuberculosis is low for persons under 20 years of age and rises with age; highest in males over 50. Most post-primary tuberculosis is endogenous, especially in low-incidence areas, i.e., arises from old latent foci remaining from initial infection. Epidemics have been reported among children in crowded classrooms or other groups congregated in enclosed spaces.

Prevalence of infection, as manifested by tuberculin testing, increases with age; usually higher in cities than in rural areas. Rapid decline in developed countries in recent decades; in U.S.A., less than 3% of males aged 17 to 20 years now react positively to 5 TU of PPD (purified protein derivative). In areas where human infection with atypical mycobacteria is prevalent, e.g., southeastern U.S.A., cross reactions may complicate the interpretation of the tuberculin reaction.

Infection with the bovine tubercle bacillus in man is rare in the U.S.A. and many other countries, but is still a problem in some.

3. Infectious agent—*Mycobacterium tuberculosis*, the human tubercle bacillus, and *M. bovis* in cattle, swine and other animals. Atypical mycobacteria occasionally produce disease indistinguishable from pulmonary tuberculosis except by culture of the organisms.

4. Reservoir—Primarily man; in some areas, also diseased cattle.

5. Mode of transmission—Exposure to bacilli in airborne droplet nuclei from sputum of infected persons. Prolonged household exposure to an active case may lead to infection of contacts and frequently active disease. Indirect contact through contaminated articles or dust may occur, but is not important; direct invasion through mucous membranes or breaks in the skin is extremely rare. Bovine tuberculosis results from exposure to tuberculous cows, usually by ingestion of unpasteurized milk or dairy products and sometimes by airborne spread to farmers and animal handlers.

6. Incubation period—From infection to demonstrable primary lesion, about 4 to 12 weeks; to progressive pulmonary or extrapulmonary tuberculosis may be years.

7. Period of communicability—As long as infectious tubercle bacilli are being discharged. Some untreated or inadequately treated patients may be intermittently sputum-positive for years. The degree of communicability depends on numbers of bacilli discharged, the virulence of the bacilli and opportunities for their aerosolization by coughing, sneezing or singing. Antimicrobial therapy generally reduces communicability within a few weeks. Extrapulmonary tuberculosis without a discharge is not directly communicable.

8. Susceptibility and resistance—Susceptibility is general; highest in children under 3 years, lowest in later childhood; then again high in adolescents and young adults; undernourished, neglected and fatigued persons or those with silicosis, diabetes, myxedema, partial gastrectomies or those on corticosteroid or immunosuppressive therapy, those with hematologic or reticuloendothelial disease such as leukemia or Hodgkin's disease, and alcoholics may be especially susceptible. The most hazardous period is the first 6 to 12 months after infection. Relapse of long latent infection, particularly in older persons, accounts for a large proportion of active cases.

9. Methods of control—

A. Preventive measures:

1) Poor social conditions which increase the risk of becoming infected, such as overcrowding, should be

improved; education of the public in mode of spread and methods of control.

2) Availability of medical, laboratory, and X-ray facilities, for examination of patients, contacts and suspects, and for early treatment of cases; beds for those needing hospitalization.

3) Public health nursing service for home supervision of patients and to encourage and arrange for examination of contacts.

4) Preventive treatment, defined as treatment of inactive disease by administration of isoniazid in therapeutic dosage for 1 year, has been shown to be effective for certain groups such as: contacts of active cases who have recently converted to a "positive" skin test; household associates of active cases; and for other populations in which the risk of tuberculosis is unusually great, e.g., optimally for all tuberculin positive young people and especially those whose risk is increased due to underlying disease, prolonged corticosteroid therapy, or immunosuppressive therapy.

A course of isoniazid will reduce the risk of relapse in arrested cases never previously treated with effective antibacterial drugs. (For purposes of this recommendation, tuberculin positivity is a response of 10 mm or greater induration 48 to 72 hours after a properly applied Mantoux test, using 5 TU of PPD). Because of the increased risk of isoniazid-associated hepatitis, routine preventive treatment of persons over 35 years of age is precluded, except in cases where the presence of additional risk factors increase the likelihood of subsequent tuberculous disease sufficiently to warrant offering preventive therapy regardless of age. (See par. 8 above.) Isoniazid therapy is contraindicated where there is a history of previous isoniazid-associated hepatic injury; severe adverse reactions to isoniazid, such as drug fever, chills, rash, and arthritis; acute liver disease of any etiology. Monitoring tests for incipient hepatitis are not indicated, but are mandatory in the event of overt signs and symptoms of hepatitis.

However, a policy of preventive treatment, even of special risk groups, is unrealistic and unsuitable for mass application in a community health program unless the treatment program for patients suffering from infectious tuberculosis is widespread and well organized, and achieves a high rate of cure.

5) BCG vaccination of uninfected (tuberculin-negative) persons induces tuberculin sensitivity in over 90% of individuals and confers variable protection. Some controlled trials have provided evidence that protection may persist for at least 12 years in high incidence countries. Where risk of infection is low, as presently in most parts of the U.S.A., mass vaccination has little role except in certain groups of high risk, e.g., medical personnel often exposed to undiagnosed cases. In many parts of the world, vaccine is used routinely as part of the program of control. In some countries, notably New Zealand, most 14 year old school children are vaccinated with BCG. Vaccine may be used for newborn infants, especially of mothers with active pulmonary tuberculosis, and also for household contacts of active cases, as well as for persons obviously at high risk of infection, as in "ghetto" populations. BCG is contraindicated for persons with immuno-deficiency diseases.

6) Elimination of tuberculosis among dairy cattle by tuberculin testing and slaughter of reactors; pasteurization of milk.

7) Measures to prevent chronic pulmonary damage due to inhalation of dangerous concentrations of dust in industrial plants and mines.

8) Examination of sputum of persons who because of chest symptoms present themselves to health services, gives a high yield of infectious tuberculosis. This is an effective case finding tool of favorable cost effectiveness in many developing countries.

9) In the U.S.A. screening by tuberculin test of groups that have a high risk of tuberculosis: greatest emphasis should be placed on contacts of active cases, patients in general and mental hospitals, recent immigrants from areas where tuberculosis is prevalent, and impoverished segments of the population; also those who constitute a special hazard to others if infected, such as school personnel. X-ray examination should be restricted to reactors.

10) Periodic X-ray screening of tuberculin-positive populations.

11) In areas where tuberculosis is still prevalent, tuberculin testing surveys, as at school entrance and at 14 years of age employing the bio-equivalent of 5 TU of PPD intracutaneously, may help to identify foci of infection.

B. *Control of patient, contacts and the immediate environment:*

1) *Report to local health authority:* Obligatory case report in most states and countries, Class 2B (see Preface). Case report should indicate if bacteriologically positive or if based on clinical or X-ray findings. Health departments should maintain a current register of active cases.

2) *Isolation:* Control of infectivity is best achieved by prompt, specific drug therapy, which usually reduces infectiousness rapidly and produces sputum conversion within a few weeks. Hospital treatment is desirable only for patients with severe illness where it is necessary to establish a therapeutic program, and for those whose medical or social circumstances make it undesirable to treat them at home. Patients treated at home or ambulatorily, should be instructed in personal hygiene, especially in the need to cover the mouth and nose when coughing or sneezing, and in the careful handling and disposal of sputum. Children with primary tuberculosis need not be isolated.

3) *Concurrent disinfection:* Handwashing and good housekeeping practices should be maintained according to regular, routine policy. There are no special precautions necessary for handling fomites (dishes, laundry, bedding, clothes and personal effects). Microbial decontamination of air by ventilation and ultra-violet light.

4) *Quarantine:* None.

5) *Immunization of contacts:* Preventive treatment of close contacts (see 9A4 preceding) is indicated. BCG vaccination of tuberculin negative household contacts, especially infants and children, may be warranted under special circumstances such as continuing exposure or improbability of close follow-up. (See Section 9A5.)

6) *Investigation of contacts:* Tuberculin testing of all members of the household and intimate extra-household contacts (or all, if feasible) with X-ray examination of reactors. If negative, a repeat skin test should be performed at 2-3 months. Retest of tuberculin negative persons only if re-exposed. Preventive treatment of convertors (see 9A4) with intensive study of the contacts is indicated.

7) *Specific treatment:* Most primary infections heal without treatment; when they are recognized antimicrobial therapy, e.g., isoniazid, is indicated to

markedly reduce the risk of progressive disease or later reactivation.

Patients with active pulmonary tuberculosis should be given prompt treatment with an appropriate combination of antimicrobial drugs continued for a minimum of 12 months. Current accepted regimens include 2 or more of the following: isoniazid (INH), ethambutol (EMB), para-aminosalicylic acid (PAS), and streptomycin (SM); Rifampin (RIF) is favored by some in combined retreatment of resistant cases, but others favor its use in initial therapy. If sputum fails to become negative after 3-4 months of regular therapy or reverts to positive after a series of negatives or if clinical response is poor, examination for drug resistance is indicated. Drug resistance, usually the result of irregularity in taking drugs, necessitates a change in regimen; at least two effective drugs should be included. All of these drugs occasionally may cause adverse side reactions. Thoracic surgery, chiefly pulmonary resection, is rarely indicated.

C. *Epidemic measures:* Alertness to recognize aggregations of new infections resulting from contact with an unrecognized infectious case and intensive search for the source of infection.

D. *International measures:* X-ray screening of individuals prior to emigration. WHO Collaborating Centres (see Preface).

MYCOBACTERIOSES

Mycobacteria, other than *M. tuberculosis, M. intracellulare, M. avium, M. leprae,* and *M. bovis,* are ubiquitous in nature and may produce disease in man. These acid-fast bacilli have been variously termed atypical, unclassified or anonymous mycobacteria, and have been separated into four groups by Runyon (Group I—Photochromogens, Group II—Scotochromogens, Group III—Non-Photochromogens, and Group IV—Rapid growers). Of the numerous identified species only about a dozen are recognized as being pathogenic to man. Clinical syndromes associated with the pathogenic "species of" mycobacteria can be broadly classified as follows: **pulmonary disease resembling tuberculosis**—*M. kansasii, M. intracellulare* (the Battey bacillus), *M. avium, M. fortuitum, M. xenopi,* **lymphadenitis** (primarily cervical)—*M. scrofulaceum* (the "orange" bacillus), *M. intracellulare, M. avium;* **skin ulcers**—*M. ulcerans* (Buruli ulcer), *M. marinum (balnei).* The epidemiology of the diseases attributable to these organisms has not been well delineated but the organisms have been found to be abundant in soil and water; other factors such as host tissue damage probably predisposes to infection; there is no evidence of person-to-person transmission with the exception of skin lesion isolates. A single isolation of these bacilli from sputum, gastric or other specimen is not diagnostic, unless combined with compatible clinical findings. Where human infection with "nontuberculous" mycobacteria is prevalent, cross reactions may interfere with the routine skin test for *M. tuberculosis*. Chemotherapy is relatively effective in treating *M. kansasii* disease but not the other mycobacterioses. For selection of an efficient drug combination, sensitivity tests for first and second-line anti-tuberculosis agents should be performed. Surgery should be given more serious consideration than in tuberculosis, especially when the disease is limited, as in cervical lymphadenitis.

TULAREMIA

1. **Identification** — An infectious disease of rodents and lagomorphs (rabbits); also occurs in domestic animals and man. In man it is characterized by sudden and dramatic onset of chills and fever. Clinical forms include ulcero-glandular, glandular, oculo-glandular, typhoidal, and pulmonary. In the glandular forms, the lymph nodes become swollen and tender and often suppurate. Fatality in untreated cases is about 5%; with treatment, negligible.

Diagnosis is by inoculation of laboratory animals with material from lesions or with blood or sputum, by recovery of the infectious agent on glucose cystine blood agar or cysteine heart agar plus blood and by development of an agglutination reaction with patient's serum.

2. **Occurrence** — Throughout North America and in many parts of continental Europe, USSR, and in Japan. Occurs in U.S.A. every month of the year; incidence may be higher in early winter during rabbit hunting season.

3. **Infectious agent** — *Francisella tularensis (Pasteurella tularensis, Bacterium tularense).*

4. **Reservoir** — Numerous wild animals, especially rabbits, hares,

muskrats and some domestic animals; also wood ticks and the common dog tick.

5. **Mode of transmission** — Inoculation of skin, conjunctival sac or anal mucosa with blood or tissue while handling infected animals, as in skinning, dressing, or performing necropsies; or by fluids from infected flies, ticks or other animals or through the bite of arthropods including a species of deer fly, *Chrysops discalis* and in Sweden, the mosquito *Aedes cinereus*. Also by bite of reservoir wood ticks, *Dermacentor andersoni;* dog ticks, *D. variabilis;* Lone Star ticks, *Amblyomma americanum;* and rabbit ticks, *Haemaphysalis leporis-palustris;* and by ingestion of insufficiently cooked rabbit or hare meat and drinking of contaminated water or by inhalation of dust from contaminated soil, grain or hay. Rarely, from bites of coyotes, skunks, hogs, cats, and dogs whose mouths presumably are contaminated from eating infected rabbits. Laboratory infections are common and frequently appear as a primary pneumonia.

6. **Incubation period** — One to 10 days, usually 3 days.

7. **Period of communicability** — Not directly transmitted from man to man. The infectious agent may be found in the blood during the first 2 weeks of disease, and in lesions for a month from onset; sometimes longer. Flies are infective for 14 days and ticks throughout their lifetime (about 2 years). Rabbits kept constantly frozen at -15°C (5°F) may remain infective more than 3 years.

8. **Susceptibility and resistance** — All ages are susceptible; long term immunity follows recovery. Through abrasions and contact with contaminated material an immune person may acquire a local tularemic papule which harbors virulent organisms but causes no constitutional reaction.

9. **Methods of control** —

   A. *Preventive measures:*
      1) Education of the public to avoid bites of flies, mosquitoes and ticks or the handling of such arthropods when working in endemic areas; and to avoid drinking raw water and swimming in waters where infection prevails among wild animals.
      2) Use of rubber gloves when skinning or handling potentially infectious wild animals, especially rabbits, or when conducting laboratory experiments. Thorough cooking of the meat of wild rabbits.
      3) Prohibition of interstate or inter-area shipment of infected animals or their carcasses.
      4) Killed vaccines are of limited value. Live vaccines are

used extensively in USSR and to a limited extent in the U.S.A. Administration of a viable vaccine intradermally by the multiple-puncture method has materially reduced the incidence of laboratory-acquired disease. This vaccine can be obtained from the Center for Disease Control, Atlanta, Georgia (see Preface).

B. *Control of patient, contacts, and the immediate environment:*

    1) Report to local health authority: In selected endemic areas (U.S.A.); in many countries, not a reportable disease, Class 3A (see Preface).

    2) Isolation: None.

    3) Concurrent disinfection: Of discharges from ulcers, lymph nodes, or conjunctival sacs.

    4) Quarantine: None.

    5) Immunization of contacts: Not indicated.

    6) Investigation of contacts: Important in each case, with search for the origin of infection.

    7) Specific treatment: Streptomycin is the drug of choice; the tetracyclines and chloramphenicol are effective when continued until temperature is normal for 4-5 days. Fully virulent streptomycin-resistant organisms have been described.

C. *Epidemic measures:* Search for sources of infection related to arthropods, to animal hosts, and to water, soil and crops. Control measures as indicated in 9A above.

D. *International measures:* None.

TYPHOID FEVER
(Enteric Fever, Typhus abdominalis)

1. **Identification**—A systemic infectious disease characterized by continued fever, headache, malaise, anorexia, a relative bradycardia, enlargement of spleen, rose spots on trunk, constipation more commonly than diarrhea, and involvement of the lymphoid tissues. Many mild and atypical infections occur. Ulceration of Peyer's patches in the ileum can produce intestinal hemorrhage or perforation, especially late in untreated cases. Non-sweating fever, mental

dullness and slight deafness may be observed. A usual fatality rate of 10% is reduced by antibiotic therapy to 2-3% or less.

Typhoid bacilli are found in the bone marrow and blood early in the disease and in feces or urine after the 1st week. The agglutination reaction becomes positive during 2nd week.

2. Occurrence — Worldwide. Prevalent in many countries of the Far East, Middle East, eastern Europe, Central and South America, and Africa. In Mexico there was a material increase in incidence in 1972, most with antibiotic resistant organisms (also reported from Southeast Asia). In the U.S.A. the number of sporadic cases has been relatively constant for several years, although there has been an increase of cases in travelers arriving in or returning from foreign countries.

3. Infectious agent — *Salmonella typhi*, the typhoid bacillus. About 50 types can be distinguished by Vi-Phages.

4. Reservoir — Man, both patients and carriers. Family contacts may be transient carriers. In most parts of the world fecal carriers are more common than urinary carriers. The carrier state is most common among persons infected during middle age, especially females. Long-term carriers frequently have a typhoid cholecystitis. Urinary carriers are seen frequently in areas where *Schistosoma haematobium* infections also occur.

5. Mode of transmission — By food or water contaminated by feces or urine of a patient or carrier. Improperly cooked starchy foods and pastries in which the bacilli multiply are common offenders. Unsafe raw fruits and vegetables are important vehicles in some parts of the world, while milk and milk products are principal vehicles in others. Contamination is usually by hands of carriers or missed cases. Under some conditions flies are important vectors. Outbreaks have been traced to imported canned meats, the organisms apparently entering through minute leaks in the cans during the process of cooling in contaminated water. Shellfish, in which pathogens present in the water are concentrated, have been incriminated in typhoid fever.

6. Incubation period — Dependent on size of infecting dose; usual range 1 to 3 weeks.

7. Period of communicability — As long as typhoid bacilli appear in excreta; usually from 1st week throughout convalescence; variable thereafter. About 10% of the patients will discharge bacilli for 3 months after onset of symptoms; 2 to 5% become permanent carriers.

8. Susceptibility and resistance — Susceptibility is general but is increased in individuals with gastric achlorhydria. Resistance to small infecting doses follows recovery from clinical disease or from inapparent infections or from active immunization. In endemic areas attack rates usually decline with age.

9. **Methods of control—**

   A. *Preventive measures:*
   1) Protection, purification and chlorination of public water supplies; provision of safe private supplies. For individual or small group protection, and while traveling or in the field, water is preferably boiled; chlorine or iodine disinfecting tablets or hypochlorite bleach can be added directly to water, the amount depending on turbidity of water and amount to be treated.
   2) Sanitary disposal of human excreta.
   3) Fly control by screening, spraying with residual insecticides and use of insecticidal baits and traps. Control of fly breeding by provisions for adequate garbage collection, elimination of open garbage dumps with substitution of landfill operations, and provision for proper disposal of feces.
   4) Boiling or pasteurization of milk and dairy products, including cheese. Sanitary supervision of commercial production, transport, processing, and delivery. Proper storage and refrigeration in stores and homes.
   5) Limiting the collection and marketing of shellfish to supplies from approved sources. Use of chlorinated water for cooling during the processing of canned foods.
   6) Sanitary supervision of processing, preparation and serving of foods in public eating places, especially foods eaten raw. Special attention to the provision and use of hand-washing facilities. If uncertain as to whether such sanitary practices are in use, select foods that are cooked and served hot.
   7) Identification and supervision of typhoid carriers. Sewage culture may help in locating carriers. If the carrier state lasts for 1 year, carriers may be released from supervision and restriction of occupation (see par. 8 below) only after 6 consecutive negative cultures of authenticated specimens of feces and urine taken 1 month apart (cf. 9B2 following). Stool specimens should be used for culture rather than rectal swabs. At least one of the 6 consecutive negative specimens should be a purged specimen. Prolonged antibiotic therapy, es-

pecially with oral ampicillin may end the carrier state; if not, a two week course of intravenous ampicillin should be administered. For persons in whom antibiotic therapy fails, cholecystectomy is recommended if there is evidence of chronic gallbladder disease.

8) Instruction of convalescents and chronic carriers in personal hygiene, particularly as to sanitary disposal of excreta, hand washing after defecation and before handling food, and exclusion from occupation as food handlers or as attendants in the care of patients or children.

9) Education of the the general public, and particularly of food handlers, concerning sources of infection and modes of transmission.

10) Immunization with a vaccine of high antigenicity, given in a primary series of 2 injections several weeks apart. Vaccination is protective only against small infecting inocula. Current practice is to vaccinate persons subject to unusual exposure from occupation or travel, those living in areas of high endemicity and institutional populations where maintenance of good sanitation may be difficult. Periodic single reinforcing injections are desirable, commonly once in 3 years.

B. *Control of patient, contacts and the immediate environment:*

1) *Report to local health authority:* Obligatory case report in most states and countries, Class 2A (see Preface).

2) *Isolation:* In a flyproof room with enteric isolation procedures. Hospital care is desirable during acute illness or for carriers treated intravenously with ampicillin. Release from supervision by local health authority should be based on not less than 3 negative cultures of feces and urine taken at least 24 hours apart and not earlier than 1 month after onset; if any one of this series is positive, repeat at least 3 negative cultures at intervals of 1 month during the 12 month period following onset (cf. 9A8 above).

3) *Concurrent disinfection:* Of feces and urine and articles soiled therewith. In communities with modern and adequate sewage disposal systems, feces and urine can be disposed of directly into sewers without preliminary disinfection. Terminal cleaning.

4) *Quarantine:* None.

5) *Management of contacts:* Administration of typhoid vaccine to family, household and nursing contacts who

have been or may be exposed to cases or carriers is of doubtful value. Family contacts should not be employed as food handlers during period of contact or until repeated negative feces and urine cultures are obtained.

6) *Investigation of contacts and sources of infection:* Actual or probable source of infection of every case should be determined by search for common and individual sources, unreported cases and carriers, or contaminated food, water, milk or shellfish. All members of travel groups in which a case has been identified should be followed-up. Presence of Vi-agglutinins in blood of suspected carriers is suggestive of the carrier state. Identification of the same phage type in organisms from patients and carriers suggests the chain of transmission.

7) *Specific treatment:* Chloramphenicol is the drug of choice; for strains not sensitive to it two other drugs, ampicillin and the combination of trimethroprim and sulfamethoxasole (co-trimoxazole) are of proven value. All *S. typhi* isolates should be checked for drug resistance. Cases thought to have originated during foreign travel should be treated with ampicillin, or cotrimoxazole, pending sensitivity testing. Some strains, resistant to both chloramphenicol and ampicillin, are sensitive to co-trimoxazole.

C. *Epidemic measures:*

1) Intensive search for case or carrier who is source of infection and for the vehicle (water or food) by which infection is carried.

2) Exclusion of suspected food.

3) Boiling of milk or pasteurization or exclusion of milk supplies or other foods suspected on epidemiologic evidence, until safety is assured.

4) Suspected water supplies should be adequately chlorinated under competent supervision or not used. All drinking water must be chlorinated, treated with iodine or boiled before use.

5) Use of vaccine is not recommended in the face of an outbreak as it renders the serological diagnosis of suspected illness more difficult.

D. *International measures:*

1) Inoculation with typhoid vaccine is advised for international travelers to endemic areas. Not a legal requirement of any country.

2) WHO Collaborating Centres (see Preface).

TYPHUS FEVER, EPIDEMIC LOUSE-BORNE
(Typhus exanthematicus, Classical typhus fever)

1. Identification — Onset is variable, often sudden and marked by headache, chills, prostration, fever and general pains; a macular eruption appears on 5th or 6th day, toxemia is usually pronounced, and the disease terminates by rapid lysis after about 2 weeks of fever. In the absence of specific therapy, the fatality rate varies from 10 to 40% and increases with age. Mild infections may occur with or without eruption, especially in vaccinated persons. The disease may recrudesce years after the primary attack (Brill-Zinsser disease); this differs from the first attack in that it need not be associated with lousiness, is milder and has fewer complications and a lower lethality.

The complement-fixation reaction with group-specific typhus antigen becomes positive, usually in the 2nd week. The Weil-Felix reaction with Proteus OX-19 also becomes positive, but is less helpful because it may be positive in other diseases.

2. Occurrence — In colder areas where people may live under unhygienic conditions and are louse-infested, especially as in war and famine. Endemic centers exist in mountainous regions of Mexico, Central and South America, the Balkans and eastern Europe, Africa and numerous countries of Asia. A few cases of Brill-Zinsser disease occur annually in U.S.A., but the last outbreak of louse-borne typhus occurred in 1921.

3. Infectious agent — *Rickettsia prowazeki.*

4. Reservoir — Man is the reservoir and is responsible for maintaining the infection during inter-epidemic periods.

5. Mode of transmission — The body louse, *Pediculus humanus humanus,* is infected by feeding on the blood of a patient with febrile typhus fever. Patients with recrudescent typhus (Brill-Zinsser disease) can infect lice and probably serve as foci for new outbreaks in louse-infested communities. Infected lice excrete rickettsiae in their feces and usually defecate at time of feeding. Man is infected by rubbing feces or crushed lice into the wound made by the bite or into superficial abrasions. Inhalation of dried infective louse feces as dust from dirty clothes may account for some infections.

6. Incubation period — From 1 to 2 weeks, commonly 12 days.

7. Period of communicability — The disease is not directly transmitted from man to man. Patients are infective for lice during the febrile illness and possibly for 2 or 3 days after the temperature returns to normal. The living louse is infective as soon as it begins to pass rickettsiae in its feces (within 2 to 6 days after the infected blood meal); it is infective earlier if crushed. The louse invariably dies within 2 weeks after infection; rickettsiae may remain viable in the dead louse for weeks.

8. **Susceptibility and resistance**— Susceptibility is general. The disease in children and in vaccinated adults is mild and may go unrecognized. One attack usually confers permanent immunity.

9. **Methods of control**—

    A. *Preventive measures:*

        1) Immunization of susceptible persons or groups of persons entering typhus areas, particularly military or labor forces, or of residents at unusual risk. The usual vaccine contains rickettsiae grown in yolk sacs of developing chick embryos, inactivated by formalin and extracted with ether or other suitable solvent. It is administered in 2 subcutaneous injections at an interval of 4 or more weeks. A booster dose repeated at yearly intervals is indicated where typhus is a hazard. For children under 10 years of age, a reduced dose (0.25 ml) is recommended. In immunized persons, the course of the disease is modified and lethality is lowered. A live vaccine prepared from the attenuated strain E of *R. prowazeki* has showed promise.

        2) Application by hand or power blower of residual insecticide powder (10% DDT or 1% lindane) at appropriate intervals to clothes and persons of populations living under conditions favoring lousiness. Lice become resistant to DDT, in which case 1% Malathion or other effective lousicide should be substituted.

        3) Improvement of living conditions with provisions for frequent bathing and washing of clothes.

        4) Individual prophylaxis of persons subject to unusual risk through residual insecticide applied at appropriate intervals to clothing by dusting or impregnation.

    B. *Control of patient, contacts, and the immediate environment:*

        1) *Report to local health authority:* Case report universally required by International Health Regulations, 1969, WHO, Class 1 (see Preface).

        2) *Isolation:* Not required after proper delousing of patient, clothing, living quarters and household contacts.

3) *Concurrent disinfection:* Appropriate insecticide powder applied to clothing and bedding of patient and contacts; laundering of clothing and bedclothes; treatment of hair for louse eggs (nits) with effective chemical agents. Lice tend to leave abnormally hot or cold bodies in search of a normothermic clothed body (see 9A2 above). If death from typhus fever occurs before delousing, delouse the body and clothing by thorough application of an insecticide.

4) *Quarantine:* Louse-infested susceptibles exposed to typhus fever ordinarily should be quarantined for 15 days; with application of an insecticide with residual effect, these susceptibles may be released.

5) *Immunization of contacts:* All immediate contacts.

6) *Investigation of contacts:* Every effort should be made to trace the infection to the immediate source.

7) *Specific treatment:* The tetracyclines or chloramphenicol orally in a loading dose followed by daily doses until the patient becomes afebrile (usually 2 days) and for 1 additional day.

C. *Epidemic measures:*
1) Delousing: The most important measure for rapid control of typhus, where reporting has been good and cases are few, is application of an appropriate insecticide with residual effect to all contacts. Where infection is known to be widespread, systematic application of residual insecticide to all persons in the community is indicated.

2) Immunization: Of persons in contact with cases; immunization may be offered to an entire community.

D. *International measures:*
1) Telegraphic notification by governments to WHO and to adjacent countries of the occurrence of an outbreak of louse-borne typhus fever in an area previously free of the disease.

2) International travelers: While no country currently requires immunization against typhus for entry, immunization is recommended for all persons who will work in or visit remote areas where typhus is present.

3) As of January 1, 1971, epidemic louse-borne typhus ceased to be a quarantinable disease under international

regulations, but the measures outlined in paragraph (1) above should be continued because it is a *Disease under Surveillance of WHO*, in accordance with a Resolution of the 22nd World Health Assembly. WHO Collaborating Centers (see Preface).

TYPHUS FEVER, FLEA-BORNE
(Murine typhus, Endemic typhus fever)

1. Identification — The clinical course of flea-borne typhus fever resembles that of epidemic louse-borne typhus, but tends to be milder. The fatality rate for all ages is about 2% but increases with age.

Absence of louse infestation, seasonal distribution, and sporadic occurrence of the disease help to differentiate it from classical (epidemic) or louse-borne typhus. The complement-fixation reaction with group-specific typhus antigen becomes positive, usually in the 2nd week. The Weil-Felix reaction with Proteus OX-19 also becomes positive, but is less helpful because it may be positive in other diseases. Differentiation from louse-borne typhus is by serologic tests, using washed type-specific rickettsial antigens.

2. Occurrence — Worldwide. Found in areas where people and rats occupy the same buildings and where plagues of mice occur. Formerly, several thousand cases occurred yearly in U.S.A., concentrated in the southeastern states; currently fewer than 50 cases are reported annually. Seasonal peak is in late summer and autumn. Cases tend to be scattered with no apparent connection to each other.

3. Infectious agent — *Rickettsia typhi (Rickettsia mooseri)*.

4. Reservoir — Infection is maintained in nature by a rat-flea-rat cycle. Rats are the reservoir, commonly *Rattus rattus* and *R. norvegicus;* infection in rats is inapparent. Oppossums, cats and possibly other wild or domestic animals may be a reservoir or serve to transport infective fleas when in proximity to humans. The cat flea, *Ctenocephalides felis* has been implicated as a possible vector.

5. Mode of transmission — Infective rat fleas (usually *Xenopsylla cheopis)* defecate rickettsiae while sucking blood, and contaminate the bite site and other fresh skin wounds. An occasional case may follow inhalation of dried infective flea feces.

6. **Incubation period** — From 1 to 2 weeks, commonly 12 days.

7. **Period of communicability** — Not directly transmitted from man to man. Once infected, fleas remain so for life (up to 1 year).

8. **Susceptibility and resistance** — Susceptibility is general. One attack confers immunity.

9. **Methods of control** —

   A. Preventive measures:
1) Application of insecticide powders with residual action to rat runs, burrows and harborages.
2) Rodent control measures should be delayed until flea populations have been reduced by insecticides, to avoid increased exposure of humans. (See Plague, 9B5, p. 228).

   B. Control of patient, contacts, and the immediate environment:
1) *Report to local health authority:* Case report obligatory in most states and countries, Class 2B (see Preface).
2) *Isolation:* None.
3) *Concurrent disinfection:* None.
4) *Quarantine:* None.
5) *Immunization of contacts:* None.
6) *Investigation of contacts and source of infection:* Search for rodents around premises or home of patient.
7) *Specific treatment:* As for epidemic typhus. See Typhus, Epidemic Louse-borne, 9B7, (p. 356).

   C. Epidemic measures: In endemic areas with numerous cases, widespread use of DDT or other residual insecticide effective against rat fleas will probably reduce the flea index of rats and the incidence of infection in rats and man.

   D. International measures: WHO Collaborating Centres (see Preface).

TYPHUS, SCRUB
(Tsutsugamushi disease, Mite-borne typhus fever)

1. **Identification**—A rickettsial disease often characterized by a primary "punched out" skin ulcer (eschar) corresponding to site of attachment of an infected mite. The acute febrile onset follows within several days, along with headache, profuse sweating, conjunctival injection and lymphadenopathy. Late in the first week of fever a dull red maculopapular eruption appears on the trunk, extends to the extremities and disappears in a few days. Cough and X-ray evidence of pneumonitis are common. Without antibiotic therapy, fever lasts for about 14 days. The fatality rate in untreated cases varies from 1 to 40%, according to locality, strain of rickettsia, or previous exposure to disease. It is consistently higher among older persons. The benign disease seen in some areas of Japan is called Shishito Fever.

Diagnosis is by isolation of the infectious agent by inoculating the patient's blood into mice. Fluorescent antibody and complement-fixation tests supplement the Weil-Felix reaction (Proteus OXK) in serologic diagnosis.

2. **Occurrence**—Central, eastern and southeastern Asia; from southeastern Siberia to northern Australia, as far west as central Pakistan and to as high as 10,000 feet above sea level in the Himalayan mountains. A place disease acquired by man in one of innumerable small, sharply delimited "typhus islands", some covering an area of only a few square feet, where rickettsiae, vectors and suitable rodents exist simultaneously. Occupation greatly influences sex distribution, but mainly restricted to adult workers who frequent scrub or overgrown terrain, or other mite-infested areas such as forest clearings, reforested areas, or even newly irrigated desert regions. Epidemics occur when susceptibles are brought into endemic areas, especially in military operations in which 20 to 50% of men have been infected within weeks or months.

3. **Infectious agent**—*Rickettsia tsutsugamushi (Rickettsia orientalis)*, which occur as multiple, serologically distinct strains.

4. **Reservoir**—Infected larval stages of trombiculid mites; *Leptotrombidium akamushi, L. deliensis* and related species (varying with locality) are the most common vectors for humans. Infection is maintained in mites by transovarian passage and possibly by a mite-wild rodent-mite cycle.

5. **Mode of transmission**—By the bite of infected larval mites; nymphs and adults do not feed on vertebrate hosts.

6. Incubation period—Usually 10 to 12 days; varies from 6 to 21.

7. Period of communicability—Not directly transmitted from man to man.

8. Susceptibility and resistance—Susceptibility is general. An attack confers prolonged immunity against the homologous strain of *R. tsutsugamushi* but only transient immunity against heterologous strains. Heterologous infection within a few months results in mild disease, but after a year produces the typical illness. Second and even third attacks of naturally acquired scrub typhus occur among persons who spend their lives in endemic areas. No currently available vaccine is effective.

9. Methods of control—

A. Preventive measures:
    1) Prevent contact with infected mites by personal prophylaxis against the mite vector, achieved by impregnating clothes and blankets with miticidal chemicals (benzyl benzoate), and application of mite repellents (diethyltoluamide), to exposed skin surfaces.

    2) The elimination of mites from the specific sites is best accomplished by application of chlorinated hydrocarbons such as lindane, dieldrin, or chlordane to ground and vegetation in environs of camps, mine buildings and other populated zones in endemic areas.

B. Control of patient, contacts, and the immediate environment:
    1) Report to local health authority: In selected endemic areas, (clearly differentiate from flea-borne and louse-borne typhus). In many countries not a reportable disease, Class 3A (see Preface).

    2) Isolation: None.

    3) Concurrent disinfection: None.

    4) Quarantine: None.

    5) Immunization of contacts: None.

    6) Investigation of contacts: None. (see C2 below).

    7) Specific treatment: One of the tetracycline antibiotics orally in a loading dose, followed by divided doses daily until patient is afebrile (average 30 hours). If treatment is started within the first 3 days, recrudescence is likely unless a 2nd course of antibiotic is given after an interval of 6 days.

C. Epidemic measures:
1) Rigorously employ procedures described in 9A1 and 9A2 in the affected area.
2) Daily observation of all persons at risk for fever and appearance of primary lesions; institute treatment upon first indication of illness.

D. International measures: WHO Collaborating Centres (see Preface).

URETHRITIS, NON-GONOCOCCAL
(Non-specific urethritis)

1. Identification—Usually a venereally transmitted urethritis of males not associated with the gonococcus. Clinical manifestations are either indistinguishable from gonorrhea or somewhat milder and include an opaque discharge of moderate quantity, urethral itching, dysuria, and burning on urination. Clinical course frequently is intermittent and characterized by remission and exacerbation; may be acquired concurrently with gonorrhea and appear after the gonorrhea has been successfully treated.

Non-gonococcal urethritis (NGU) is usually diagnosed by failure to demonstrate *Neisseria gonorrhea* by repeated smear or culture. Chlamydia infections can be confirmed by techniques for identification of other chlamydia (TRIC agents) (See Inclusion Conjunctivitis, p. 84). For other agents see par. 3 below and appropriate sections.

2. Occurrence—A common disease usually of venereal origin that is of unknown extent in the U.S.A.; in the United Kingdom it is more frequent and is increasing more rapidly in the general population than gonorrhea.

3. Infectious agent—Several agents identified; *Chlamydia (Bedsonia) trachomatis* has been identified in approximately 50% of cases. *Herpes virus type 2, Candida* species and *Trichimonas vaginalis* are involved in approximately 5% of cases; no recognized pathogen in the remainder.

4. Reservoir—Man is the only known reservoir; several animal species possibly may be.

5. Mode of transmission—Probably by sexual intercourse.

6. **Incubation period** — Not precisely known; generally thought to be 5-7 days or longer.

7. **Period of communicability** — Unknown.

8. **Susceptibility and resistance** — Susceptibility is general. No acquired immunity has been demonstrated.

9. **Methods of control** —

   A. *Preventive measures:* Health and sex education; good sex hygiene.

   B. *Control of patient, contacts, and the immediate environment:*
      1) *Report to local health authority:* NGU is not now a reportable disease in the United States, Class 5 (see Preface).
      2) *Isolation:* None. Appropriate antibiotic therapy renders discharge non-infectious for *C. trachomatis.*
      3) *Concurrent disinfection:* Care in disposal of articles contaminated with urethral discharges.
      4) *Quarantine measures:* None.
      5) *Immunization of contacts:* Not applicable.
      6) *Investigation of contacts:* Since no specific agent has been definitely proved to cause NGU, investigation and epidemiologic treatment of contacts, as with gonorrhea (p. 131) is not indicated as a public health measure. In individual cases, concurrent treatment of consorts appears to be the only practical approach to management.
      7) *Specific treatment:* Tetracycline, two grams daily for 7-10 days or one gram daily for 21 days, has been shown to be effective in both *C. trachomatis* positive and negative cases. *C. trachomatis* shedding is interrupted in both men and women following such therapy.

   C. *Epidemic measures:* See 9B6 above.

   D. *International measures:* None.

VERRUCA VULGARIS
(Warts)

1. **Identification** — A viral disease manifested by firm papules with horny surfaces; they vary in appearance depending upon area of the body affected. On the forehead or knees, plane warts are smooth, flat and usually flesh-colored. In the genital area they are moist, fast-growing and may attain huge dimensions; must be differentiated from condylomata lata of syphilis. On the soles of the feet, plantar warts are usually tender, circular lesions with a speckled core.

2. **Occurrence** — Worldwide.

3. **Infectious agent** — The human wart virus, a papova virus.

4. **Reservoir** — Man.

5. **Mode of transmission** — Usually by direct contact, but contaminated floors and fomites are frequently implicated. Warts may be autoinoculated by razors in shaving.

6. **Incubation period** — About 4 months; range is 1-20 months.

7. **Period of communicability** — Unknown, but probably as long as visible lesions persist.

8. **Susceptibility and resistance** — Plane warts and hand warts are most frequently seen in young children, genital warts in sexually active young adults, and plantar warts in school-age children and teenagers. Regression of multiple verrucae is often simultaneous, but seems to be unrelated to circulating antibody titers or other immunological factors.

9. **Methods of control** —

   A. *Preventive measures:* Avoidance of contact with affected persons or contaminated floors where possible.

   B. *Control of patient, contacts, and the immediate environment:* Treatment of the affected individual will decrease the amount of wart virus available for transmission.
      1) Report to local health authorities: None.
      2) Isolation: None.
      3) Concurrent disinfection: None.
      4) Quarantine: None.
      5) Immunization of contacts: None.
      6) Investigation of contacts and source of infection: None.
      7) Specific treatment: Verrucae nearly always regress spontaneously within a period of months. If treatment is indicated, freezing with liquid nitrogen is best for lesions

on most of the body surface. Salicylic acid plasters and curretage is best for plantar warts, and 25% podophyllin in tincture of benzoin for genital warts except in pregnant females.

WHOOPING COUGH
(Pertussis)

1. Identification—An acute bacterial disease involving the tracheo-bronchial tree. The initial catarrhal stage has an insidious onset with an irritating cough which gradually becomes paroxysmal, usually within 1 to 2 weeks, and lasts for 1 to 2 months. Paroxysms are characterized by repeated violent cough; each series of paroxysms has many coughs without intervening inhalation, followed by a characteristic crowing or high pitched inspiratory whoop, frequently ending with the expulsion of clear, tenacious mucus. Young infants and adults often do not have the typical paroxysm. Fatality in U.S.A. is low. Approximately 70% of deaths are among children under 1 year of age, most in those under 6 months.

The infectious agent may be recovered in a majority of cases from nasopharyngeal swabs obtained during the catarrhal and early paroxysmal stages. Strikingly high white blood counts with a strong preponderance of lymphocytes are found as the whooping stage develops.

Parapertussis is an allied disease clinically indistinguishable from pertussis. It is usually milder and occurs relatively infrequently. Identification is by immunologic differences between *Bordetella parapertussis and B. pertussis*. A similar clinical syndrome can be produced by viruses, especially adenovirus.

2. Occurrence—A common disease among children everywhere, regardless of race, climate, or geographic location. In large communities, incidence is generally highest in late winter and early spring; in smaller communities, seasonal incidence is variable. There has been a marked decline in incidence and mortality during the past two decades, chiefly in communities fostering active immunization and where good nutrition and medical care, and effective public health programs are available.

In unimmunized populations, beset by poverty, malnutrition and multiple infections with parasitic and microbial pathogens, pertussis is among the most lethal diseases of children.

3. **Infectious agent** — *Bordetella pertussis*, the pertussis bacillus.

4. **Reservoir** — Man.

5. **Mode of transmission** — Primarily by direct contact with discharges from respiratory mucous membranes of infected persons, by the airborne route, probably by droplets, or by indirect contact with articles freshly soiled with the discharges of infected persons.

6. **Incubation period** — Commonly 7 days, almost uniformly within 10 days, and not exceeding 21 days.

7. **Period of communicability** — Highly communicable in the early catarrhal stage, before paroxysmal cough. Thereafter, communicability gradually decreases and becomes negligible for ordinary nonfamilial contacts in about 3 weeks, despite persisting spasmodic cough with whoop. For control purposes, the communicable stage extends from 7 days after exposure to 3 weeks after onset of typical paroxysms in patients not treated with antibiotics; when treated, either with erythromycin or ampicillin, the period of infectiousness extends only 5 to 7 days after onset of therapy.

8. **Susceptibility and resistance** — Susceptibility is general; there is no evidence of temporary passive immunity in young infants born of immune mothers. Predominantly a childhood disease; incidence is highest under 7 years of age. Numerous inapparent and missed atypical cases occur. One attack confers definite and prolonged immunity, although exposed adults occasionally have second attacks. Morbidity and mortality are higher in females than in males, at all ages.

9. **Methods of control** —

   A. *Preventive measures:*

      1) Active immunization is recommended with a vaccine consisting of a suspension of killed bacteria adsorbed on aluminum salts. There is no advantage to nonadsorbed ("plain") preparations, either for primary immunization or booster shots. A primary series of three injections should be administered one month apart to all children, beginning at one to two months of age; give routine booster injections at 18 months and five or six years. This schedule does not need to be restarted because of delay, no matter how long. Pertussis vaccination does

not provide complete and permanent immunity. The vaccine is generally administered together with diphtheria and tetanus toxoids as a triple vaccine known as DTP. In Australia pertussis is omitted after two years of age. Active immunization will not protect against disease resulting from exposure prior to first immunizing injection. Passive immunization through use of regular immune serum globulin, special pertussis hyperimmune globulin, or convalescent serum is of no value in preventing pertussis, even if given immediately after exposure.

2) Education of the public, and particularly parents of infants, as to the dangers of whooping cough and as to the advantages of immunization in infancy.

B. *Control of patient, contacts, and the immediate environment:*

1) *Report to local health authority:* Case report obligatory in most states and countries, Class 2B (Preface).

2) *Isolation:* Isolate known cases. Exclude suspected cases from the presence of young non-immune children, especially infants who are at high risk.

3) *Concurrent disinfection:* Discharges from nose and throat and articles soiled therewith. Terminal cleaning.

4) *Quarantine:* Non-immune children should be excluded from schools and public gatherings for 14 days after last exposure to a household case.

5) *Protection of contacts:* Passive immunization is not effective and it is too late for the initiation of active immunization to protect against a prior exposure. Previously immunized children under three years of age (who have not received the full course of five immunizations) should be boosted as soon after exposure as possible. Non-immunized infant contacts should receive chemoprophylaxis (erythromycin or ampicillin) for ten days after contact is broken or for duration of communicability in infected contacts if separation cannot be effected. (See 9B7 below).

6) *Investigation of contacts:* A search for early, missed or atypical cases is indicated where a nonimmune infant or young child is or might be at risk.

7) *Specific treatment*—Erythromycin or ampicillin is used in infants and young children as primary treatment for whooping cough; there are no data to suggest that immune human serum globulin is effective. Intensive

care by experienced nurses is of prime importance. Antibiotics may shorten period of communicability and duration of symptoms.

C. *Epidemic measures:* A search for unrecognized and unreported cases to protect preschool children from exposure and to assure adequate medical care for exposed infants.

D. *International measures:* Active immunization of susceptible infants and young children traveling to other countries, if not already protected; review need of booster dose for those previously inoculated. WHO Collaborating Centres (see Preface).

WOLHYNIAN FEVER
(Trench fever, Five-day fever, Quintana fever)

1. Identification — A nonfatal, febrile, self-limited, often relapsing ricksettsial disease of protean manifestations and greatly varying severity; characterized by headache, malaise, and pain and tenderness especially in the shins; onset either sudden or slow with fever, which may be relapsing, typhoid-like, or limited to a single short febrile episode lasting for several days. Splenomegaly is common. A transient macular rash may be present at some time. Subsequent course is extremely variable. Inapparent infection may occur; rickettsemia may last for months with or without repeated recurrence of symptoms. Relapses can occur many years after primary infection.

Laboratory diagnosis is by culture of causative organism from patient's blood on blood agar under 5% CO_2 tension in air. Microcolonies are visible after 2 weeks of incubation at 37°C. Infection evokes antibodies detectable by complement-fixation, passive hemagglutination, and immunofluorescence tests.

2. Occurrence — Epidemics occurred in World Wars I and II in Europe among troops living under crowded, unhygienic conditions. Sporadic cases in areas of endemic foci probably go unrecognized.

Endemic foci of infection have been detected in Poland, Russia, Mexico, Ethiopia and North Africa. The organism probably can be found wherever man and the human body louse coexist.

3. **Infectious agent**—*Rickettsia quintana* (probably identical with *R. weiglii*, *R. pediculi* and *R. wolhynica*).

4. **Reservoir**—Man. Intermediate host is the body louse, *Pediculus humanus humanus*, in which the organism multiplies for the duration of the insect's life, extracellularly and within the gut lumen. No transovarial transmission in the louse.

5. **Mode of transmission**—Not directly transmitted from man to man. Man is infected by inoculation of infected louse feces through skin damaged by either the bite of the louse or other means. Infected lice begin to excrete infectious feces 5-12 days after ingesting infective blood and continue for duration of life (average life span approximately 5 weeks after hatching from egg). Nymphal stages may become infected. Lice tend to leave abnormally hot (febrile) or cold (dead) bodies in search of a normothermic clothed body.

6. **Incubation period**—Generally 7-30 days.

7. **Period of communicability**—Symptomless rickettsemia may last for weeks, months or years. Recurrence of rickettsemia can occur with or without symptoms.

8. **Susceptibility and resistance**—Susceptibility is general. After infection, the degree of protective immunity to either infection or disease is unknown.

9. **Methods of control**—

   A. *Preventive measures:* Delousing procedures will destroy the vector and prevent transmission to man. Dusting of clothing and body with an effective lousicide.

   B. *Control of patient, contacts, and the immediate environment:*
   1) *Report to local health authority:* Cases should be reported so that an evaluation of louse infestation in the population may be made and appropriate measures taken, since lice also transmit epidemic typhus and relapsing fever. Class 3B (see Preface).
   2) *Isolation:* None.
   3) *Concurrent disinfection:* Louse-infested clothing should be treated to kill the lice.
   4) *Quarantine:* None.
   5) *Immunization of contacts:* None.
   6) *Investigation of contacts and source of infection:* Search for the presence of the human body louse in clothing and on the bodies of people at risk.
   7) *Specific treatment:* Tetracyclines and chloramphenicol

not yet adequately tested in clinical cases; probably effective.

C. *Epidemic measures:* Systematic application of residual insecticide to all persons in the affected population and their clothing (see 9A above).

D. *International measures:* WHO Collaborating Centres (see Preface).

YAWS
(Frambesia tropica, Pian, Bouba, Parangi)

1. **Identification**—A chronic relapsing non-venereal treponematosis characterized by hypertrophic granulomatous or ulcerative destructive lesions of the skin and cartilage (gangosa), and by destructive and hypertrophic changes in bone. In several weeks to months, and often before the initial lesion has healed, mild constitutional symptoms appear; also a generalized eruption of papules, some developing into typical frambesial (raspberry) lesions which occur in successive crops and last several months. Papillomata on the palms and soles (crab yaws), and also hyperkeratoses may appear in both early and late stages. The late stage, characterized by destructive lesions of skin and bone, often develops some years after the last early lesions. Early and late lesions tend to heal spontaneously but may relapse. Between these active phases, infection is latent; thus there is a latent early stage from which early relapses occur, and a latent late stage with late lesions and relapses. The central nervous system, eyes, aorta and viscera are not involved. Congenital transmission of yaws has not been observed. The disease is rarely, if ever, fatal.

Diagnosis is confirmed by dark-field examination of exudates from lesions. Serologic tests for syphilis are reactive with the same frequency in yaws as in syphilis; they become positive during the initial stage, remain positive during the early stage and can become negative after many years of latency, even without specific therapy.

2. **Occurrence**—Primarily in the rural tropics and subtropics; the lowest social and economic groups have the highest rates. Pre-

dominantly a childhood disease; occurrence in males is greater than in females. Particularly common in tropical Africa, the Philippines, Southeast Asia, Indonesia and throughout the South Pacific Islands; endemic foci are found in the Caribbean area and in part of Brazil, Colombia, Venezuela, Peru, Ecuador, Panama, Haiti, and Guyana. The incidence of yaws is decreasing in many areas.

3. **Infectious agent**—*Treponema pertenue,* a spirochete.

4. **Reservoir**—Man and possibly higher primates.

5. **Mode of transmission**—Principally by direct contact with exudates of early skin lesions of infected persons. Indirect transmission by contamination from scratching, piercing articles and by flies on open wounds is probable, but of undetermined importance.

6. **Incubation period**—From 2 weeks to 3 months.

7. **Period of communicability**—Variable; may extend intermittently over several years while moist lesions are present; the infectious agent is not usually found in late ulcerative lesions.

8. **Susceptibility and resistance**—No evidence of natural or racial resistance. Infection results in immunity to homologous and heterologous strains; heterologous immunity develops slowly and probably is not complete until 1 year. The role of superinfection in nature is not well defined and may not be important. Immunity to yaws appears to protect against syphilis.

9. **Methods of control**—

A. *Preventive measures:* The following are applicable to yaws and to other nonvenereal treponematoses. By present techniques the infectious agents in all are morphologically identical, but it is unlikely that the differences in clinical syndromes result only from epidemiologic factors.
   1) General health promotional measures; health education of the public about treponematosis; better sanitation, including liberal use of soap and water, and improvement of social and economic conditions over a period of years will reduce incidence.
   2) Organization of intensive control activities on a community basis, to include analysis of the specific local problem, clinical examination of entire populations, and mass treatment of patients with active lesions, latent cases and contacts, where a high prevalence justifies such measures. Periodic surveys and continuous surveillance are essential to successful results.

3) Provision of facilities for early diagnosis and treatment as part of a continuing plan, whereby the mass control campaign (9A2 above) is eventually consolidated into permanent local health services providing early diagnosis and treatment to patients, and contact investigation and continuing health education to the community.

4) Treatment of disfiguring and incapacitating late manifestations; surveys for latent cases, since many relapse and develop infective lesions which may help maintain the disease in the community.

B. *Control of patient, contacts, and the immediate environment:*

1) *Report to local health authority:* In selected endemic areas; in many countries not a reportable disease, Class 3B (see Preface). Differentiation of venereal and non-venereal treponematoses, with proper reporting of each, has particular importance in evaluation of mass campaigns and in the consolidation period thereafter.

2) *Isolation:* None; avoid intimate contact, flies and contamination of the environment until lesions are healed.

3) *Concurrent disinfection:* Care in disposal of discharges and articles contaminated therewith.

4) *Quarantine:* None.

5) *Immunization of contacts:* Not applicable; prompt institution of a course of treatment (see 9B7 below).

6) *Investigation of contacts:* All familial contacts should be treated; those with no active disease should be regarded as latent cases. In areas of low prevalence, treat all active cases, all children, and close contacts of infectious cases.

7) *Specific treatment:* Penicillin. For patients with active disease a single intramuscular injection of benzathine penicillin G (Bicillin) (1.2. million units); half-doses for children under 15 and for latent cases and contacts.

C. *Epidemic measures:* Active mass treatment programs in areas of high prevalence. Essential features are that (1) a high percentage of the population be examined through field surveys; (2) treatment of active cases be extended to the segments of the population with demonstrated prevalence of active yaws; and (3) periodic surveys be made at yearly intervals for 1 to 3 years, with surveillance and integration of activities into the established rural public health activities of the country.

D. *International measures:* To protect countries against risk of reinfection where active mass treatment programs are in progress, adjacent countries in the endemic area should institute suitable measures against yaws. Movement of infected persons across frontiers may need supervision. (See Syphilis 9D, p. 318). WHO Collaborating Centers (see Preface).

∞

YERSINIOSIS
(Pseudotuberculosis, enterocolitis)

1. **Identification**—An acute enteric disease caused by two biochemically and serologically distinct agents, *Yersinia enterocolitica* and *Y. pseudotuberculosis*. Signs and symptoms often are similar or indistinguishable and include diarrhea, enterocolitis, acute mesenteric lymphadenitis mimicking appendicitis, low-grade fever, headache, pharyngitis, anorexia, vomiting, erythema nodosum, arthritis, cutaneous ulceration, abscesses and septicemia. *Y. enterocolitica* more commonly presents with a gastro-enterocolitis syndrome (diarrhea), and *Y. pseudotuberculosis* with abdominal pain (mesenteric lymphadenopathy). Infection with *Y. pseudotuberculosis* has greater lethality.

In generalized infections blood cultures usually yield positive results. The organisms of *Y. enterocolitica* can be recovered on usual enteric media from feces or excised tissue from many patients with Yersinia-associated gastro-intestinal symptoms. Enrichment of specimens in buffered saline at 4°C may help recover the organism in some instances. No selective medium is available for isolation of *Y. pseudotuberculosis*. Serologic agglutination tests may be useful in the absence of bacterial isolation; these tests may be subgroup as well as species specific, and diagnostic criteria in reported series have been variable.

2. **Occurrence**—Worldwide. Frequently reported from Western Europe and Scandinavian countries; sporadically from U.S.S.R., Japan, Central Africa, Southeast Asia, India, Australia, Mongolia, Brazil and North America. Since the 1960's the *Yersinae* have been recognized as important etiological agents of gastroenteritis and mesenteric lymphadenitis. *Y. pseudotuberculosis* is primarily a zoonotic disease of wild and domesticated birds and mammals, with man as an accidental host. *Y. enterocolitica* has been recovered from

a wide variety of animals without signs of disease. In chinchillas fatal outbreaks have been reported. The number of human cases that are recognized is small and largely dependent on the skill and experience of the diagnostician and/or microbiologist. Two epidemics involving adolescents in hospitals and schools have occurred respectively in Canada and Japan; they were caused by *Y. enterocolitica* and were thought to have been spread person-to-person. The first recognized epidemic of enteritis caused by *Y. enterocolitica* in the United States occurred in 1973 among four rural families with poor sanitary facilities; sixteen of twenty-one persons in these families became ill; two died.

3. **Infectious agents** — *Yersinia pseudotuberculosis* is comprised of 6 O-groups (I-VI), 4 O-subgroups (I, II, IV, V, all with A and B subgroups), 14 O-factors (2-14), one "R" factor (1) common to all groups and 5 H factors (a-e). More than 90% of the infections in man and animals caused by *Y. pseudotuberculosis* have been O-group I strains. *Y. enterocolitica* comprises more than 34 serotypes. Most human strains in European series have been serotypes 3 and 9; within the United States and Canada serotypes 3, 5b, 6, 8, 9, 10/11, and 20 have been identified.

4. **Reservoir** — The principal reservoirs for these *Yersinia* have not been conclusively established. *Y. pseudotuberculosis* is a widespread disease in many species of avian and mammalian hosts. *Y. enterocolitica* has been recovered from animals not presenting symptoms, and recently from African and New World primates with acute enteric disease. While the source of infection in man remains obscure despite extensive epidemiological investigations, there nevertheless have been two outbreaks associated with sick pet puppies and one with a pet kitten in which the same serotypes as in the human cases were identified.

5. **Mode of transmission** — Although the mode of transmission of these agents has not been defined, the fecal-oral route seems likely. Transmission may occur directly by contact with infected persons or animals (hand-to-mouth mode), or indirectly by eating and drinking of fecally contaminated raw foodstuffs and water. Fecally soiled linens and wastes may be vehicles for epidemics in hospitals.

6. **Incubation period** — Probably 3 to 7 days, generally less than 10 days.

7. **Period of communicability** — In the acute infectious stage there is fecal shedding as long as symptoms exist. A chronic carrier state exists.

8. **Susceptibility and resistance** — Susceptibility is general, but the disease is more common and severe in adolescents and the aged.

Y. pseudotuberculosis exhibits a predilection for male adolescents while *Y. enterocolitica* attacks all groups of both sexes. In active infections high titers of circulating antibodies are found, but gradually disappear in 2 to 6 months.

9. Methods of control—

A. *Preventive measures:*
   1) Sanitary disposal of human and dog feces.
   2) Protection of the water supply from animal feces or appropriate purification.
   3) Hand washing prior to food-handling and eating.
   4) Sanitary preparation of food, especially those consumed raw.

B. *Control of patient, contacts, and the immediate environment:*
   1) *Report to local health authority:* Obligatory report of epidemics, no individual case report, Class 4 (see Preface).
   2) *Isolation:* Removal of infected person from food handling, patient care, or occupations involving care of young children. Enteric precautions for patients in hospitals.
   3) *Concurrent disinfection:* In communities with modern and adequate sewage disposal systems, feces can be discharged directly into sewers without preliminary disinfection.
   4) *Quarantine:* None.
   5) *Immunization of contacts:* None.
   6) *Investigation of contacts:* Search for unrecognized mild cases and convalescent carriers among contacts is time consuming and is rarely indicated except for those contacts who are food handlers serving the public or employed in some aspect of nursing care of children or the elderly. Consider the possibility that all pets and domestic animals are zoonotic sources of infection.
   7) *Specific treatment:* Organisms are sensitive to most antibiotics, with occasional resistance to penicillin and its semi-synthetic derivatives. Therapy may be helpful for gastrointestinal symptoms; definitely indicated for septicemia or other somatic disease. In individuals demonstrating symptoms, ampicillin, streptomycin, tetracycline, kanamycin or chloramphenicol may be useful.

C. *Epidemic measures:*
   1) Any group of cases of acute diarrheal disorders should

be reported at once to the local health authority even in the absence of specific identification of the disease.

2) Investigation of general sanitation; attention to close contacts with animals, especially pet dogs and cats.

D. International measures: None.

Definitions
and
Index

DEFINITIONS

(Technical meaning of terms used in the text)

1. *Carrier*—An infected person (or animal) that harbors a specific infectious agent in the absence of discernible clinical disease and serves as a potential source of infection for man. The carrier state may occur in an individual with an infection that is inapparent throughout its course (commonly known as *healthy* or *asymptomatic carrier)*, or during the incubation period, convalescence, and post-convalescence of an individual with a clinically recognizable disease (commonly known as *incubatory carrier* or *convalescent carrier)*. Under either circumstance the carrier state may be of short or long duration *(temporary* or *transient carrier* or *chronic carrier)*.

2. *Chemoprophylaxis*—The administration of a chemical, including antibiotics, to prevent the development of an infection or the progression of an infection to active manifest disease. *Chemotherapy*, on the other hand, refers to use of a chemical to cure a clinically recognizable infectious disease or to limit its further progress.

3. *Cleaning*—The removal by scrubbing and washing, as with hot water, soap or suitable detergent or by vacuum cleaning, of infectious agents and of organic matter from surfaces on which and in which infectious agents may find favorable conditions for surviving or multiplying.

4. *Communicable disease*—An illness due to a specific infectious agent or its toxic products which arises through transmission of that agent or its products from a reservoir to a susceptible host, either directly, as from an infected person or animal, or indirectly, through an intermediate plant or animal host, vector, or the inanimate environment (see 45, Transmission of infectious agents).

5. *Communicable period*—The time or times during which an infectious agent may be transferred directly or indirectly from an infected person to another person, from an infected animal to man, or from an infected man to an animal, including arthropods.

   In diseases such as diphtheria and scarlet fever in which mucous membranes are involved from the first entry of the pathogen, the period of communicability is from the date of first exposure to a source of infection until the infecting microorganism is no longer disseminated from the involved mucous membranes, i.e., from the period before the prodromata until termination of a carrier state, if the latter develops. Most diseases are not communicable during the early incubation period or after full recovery.

In diseases such as tuberculosis, syphilis and gonorrhea, and some of the salmonelloses, the communicable state may exist at any time over a long and sometimes intermittent period when unhealed lesions permit the discharge of infectious agents from the surface of the skin or through any of the body orifices.

In diseases transmitted by arthropods, such as malaria and yellow fever, the periods of communicability are those during which the infectious agent occurs in infective form in the blood or other tissues of the infected person in sufficient numbers to permit vector infection. A period of communicability is also to be distinguished for the arthropod vector, namely, that time during which the agent is present in the tissues of the arthropod in such form and locus *(infective state)* as to be transmissible.

6. *Contact*—A person or animal that has been in such association with an infected person or animal or a contaminated environment as to have had opportunity to acquire the infection.

7. *Contamination*—The presence of an infectious agent on a body surface; also on or in clothes, bedding, toys, surgical instruments or dressings, or other inanimate articles or substances including water, milk and food. Pollution is distinct from contamination and implies the presence of offensive, but not necessarily infectious matter, in the environment. Contamination on a body surface does not imply a carrier state.

8. *Disinfection*—Killing of infectious agents outside the body by chemical or physical means, directly applied.

Concurrent disinfection is the application of disinfective measures as soon as possible after the discharge of infectious material from the body of an infected person, or after the soiling of articles with such infectious discharges, all personal contact with such discharges or articles being minimized prior to such disinfection.

Terminal disinfection is the application of disinfective measures after the patient has been removed by death or to a hospital, or has ceased to be a source of infection, or after hospital isolation or other practices have been discontinued. Terminal disinfection is rarely practiced; terminal cleaning generally suffices (see 3, Cleaning), along with airing and sunning of rooms, furniture and bedding. It is necessary only for diseases spread by indirect contact; steam sterilization or incineration of bedding and other items is desirable after smallpox.

9. *Disinfestation*—Any physical or chemical process serving to destroy or remove undesired small animal forms, particularly

arthropods or rodents, present upon the person, the clothing, or in the environment of an individual, or on domestic animals (see 25, Insecticide, and 40, Rodenticide). Disinfestation includes delousing for infestation with *Pediculus humanus humanus,* the body louse. Synonyms include the term *disinsection* when insects only are involved.

10. *Endemic*—The constant presence of a disease or infectious agent within a given geographic area; may also refer to the usual prevalence of a given disease within such area. *Hyperendemic* expresses a persistent intense transmission, e.g., malaria.

11. *Epidemic*—The occurrence in a community or region of cases of an illness (or an outbreak) clearly in excess of normal expectancy and derived from a common or a propagated source. The number of cases indicating presence of an epidemic will vary according to the infectious agent, size and type of population exposed, previous experience or lack of exposure to the disease, and time and place of occurrence; epidemicity is thus relative to usual frequency of the disease in the same area, among the specified population, at the same season of the year. A single case of a communicable disease long absent from a population (as smallpox in a traveler through New York City in 1962) or first invasion by a disease not previously recognized in that area (as American trypanosomiasis in Arizona) is to be considered sufficient evidence of a potential epidemic to require immediate reporting and full field investigation. (See 37, Report of a disease, par. 3.)

12. *Fatality Rate*—Usually expressed as a percentage of the number of persons diagnosed as having a specified disease who die as a result of that illness. The term is frequently applied to a specific outbreak of acute disease in which all patients have been followed for an adequate period of time to include all attributable deaths. The *fatality rate* must be clearly differentiated from *mortality rate* (see Definition 29). Synonym—fatality percentage.

13. *Fumigation*—Any process by which the killing of animal forms, especially arthropods and rodents, is accomplished by the use of gaseous agents (see 25, Insecticide, and 40, Rodenticide).

14. *Health Education*—Health education is the process by which individuals and groups of people learn to promote, maintain or restore health. To be effective, the methods and procedures used to achieve this aim must take account of the ways in which people develop various forms of behavior, of the factors that lead them to maintain or to alter their acquired behavior, and of

the ways in which people acquire and use knowledge. Therefore, education for health begins with people as they are, with whatever interests they may have in improving their living conditions. Its aim is to develop in them a sense of responsibility for health conditions, as individuals and as members of families and communities. In communicable disease control, health education commonly includes an appraisal of what is known by a population about a disease, an assessment of habits and attitudes of the people as they relate to spread and frequency of the disease, and the presentation of specific means to remedy observed deficiencies. Synonyms: Education; education for health; education of the public.

15. *Host*—A man or other living animal, including birds and arthropods, which affords subsistence or lodgment to an infectious agent under natural conditions. Some protozoa and helminths pass successive stages in alternate hosts of different species. Hosts in which the parasite attains maturity or passes its sexual stage are *primary* or *definitive hosts;* those in which the parasite is in a larval or asexual state are *secondary* or *intermediate hosts.* A transport host is a carrier in which the organism remains alive but does not undergo development.

16. *Immune person*—A person (or animal) that possesses specific protective antibodies or cellular immunity as a result of previous infection or immunization, or is so conditioned by such previous specific experience as to respond adequately with production of antibodies sufficient to prevent clinical illness following exposure to the specific infectious agent of the disease. Immunity is relative; an ordinarily effective protection may be overwhelmed by an excessive dose of the infectious agent or via an unusual portal of entry; may also be impaired by immuno-suppressive drug therapy or concurrent disease (cf. 39, Resistance).

17. *Inapparent infection*—The presence of infection in a host without occurrence of recognizable clinical signs or symptoms. Inapparent infections are only identifiable by laboratory means. Synonym: *Subclinical* infection.

18. *Incidence rate*—A quotient (rate), with the number of cases of a specified disease diagnosed or reported during a defined period of time as the numerator, and the number of persons in the population in which they occurred as the denominator. This is usually expressed as cases per 1,000 or 100,000 per annum. This rate may be expressed as age- or sex-specific or as specific for any other population characteristic or subdivision (see 28, Morbidity rate).

Attack rate, or *case rate,* is an incidence rate often used for particular groups, observed for limited periods and under special circumstances, as in an epidemic. The *secondary attack rate* in communicable disease practice expresses the number of cases among familial or institutional contacts occurring within the accepted incubation period following exposure to a primary case, in relation to the total of such contacts; may be restricted to susceptible contacts when determinable. *Case rate* expresses the incidence of manifest and inapparent cases.

19. *Incubation period*—The time interval between exposure to an infectious agent and appearance of the first sign or symptom of the disease in question.

20. *Infected person*—A person who harbors an infectious agent and who has either manifest disease (see 32, Patient or sick person) or inapparent infection (see 1, Carrier). An *infectious person* is one from whom the infectious agent can be naturally acquired.

21. *Infection*—The entry and development or multiplication of an infectious agent in the body of man or animals. Infection is not synonymous with infectious disease; the result may be inapparent (see 17, Inapparent infection) or manifest (see 23, Infectious disease). The presence of living infectious agents on exterior surfaces of the body, or upon articles of apparel or soiled articles, is not infection, but contamination of such surfaces and articles (see 7, Contamination).

22. *Infectious agent*—An organism, chiefly a microorganism but including helminths, that is capable of producing infection or infectious disease.

23. *Infectious disease*—A disease of man or animals resulting from an infection (see 21).

24. *Infestation*—For persons or animals the lodgment, development and reproduction of arthropods on the surface of the body or in the clothing. Infested articles or premises are those which harbor or give shelter to animal forms, especially arthropods and rodents.

25. *Insecticide*—Any chemical substance used for the destruction of arthropods, whether applied as powder, liquid, atomized liquid, aerosol, or as a "paint" spray; residual action is usual. The term *larvicide* is generally used to designate insecticides applied specifically for destruction of immature stages of arthropods; *imagocide* or *adulticide,* to designate those applied to destroy mature or adult forms.

26. *Isolation*—The separation, for the period of communicability, of infected persons or animals from others, in such places and

under such conditions as to prevent the direct or indirect conveyance of the infectious agent from those infected to those who are susceptible or who may spread the agent to others (cf. 35, Quarantine).

27. *Molluscicide*—A chemical substance used for the destruction of snails and other molluscs.

28. *Morbidity rate*—An *incidence rate* (see Definition 18) used to include all persons in the population under consideration who become ill during the period of time stated.

29. *Mortality rate*—A rate calculated in the same way as an incidence rate (see Definition 18), using as a numerator the number of deaths occurring in the population during the stated period of time, usually a year. A *total* or *crude* mortality rate utilizes deaths from all causes, usually expressed as deaths per 1,000 while a *disease-specific* mortality rate includes only deaths due to one disease and is usually reported on the basis of 100,000 persons.

30. *Nosocomial Infection*—An infection originating in a medical facility, e.g., occurring in a hospitalized patient in whom it was not present or incubating at the time of admission, or is the residual of an infection acquired during a previous admission. Includes infections acquired in the hospital but appearing after discharge; it also includes infections among staff.

31. *Pathogenicity*—The capability of an infectious agent to cause disease in a susceptible host.

32. *Patient or sick person*—A person who is ill; here limited to a person suffering from a recognizable attack of a communicable disease.

33. *Personal hygiene*—Those protective measures, primarily within the responsibility of the individual, which promote health and limit the spread of infectious diseases, chiefly those transmitted by direct contact. Such measures encompass (a) keeping the body clean by sufficiently frequent soap and water baths, (b) washing hands in soap and water immediately after voiding bowels or bladder and always before handling food and eating, (c) keeping hands and unclean articles, or articles that have been used for toilet purposes by others, away from the mouth, nose, eyes, ears, genitalia, and wounds, (d) avoiding the use of common or unclean eating, drinking cups, towels, handkerchiefs, combs, hairbrushes, and pipes, (e) avoiding exposure of other persons to spray from the nose and mouth as in coughing, sneezing, laughing or talking, and (f) washing hands thoroughly after handling a patient or his belongings.

34. Prevalence rate—A quotient (rate) using as the numerator the number of persons sick or portraying a certain condition, in a stated population, *at a particular time,* regardless of when that illness or condition began, and as the denominator the number of persons in the population in which they occurred. For example, the prevalence rate of ringworm of the foot in a class of boys when examined on a certain day could be 25 per 100. Or, the prevalence rate of a positive serological test in a survey during which blood samples were collected from a population could be 10 per 1,000.

35. Quarantine—
   a. **Complete quarantine:** The limitation of freedom of movement of such well persons or domestic animals as have been exposed to a communicable disease, for a period of time not longer than the longest usual incubation period of the disease, in such manner as to prevent effective contact with those not so exposed (cf. 26, Isolation).
   b. **Modified quarantine:** A selective, partial limitation of freedom of movement of persons or domestic animals, commonly on the basis of known or presumed differences in susceptibility, but sometimes because of danger of disease transmission. It may be designed to meet particular situations. Examples are exclusion of children from school; or exemption of immune persons from provisions applicable to susceptible persons, such as barring non-immune contacts from acting as food handlers; or restriction of military populations to the post or to quarters.
   c. **Personal surveillance:** The practice of close medical or other supervision of contacts in order to promote prompt recognition of infection or illness but without restricting their movements.
   d. **Segregation:** The separation for special consideration, control or observation of some part of a group of persons or domestic animals from the others to facilitate control of a communicable disease. Removal of susceptible children to homes of immune persons, or establishment of a sanitary boundary to protect uninfected from infected portions of a population, are examples.

36. Repellent—A chemical applied to the skin or clothing or other places to discourage (1) arthropods from alighting on and attacking an individual, and (2) other agents, such as worm larvae, from penetrating the skin.

37. Report of a disease—An official report notifying appropriate authority of the occurrence of a specified communicable or other disease in man or in animals. Diseases in man are reported to the local health authority; those in animals to the livestock sanitary or agriculture authority. Some few diseases in animals, also transmissible to man, are reportable to both authorities. Each health jurisdiction declares a list of reportable diseases appropriate to its particular needs (see Preface). Reports also should list suspect cases of diseases of particular public health importance, ordinarily those requiring epidemiologic investigation or initiation of special control measures.

When a person is infected in one health jurisdiction and the case is reported from another, the authority receiving the report should notify the other jurisdiction, especially when the disease requires examination of contacts for infection, or if food or water or other common vehicles of infection may be involved.

In addition to routine report of cases of specified diseases, special notification is required of all epidemics or outbreaks of disease, including diseases not on the list declared reportable (see 11, Epidemic).

38. *Reservoir of infectious agents*—Any human beings, animals, arthropods, plants, soil or inanimate matter in which an infectious agent normally lives and multiplies, and on which it depends primarily for survival and reproduces itself in such manner that it can be transmitted to a susceptible host.

39. *Resistance*—The sum total of body mechanisms which interpose barriers to the progress of invasion or multiplication of infectious agents or to damage by their toxic products.

   a. **Immunity**—That resistance usually associated with possession of antibodies having a specific action on the microorganism concerned with a particular infectious disease or on its toxin. *Passive immunity* is attained either naturally by maternal transfer, or artificially by inoculation of specific protective antibodies [convalescent or hyperimmune serum, or immune serum (gamma) globulin (human)]; it is of brief duration (days to months). *Active immunity* is attained either naturally by infection with or without clinical manifestations, or artificially by inoculation of fractions or products of the infectious agent or of the agent itself in killed, modified or variant form. It lasts months to years. Active immunity depends on *cellular immunity* which is conferred by T-lymphocyte sensitization, and *humoral immunity* which is based on B-lymphocyte response.

   b. **Inherent resistance**—An ability to resist disease independent of antibodies or of specifically developed tissue response; it commonly resides in anatomic or physiologic characteristics of the host and may be genetic or acquired, permanent or temporary. Synonym: Non-specific immunity.

40. *Rodenticide*—A chemical substance used for the destruction of rodents, generally through ingestion (cf. 13, Fumigation).

41. *Source of infection*—The person, animal, object or substance from which an infectious agent passes immediately to a host. Source of *infection* should be clearly distinguished from source of *contamination,* such as overflow of a septic tank contaminating a water supply, or an infected cook contaminating a salad. (Cf. 38, Reservoir.)

42. *Surveillance of disease*—As distinct from surveillance of persons, (see 35, par. 3) surveillance of disease is the continuing scrutiny of all aspects of occurrence and spread of a disease that are pertinent to effective control. Included are the systematic collection and evaluation of (a) morbidity and mortality reports, (b) special reports of field investigations of epidemics and of individual cases, (c) isolation and identification of infectious agents by laboratories, (d) data concerning the availability, use and untoward effect of vaccines and toxoids, immune globulins, insecticides, and other substances used in control, (e) information regarding immunity levels in segments of the population, and (f) other relevant epidemiologic data. A report summarizing the above data should be prepared and distributed to all cooperating persons and others with a need to know the results of the surveillance activities. The procedure applies to all jurisdictional levels of public health from local to international.

43. *Susceptible*—A person or animal presumably not possessing sufficient resistance against a particular pathogenic agent to prevent contracting a disease if or when exposed to the agent.

44. *Suspect*—A person whose medical history and symptoms suggest that he may have or be developing some communicable disease.

45. *Transmission of infectious agents*—Any mechanism by which a susceptible human host is exposed to an infectious agent. These mechanisms are:

   a. **Direct transmission:** Direct and essentially immediate transfer of infectious agents (other than from an arthropod in which the organism has undergone essential multiplication or development) to a receptive portal of entry through which infection of man may take place. This may be by direct contact as by touching, kissing or sexual intercourse, or by the direct projection (droplet spread) of droplet spray onto the conjunctiva or onto the mucous membranes of the nose or mouth during sneezing, coughing, spitting, singing or talking (usually limited to a distance of about 1 meter or less). It may also be by direct exposure of susceptible tissue to an agent in soil, compost or decaying vegetable matter in which it normally leads a saprophytic existence, e.g., the systemic mycoses; or by the bite of a rabid animal.

b. **Indirect transmission:**

1) VEHICLE-BORNE—Contaminated materials or objects such as toys, handkerchiefs, soiled clothes, bedding, cooking or eating utensils, surgical instruments or dressings (indirect contact); water, food, milk, biological products including serum and plasma; or any substance serving as an intermediate means by which an infectious agent is transported and introduced into a susceptible host through a suitable portal of entry. The agent may or may not have multiplied or developed in or on the vehicle before being introduced into man.

2) VECTOR-BORNE—a) *Mechanical:* Includes simple mechanical carriage by a crawling or flying insect through soiling of its feet or proboscis, or by passage of organisms through its gastrointestinal tract. This does not require multiplication or development of the organism. b) *Biological:* Propagation (multiplication), cyclic development, or a combination of these (cyclopropagation) is required before the arthropod can transmit the infective form of the agent to man. An incubation period (extrinsic) is required following infection before the arthropod becomes *infective*. Transmission may be by saliva during biting, or by regurgitation or deposition on the skin of feces or other material capable of penetrating subsequently through the bite wound or through an area of trauma from scratching or rubbing. This is transmission by an infected non-vertebrate host and must be differentiated for epidemiological purposes from simple mechanical carriage by a vector in the role of a vehicle. An arthropod in either role is termed a *vector*.

3) *AIRBORNE*—The dissemination of microbial aerosols to a suitable portal of entry, usually the respiratory tract. Microbial aerosols are suspensions in the air of particles consisting partially or wholly of microorganisms. Particles in the 1 to 5 micron range are easily drawn into the alveoli of the lungs and may be retained there; many are exhaled from the alveoli without deposition.

They may remain suspended in the air for long periods of

time, some retaining and others losing infectivity or virulence. Not considered as airborne are droplets and other large particles which promptly settle out (see a. Direct transmission, above).

The following are airborne and their mode of transmission is direct:

a) *Droplet nuclei:* Usually the small residues which result from evaporation of fluid from droplets emitted by an infected host (see above). Droplet nuclei also may be created purposely by a variety of atomizing devices, or accidentally as in microbiology laboratories or in abattoirs, rendering plants or autopsy rooms. They usually remain suspended in the air for long periods of time.

b) *Dust:* The small particles of widely varying size which may arise from soil (as for example fungus spores separated from dry soil by wind or mechanical agitation), clothes, bedding, or contaminated floors.

46. *Zoonosis*—An infection or an infectious disease transmissible under natural conditions from vertebrate animals to man. May be *enzootic* or epizootic (see 10, Endemic and 11, Epidemic).

INDEX

389